90

ESSENTIALS
of
SPINAL DISORDERS

ESSENTIALS
of
SPINAL DISORDERS

Jason C Eck DO MS
Orthopedic Spine Surgeon
Center for Sports Medicine and Orthopedics
Chattanooga, Tennessee, USA

Christian P DiPaola MD
Assistant Professor
Department of Orthopedic Surgery
University of Massachusetts
Worcester, Massachusetts, USA

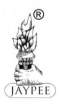

JAYPEE BROTHERS MEDICAL PUBLISHERS (P) LTD

New Delhi • London • Philadelphia • Panama

Jaypee Brothers Medical Publishers (P) Ltd

Headquarters

Jaypee Brothers Medical Publishers (P) Ltd
4838/24, Ansari Road, Daryaganj
New Delhi 110 002, India
Phone: +91-11-43574357
Fax: +91-11-43574314
Email: jaypee@jaypeebrothers.com

Overseas Offices

J.P. Medical Ltd
83, Victoria Street, London
SW1H 0HW (UK)
Phone: +44-2031708910
Fax: +02-03-0086180
Email: info@jpmedpub.com

Jaypee-Highlights Medical Publishers Inc
City of Knowledge, Bld. 237
Clayton, Panama City, Panama
Phone: +507-301-0496
Fax: +507-301-0499
Email: cservice@jphmedical.com

Jaypee Medical Inc.
The Bourse
111 South Independence Mall East
Suite 835, Philadelphia, PA 19106, USA
Phone: + 267-519-9789
Email: jpmed.us@gmail.com

Jaypee Brothers
Medical Publishers (P) Ltd
17/1-B Babar Road, Block-B
Shaymali, Mohammadpur
Dhaka-1207, Bangladesh
Mobile: +08801912003485
Email: jaypeedhaka@gmail.com

Jaypee Brothers
Medical Publishers (P) Ltd
Bhotahity, Kathmandu
Nepal
Phone: +977-9741283608
Email: kathmandu@jaypeebrothers.com

Website: www.jaypeebrothers.com
Website: www.jaypeedigital.com

© 2014, Jaypee Brothers Medical Publishers

Inquiries for bulk sales may be solicited at: jaypee@jaypeebrothers.com

Essentials of Spinal Disorders

First Edition: 2014

ISBN 978-93-5090-983-6

Printed at: Replika Press Pvt. Ltd.

Preface

Disorders of the spine are one of the most common medical complaints and can affect nearly everyone at some point during life. As a result, it is crucial for the medical professionals caring for these patients to have a solid understanding of these conditions including a thorough knowledge of spinal anatomy, applied biomechanics, and pathophysiology combined with nonoperative and surgical treatment options.

Essentials of Spinal Disorders first provides chapters reviewing the various aspects of basic science including anatomy and biomechanics as well as an overview of key physical examination points and appropriate use of imaging studies. Each of the subsequent chapters on specific spinal disorders consists of a discussion of patient presentation, pathophysiology, imaging findings, and nonoperative and surgical treatment options. It is our hope that *Essentials of Spinal Disorders* serves as a valuable resource for the practicing physicians as well as those still in training.

Jason C Eck
Christian P DiPaola

Acknowledgments

We would like to thank the publishing staff at M/s Jaypee Brothers Medical Publishers (P) Ltd, New Delhi, India, and specifically Ms Chetna Malhotra Vohra (Senior Manager–Business Development) for her work in completing this book.

Contents

Essentials of Spinal Disorders

Introduction

At some point during life, nearly everyone will be affected by back or neck pain. It remains the second most common reason for a visit to the primary care physician after the common cold. Fortunately, the majority of these cases are self-limiting and resolve relatively quickly regardless of treatment. These patients often just require reassurance that their symptoms will resolve with some basic symptomatic treatment including anti-inflammatory medications and physical therapy. Even more important, however, is to be able to recognize which of these patients requires a more extensive evaluation and treatment. There are "red flags" that can help to identify more serious etiologies of spinal disorders including increased pain at rest, extremes of age, history of infection, malignancy or trauma and progressive neurologic deficits. It is crucial for any practitioner caring for a patient with a spinal disorder to be capable of identifying these more serious conditions and guiding the patient to the most appropriate treatment.

As with other medical fields, the amount of information available regarding spinal disorders is ever expanding. It is not possible for the primary care physicians or those early in their specialty training to have a comprehensive understanding of patients with spinal disorders. Instead, being able to properly diagnose the specific spinal disorder and quickly and accurately identify the most serious etiologies is crucial for all practitioners caring for these patients.

Due to limited resources, it is not reasonable for every patient with back or neck pain to receive a comprehensive work up. In fact, many patients begin to have a resolution of their symptoms prior to seeing their physician and having the work up completed. Patients with generalized neck or back pain without radicular pain, paresthesias or weakness and without "red flags" typically do not require imaging studies or referral to a specialist initially. Advanced imaging studies should be reserved for patients with neurologic findings or "red flags" for more serious etiologies. The most serious findings include a progressive neurologic deficit or loss of bowel and bladder control. Patients with these findings typically need emergent imaging and evaluation by a spine specialist. The longer these symptoms are present, the greater the likelihood that they can become permanent.

The most common reason for generalized neck and back pain is a simple muscle strain. Often, there is no specific recollection of an injury, and they typically resolve without treatment. The majority of spinal disorders fall into the category of degenerative disorders and can include degenerative disk disease, disk herniation and spinal stenosis. These are very common disorders that become more prevalent with age. The development of degenerative spinal disorders is also more common in patients with a strong family history of spine problems due to a genetic predilection for these disorders. Additionally, patients with long-term higher physical demands, such as laborers and contact athletes, have a higher rate of degenerative spinal disorders.

In most cases spinal trauma is the result of a specific injury to the spine that the patient is able to recall. If there are underlying abnormalities in the spine such as severe osteoporosis or spondyloarthropathies, injury to the spine can occur with little to no trauma. The most important initial goals in managing patients with a suspected spine trauma are to assure that the spine is properly stabilized to prevent further injury and identifying and managing coexisting injuries.

Spinal deformities can vary from simple curves that are just observed over time to severe curves in multiple planes that can cause neurologic, cardiac and pulmonary compromise. Less common disorders of the spine include tumor and infection. The majority of spine tumors are the result of metastatic spread of disease to the spine, but primary tumors of the spine can occur, and these need to be properly identified and managed. Infections of the spine can occur from vascular or lymphatic spread from other areas of the body or by direct inoculation as found in postoperative infections. Both tumors and infections of the spine can lead to destruction of the vertebrae and subsequent instability and potential neurologic compromise.

Caring for a patient with a spinal disorder can appear to be a daunting task especially early in one's career. However, with a solid understanding of the basic principles, the practitioners can learn to properly evaluate these complex patients and assure that the patient is provided with the appropriate treatment.

The purpose of this text is to provide an overview of the evaluation and treatment of the patient with a spinal disorder. The text begins with chapters to assist with the evaluation of the patient including medical history and physical examination, biomechanics and imaging studies. The remainder of the text is devoted to more in-depth evaluation and treatment of specific spinal disorders including degenerative, traumatic, deformity, tumor, and infection. There are full-length textbooks devoted to each of these areas, and this text is not expected to be a comprehensive source of information. Instead, it is geared to those looking for succinct summary of the most important information provided in a clear, and easy-to-understand format. It is designed to be completed during a single rotation on a spine service for a resident or medical student.

CHAPTER

1

Anatomy of the Spine

The spine is a complex structure that provides structural support for the body, transmits loads, allows for motion, protects the spinal cord and exiting nerve roots, and acts as an attachment site for the muscles and ligaments. While a complete description of the complex anatomy of the spine is beyond scope of this chapter, it provides an overview of the most important aspects for the spinal surgeon.

☞ VERTEBRAE

The spine is composed of 33 vertebrae (7 cervical, 12 thoracic, 5 lumbar, 5 sacral and 4 coccygeal). The mobile spine consists of cervical spine in the neck, thoracic spine in the middle back and lumbar spine in the lower back. The sacrum is a collection of five fused vertebrae between the innominate bones that act as a connection between the spine and the pelvis. The coccyx consists of four or five ossicles that form the tailbone.

In general, the vertebrae are composed of two parts: (1) vertebral body ventrally and (2) vertebral arch dorsally as shown in Figures 1A and B. Vertebral bodies are connected to the vertebral arch by pedicles. Vertebral bodies are attachment sites for the anterior and posterior longitudinal ligaments and are separated by the intervertebral disk in between. The vertebral arch surrounds the spinal canal to protect the spinal cord and exiting nerve roots. It has several projections including dorsal spinous process, two laterally projecting transverse processes and two superior and inferior articular processes. Neighboring articular processes join to form the diarthrodial facet joints. Pars interarticularis is located between the superior and inferior articular processes and acts to resist translational motion between two adjacent vertebral bodies. Failure of the pars interarticularis results in spondylolisthesis or ventral displacement of one vertebra on another. It occurs most commonly in the lower back between L4 and L5, or L5 and S1, or in cases of cervical spine trauma at C2 from a Hangman's fracture.

The vertebrae gradually increase in size and strength cranially at C3 to caudally at L5. This allows vertebrae to withstand the increased forces applied to them as they move more caudally. There are normal curves present in the sagittal plane with lordosis in the cervical and lumbar spine and kyphosis in the thoracic spine as shown in Figure 2. These normal curves allow for improved flexibility and load-bearing capacity of the spine.

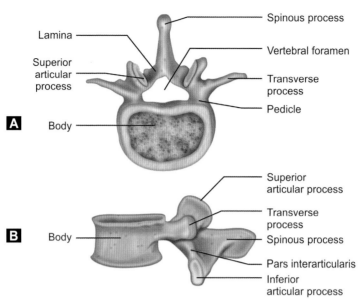

Lamina

Superior
articular
process

A Body

Spinous process

Vertebral foramen

Transverse
process

Pedicle

Superior
articular process

Transverse
process

B Body

Spinous process

Pars interarticularis

Inferior
articular process

Figs 1A and B: A typical vertebra with major anatomical features.
(A) Viewed from above; (B) From the side

The cervical and lumbar spine vertebrae are highly mobile as compared to the more rigid thoracic vertebrae that are restrained by the rib cage. The facet joints are oriented in the coronal plane in the cervical spine with a gradual change to the sagittal plane orientation in the lumbar spine. The transition zones between these regions are areas of increased stress and have higher rates of trauma.

The upper cervical vertebrae differ anatomically from remainder of the vertebrae and require special consideration. The first cervical vertebra, the atlas, is a ring composed of an anterior and posterior arch connected by two lateral masses as shown in Figure 3. The superior articular processes of the atlas articulate with the occipital condyles. Motion between these joints accounts for approximately 50% of the flexion/extension motion of the cervical spine. The second cervical vertebra, the axis, has a vertebral body with a cranially projecting process called the odontoid process or dens (Fig. 3). The odontoid process acts as a post about which the atlas can rotate. This provides approximately 50% of the axial rotation of the cervical spine.

Another variation in vertebrae anatomy is the presence of transverse foramina in the cervical vertebrae

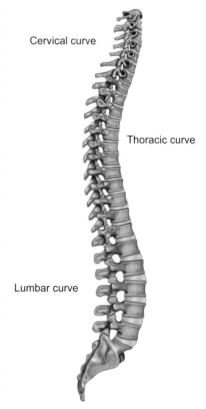

Cervical curve

Thoracic curve

Lumbar curve

Fig. 2: Sagittal view of the spine showing normal cervical and lumbar lordosis and thoracic kyphosis

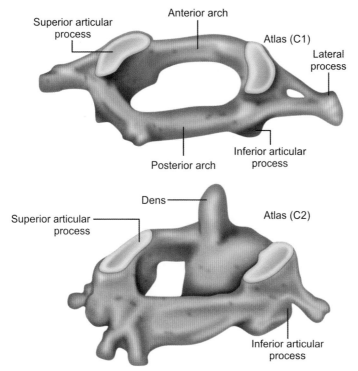

Fig. 3: Atlas and axis, the atypical upper cervical vertebrae

through which the vertebral arteries pass. These foramina are present from C1 through C6 but are inconsistently found in C7 where vertebral arteries often pass outside the vertebrae.

The thoracic vertebrae contain diarthrodial facets for connection with the ribs on vertebral bodies and transverse processes. The pedicle height increases in the thoracic spine from cranial to caudal vertebrae, but the width is the smallest from T3 to T6.[1] This is an important consideration in placing pedicle screws in the thoracic spine.

LIGAMENTS

The anterior longitudinal ligament (ALL) extends along ventral vertebral bodies from the skull to the sacrum. It gradually widens as it extends more caudally to the lumbar spine. It acts as a restraint to extension injury. The posterior longitudinal ligament (PLL) also extends from the skull to the sacrum along the posterior aspect of vertebral bodies; however, in contrast to the ALL, fibers of the PLL decrease in width as they extend caudally to the lumbar spine. In the lumbar spine there is a central band of fibers at the level of the disk space, but there is less coverage or even a void posterolaterally along the disk space. This is relevant in that majority of lumbar disk herniations occur in a posterolateral direction where there is less support from the PLL.

A connection between the vertebral arches is formed through paired sets of ligamentum flava, intertransverse ligaments, interspinous ligaments and unpaired supraspinous ligaments. The ligamentum flavum connects adjacent lamina from C2 to S1. It attaches

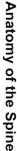

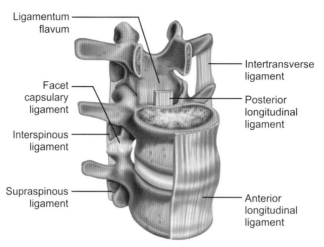

Fig. 4: Anterior and posterior longitudinal ligaments, ligamentum flavum and intertransverse, interspinous and supraspinous ligaments

from the ventral surface of cranial lamina to the superior lip of caudal lamina and helps to resist flexion injury. Redundancy or hypertrophy of this ligament can contribute to spinal stenosis. The intertransverse ligaments attach between adjacent transverse processes. They are a useful landmark as the exiting nerve roots exit beneath them. By avoiding dissection deep to the intertransverse ligaments the nerve root is safe. The interspinous ligaments attach obliquely in pairs between adjacent spinous processes with a small cleft separating them. The supraspinous ligament runs continuously from the spinous process of C7 to the end of the sacrum. In the cervical spine it continues cranially as the ligamentum nuchae to the occipital cervical protuberance. Both interspinous and supraspinous ligaments act to resist flexion injury. These ligamentous structures are illustrated in Figure 4.

As with osseous structures, ligamentous structures of the upper cervical spine differ from remainder of the spinal column. The ALL continues cranially as the anterior atlanto-occipital membrane and attaches to the basion. The ligamentum flavum continues to the skull as the posterior atlanto-occipital membrane. The transverse atlantal ligament connects on the inner surface between opposite sides of anterior arch of the atlas and posterior aspect of the odontoid process. This band-like ligament resists ventral displacement of C1 with respect to the odontoid. The alar ligaments span obliquely from the odontoid process to the anterior foramen magnum. The apical odontoid ligament attaches from the tip of the odontoid process to the basion. These upper cervical ligamentous structures are illustrated in Figure 5.

☞ INTERVERTEBRAL DISK

The intervertebral disk is the fibrocartilaginous space found between the vertebral bodies. It is composed of the inner nucleus pulposus and the outer annulus fibrosus. The nucleus pulposus is the remnant of the embryonic notochord. It is composed predominantly of type II collagen, proteoglycans and mucopolysaccharides. In younger patients it is composed of 70–90% water, but this water content decreases with age. Nucleus pulposus is responsible

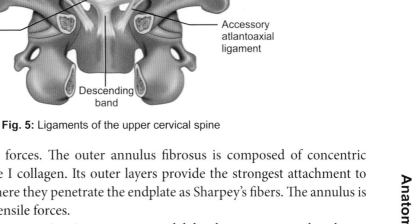

Fig. 5: Ligaments of the upper cervical spine

for resisting compressive forces. The outer annulus fibrosus is composed of concentric layers of overlapping type I collagen. Its outer layers provide the strongest attachment to the vertebral endplates where they penetrate the endplate as Sharpey's fibers. The annulus is responsible for resisting tensile forces.

The disks gradually increase in size at more caudal levels to accommodate larger vertebral bodies and to withstand increased forces. The disks in the lumbar spine are more wedge-shaped with increased height anteriorly to provide increased lumbar lordosis.

Another variation occurs in the cervical spine due to the presence of uncovertebral joints (joints of Luschka) as shown in Figure 6. These are projections of the superior portion of vertebral endplates bilaterally. They are thought to resist shearing forces. They are the important landmarks that must be removed in many cervical disk arthroplasty devices to allow for proper fit. Additionally, their removal during routine anterior cervical discectomy and fusion allows for a more direct decompression of the vertebral foramen and exiting nerve roots.

While the disk has a vascular supply in children, the mature adult disk remains avascular. As a result the disk relies on diffusion of substances for nutrition. This plays a major role in the development of degenerative disk disease. Once the degenerative cascade has begun, the disk is unable to repair itself due to the lack of blood supply. The disk receives its innervation from sinuvertebral nerves and is thought to be a major potential source of lower back pain.[2]

☛ INTERVERTEBRAL FORAMEN

Exiting nerve roots travel through the intervertebral foramen to leave the spinal column as shown in Figure 7. The cranial and caudal borders of the foramen are pedicles of neighboring vertebrae. The ventral border is the dorsolateral intervertebral disk and PLL. The dorsal border is the facet joint and ligamentum flavum. The foramen is elliptical in shape and is much taller than is wide. As a result the disk height can become significantly

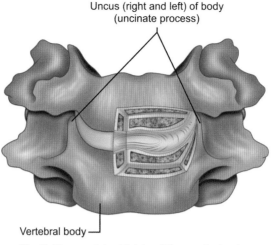

Uncus (right and left) of body
(uncinate process)

Vertebral body

Fig. 6: Uncovertebral joints of the cervical spine

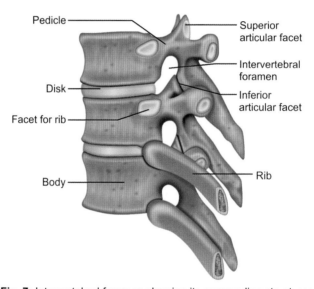

Pedicle

Superior
articular facet

Intervertebral
foramen

Disk

Inferior
articular facet

Facet for rib

Rib

Body

Fig. 7: Intervertebral foramen showing its surrounding structures

reduced and narrow the foraminal height with less impact than changing the width of the foramen. Hypertrophy of the ligamentum flavum or facet joint, thus can play a major role in the development of foraminal stenosis and radiculopathy.

☞ REFERENCES

1. Scoles PV, Linton AE, Latimer B, et al. Vertebral body and posterior element morphology: the normal spine in middle life. Spine. 1988;13(10):1082-6.
2. Bogduk N, Tynan W, Wilson AS. The nerve supply to the human lumbar intervertebral disc. J Anat. 1981;132(Pt 1):39-56.

CHAPTER

2

Spinal Imaging

Accurate diagnostic imaging of the spine is a crucial component in the evaluation of a patient with spinal disorder. Specific information obtained from the medical history and physical examination can help guide the judicious use of imaging studies. In an attempt to reduce the utilization of unnecessary imaging studies and its associated cost and radiation exposure, an understanding of the benefits and limitations of various imaging modalities is important.

The most common imaging modalities used for the evaluation of spinal disorders include conventional radiographs, myelography, computed tomography (CT), magnetic resonance imaging (MRI), scintigraphy and angiography. Each of these modalities has been discussed in further detail in this chapter to provide an understanding of their capabilities and justification for use. Additionally, the imaging of specific categories of spinal disorders including degenerative, traumatic, neoplastic and postoperative has been discussed.

IMAGING MODALITIES

Conventional Radiographs

In many cases the initial imaging study obtained is the plain radiograph due to its near universal availability in the hospital and office setting, relative low cost and ability to provide a general overview image of the osseous spine. There are commonly performed series of radiographs that are obtained for specific regions of the spine or for specific indications. In the cervical spine anteroposterior (AP) and lateral images are commonly obtained for subaxial disorders. It is important to verify that the entire cervical spine is visualized on the lateral view to include the C7-T1 disk space. Often, due to overlying shoulders, this is not possible without the addition of a swimmer's view as shown in Figures 1A and B. For upper cervical spine pathology an open-mouth odontoid view may be obtained. If there is a concern for potential instability lateral flexion and extension views may be obtained if the patient is clinically able to do this safely.

In the thoracic spine AP and lateral images are most commonly obtained. In cases of deformities including scoliosis, kyphosis or abnormal sagittal balance, a full-length AP and lateral image of the spine should be obtained. The importance of the full-length images has

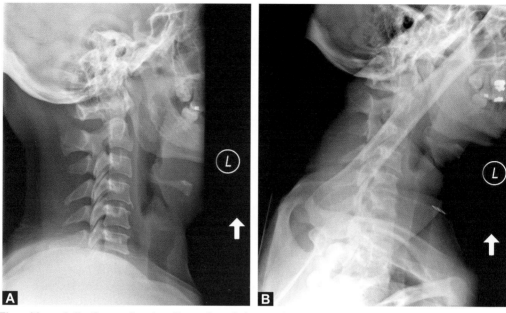

Figs 1A and B: Conventional radiographs of the cervical spine. (A) Lateral radiograph limited to the C6-C7 disk space; (B) Swimmer's view to fully visualize the C7-T1 disk space

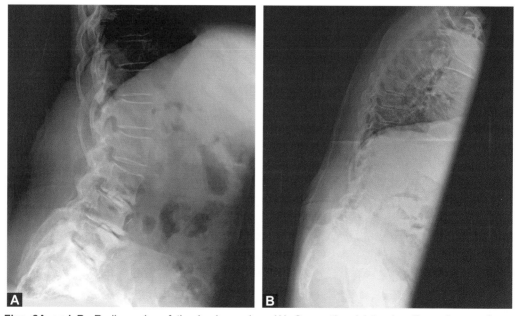

Figs 2A and B: Radiographs of the lumbar spine. (A) Conventional lateral radiograph revealing a postoperative pseudoarthrosis; (B) A full-length lateral radiograph identifying a severe positive sagittal imbalance not well appreciated on the lumbar image alone

been shown in Figures 2A and B where initial lumbar radiographs revealed the presence of a postoperative pseudoarthrosis, but a full-length lateral image was necessary to identify the severity of positive sagittal imbalance.

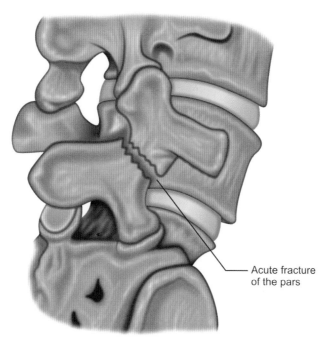

Acute fracture
of the pars

Fig. 3: Oblique view of the lumbar spine showing the "Scotty Dog" image. Spondylolisthesis can be associated with the fracture of pars interarticularis, which corresponds to the collar of a dog in the image

In the lumbar spine three views are typically obtained including AP, lateral and spot view of the lumbosacral junction. Oblique radiographs of the lumbar spine can be obtained to evaluate for spondylolysis or fracture of pars interarticularis as shown in Figure 3, but this exposes the patient to more than double the gonadal radiation. Roberts et al. reported a 5% rate of missed unilateral spondylolysis without associated spondylolisthesis on AP and lateral radiographs that were identified with oblique views.[1] Scavone et al. performed a retrospective review of 782 patients to determine the diagnostic value of the spot lateral and oblique radiographs in the lumbar spine.[2] They reported a 2.4% rate of pathology identified only on those views that would have been missed on the conventional AP and lateral images. There were no cases of spondylolisthesis in either study that were missed on lateral imaging alone. Due to the increased cost and radiation exposure each of the studies recommended against the routine use of oblique radiographs of the lumbar spine.

Despite their widespread use, plain radiographs have major limitations including inability to visualize neurologic structures and high rate of false positive findings in asymptomatic patients.

Myelography

Myelography involves the injection of a water-soluble contrast agent into the thecal sac either through a lumbar puncture or a C1-C2 puncture. This can allow for visualization of extradural compression of the neural structures by a change in normal contour of the thecal sac or nerve root sleeves. Conventional myelography is rarely used anymore without using postmyelogram CT scan. This technique has two major disadvantages over newer imaging modalities. The first is its invasiveness. While the newer water-soluble contrast agents are safer and carry less risk of adverse reactions, the technique remains invasive. In most cases the patient can be safely discharged after monitoring for several hours after the procedure. The technique has a potential risk for cerebral spinal fluid leak with spinal cephalgia, infection, neurologic injury and vascular injury.

The second limitation of this technique is its lack of specificity in diagnosis. Since neural compression is visualized indirectly by a distortion of contrast in the thecal sac, it is not possible to accurately identify the specific cause of compression.

The accuracy of myelography varies among different reports, but in a large meta-analysis of the literature by Kent et al. the rates ranged from 67% to 78% for the detection of lumbar spinal stenosis.[3] The accuracy of myelography for the detection of cervical spine stenosis varies from 67% to 92%.[4-6]

Computed Tomography

The use of CT allows for axial imaging of the spine to provide an improved, direct visualization of compressive structures. The gantry can be tilted to permit axial imaging in line with the curve of the spine. This is particularly useful in cases of severe spinal deformity to provide images through disk spaces and to detect lateral recess stenosis. In these cases MRI is more limited in its ability to obtain imaging directly through the level of the disk space because of the deformity. CT has an ability to better differentiate the compression of neural structures by soft tissues versus compression by bone as shown in Figures 4A and B.

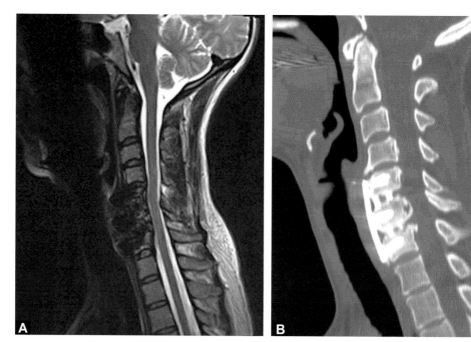

Figs 4A and B: Postoperative sagittal MRI versus postoperative CT of the cervical spine. (A) Postoperative sagittal MRI revealing some remaining central spinal stenosis; (B) Postoperative CT allowing for improved visualization of osteophytes posterior to vertebral bodies causing more severe stenosis

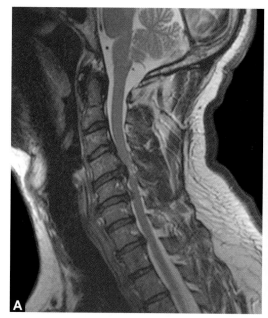
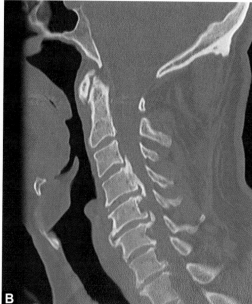

Figs 5A and B: Sagittal MRI versus sagittal CT of the cervical spine in differentiating disk herniation from ossification of the posterior longitudinal ligament (OPLL). (A) Sagittal MRI showing central stenosis severe at C4-C5 and moderate at C5-C6 and C7-T1 from suspected disk herniation; (B) Sagittal CT of the same patient identifying the presence of OPLL

This is particularly useful in differentiating disk herniation from ossification of the posterior longitudinal ligament (OPLL) as shown in Figures 5A and B. The surgical management of this patient was altered based on the additional information provided by CT scan over MRI scan. Instead of an anterior cervical discectomy and fusion the patient underwent a posterior approach to decrease the risk of durotomy associated with OPLL treated through an anterior approach. Another major benefit of CT is the ability to obtain axial imaging in patients who are unable to undergo MRI including those with certain pacemakers or stents, aneurysm clips and metallic debris in the eyes. The obvious disadvantage of CT is the associated exposure of the patient to ionizing radiation.

Magnetic Resonance Imaging

Magnetic resonance imaging has become the imaging modality of choice for the evaluation of many spinal disorders. This is due to its ability to provide high quality axial imaging of the spine with direct visualization of neural structures and other soft tissues including disks, ligaments, facet capsules and muscles. The traditional MRI sequences include axial and sagittal T1- and T2-weighted images. The addition of short inversion-time inversion recovery (STIR) sequence provides additional sensitivity for many spinal disorders including trauma and tumors.

The high prevalence of abnormal MRI findings in asymptomatic patients should be considered when making a diagnosis. Boden et al. performed prospective studies on the cervical and lumbar spine to determine the prevalence of abnormal MRI findings in

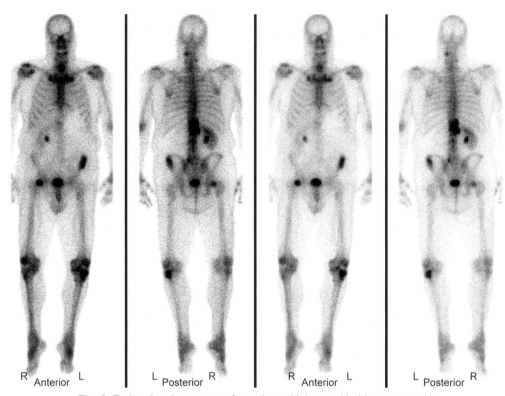

Fig. 6: Technetium bone scan of a patient with known bladder cancer with metastasis to T11 and T12 vertebral bodies

asymptomatic individuals. In the cervical spine 25% of asymptomatic individuals under the age of 40 had degenerative changes compared to 60% of those over 40 years of age.[7] In the lumbar spine 20% of asymptomatic individuals under the age of 60 had disk herniation, 36% of those over 60 years had disk herniation and 21% had stenosis as well.[8] As a result of this, all imaging findings need to be firmly associated with clinical findings prior to the formulation of diagnosis and treatment plan.

Scintigraphy

Bone scintigraphy can be used for the identification of inflammatory changes in the spine. These studies use radionuclides to detect inflammatory changes in a patient with a known history of metastatic bladder cancer to T11-T12 vertebral bodies as shown in Figure 6. The most commonly used radionuclide is technetium-99m phosphate, but others include gallium citrate and indium-111-labeled white blood cells. The disadvantages of these studies are their lack of specificity and prolonged time to normalization. As a result they cannot accurately differentiate between different types of inflammatory changes including trauma, infection and tumor. Also, they may remain positive after clinical resolution of the infectious or neoplastic disease process.

Common uses of bone scintigraphy of the spine include evaluation for metastatic disease to the spine and determination of acuity of fracture. Caution should be taken in patients with multiple myeloma or renal cell carcinoma as they are more likely to result in a

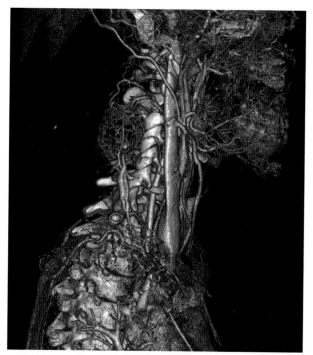

Fig. 7: A three-dimensional CT angiography of a 13-year-old patient with an aneurysmal bone cyst of the posterior elements of C3 showing abundant vascular supply to this tumor. Serial preoperative embolization reduced vascular supply to the tumor and decreased the risks of bleeding intraoperatively

false-negative study. An alternative screening examination is a plain radiographic bone survey. In patients with plain radiographic evidence of vertebral compression fracture either a bone scan or MRI can be useful in determining whether the fracture is acute or chronic. If the fracture is less than 3 months old it will remain positive on both MRI and bone scan. After 3 months from the time of injury when the fracture has healed there is no longer increased edema visible on MRI or inflammatory response visible on bone scan.

Angiography

Spinal angiography can be useful for the evaluation of vascular malformations, vascular supply to a tumor or the spinal cord, and detection of vascular injury from trauma. In addition to its diagnostic capabilities, angiography can be used for embolization for definitive treatment or to decrease the risk of bleeding with resection of vascular tumors.

Certain tumors are known to have abundant vascular supplies including renal cell carcinoma and aneurysmal bone cysts as shown in Figure 7. Prior to attempting surgical resection of tumors, angiography is recommended to evaluate the vascular supply and potential embolization of major feeding vessels to the tumor.

In cases of planned corpectomy around the thoracolumbar junction, angiography can be useful to evaluate the vascular supply to the spinal cord, specifically the artery of Adamkiewicz. Prior to disruption of segmental vessels at this level it is crucial to verify that there will be sufficient remaining vascular supply to the spinal cord to prevent postoperative paralysis.

In cases of cervical spine trauma there is a potential for vertebral artery injury. Fortunately, majority of these injuries remain asymptomatic. The indications for angiography in the setting of cervical spine trauma vary greatly among different institutions. There is a lack of agreement on when to perform this test, and what the ideal treatment should be in the case of asymptomatic injury. Angiography should be performed in all symptomatic cases and should be considered in cases of facet fracture/dislocation and fracture into the vertebral foramen as shown in Figures 8A to C.

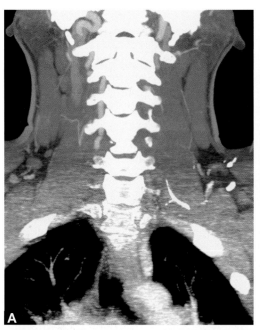
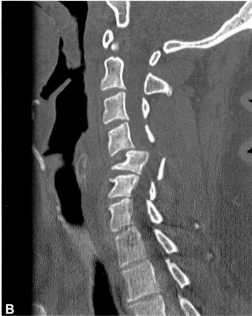
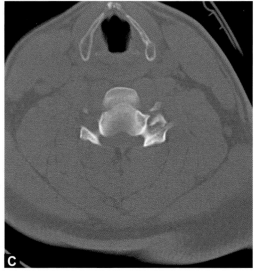

Figs 8A to C: Spinal angiography. (A) Coronal CT angiography of a patient with complete facet dislocation showing complete occlusion of left vertebral artery. The patient remained asymptomatic in regard to arterial occlusion; (B) The sagittal CT scan showing the complete dislocation of C4-C5 facets; (C) Axial CT scan showing bony fragments of fracture facets in the vertebral foramen

Degenerative Disorders

Degenerative disorders of the spine are one of the most common reasons for seeing a spine specialist. These disorders become progressively more prevalent with increasing age. It is important to understand that many individuals having changes on imaging studies remain asymptomatic and do not require treatment. Plain radiographs will reveal the loss of disk space height, endplate sclerosis and osteophyte formation with more advanced degenerative disease as shown in Figures 9A and B.

Magnetic resonance imaging has become the imaging modality of choice for majority of degenerative spinal disorders. Indications for obtaining an MRI are debated but generally include the presence of radicular symptoms, progressive neurologic deficit, failed conservative treatment for 4–6 weeks and clinical warning signs for potential infection or tumor.

Typical MRI findings include loss of disk space height, loss of fluid signal within the disk space, osteophyte formation and endplate edema as shown in Figure 10. The presence of a high intensity zone suggests a tear of outer layers of annulus fibrosus of the disk. This appears as an increased signal on T2-weigthed images on the posterior aspect of the disk as shown in Figure 11. Age-related degenerative MRI changes of the vertebral endplates have been well studied, and the associated Modic changes are summarized in Table 1.[9] Disk herniations can

Spinal Imaging

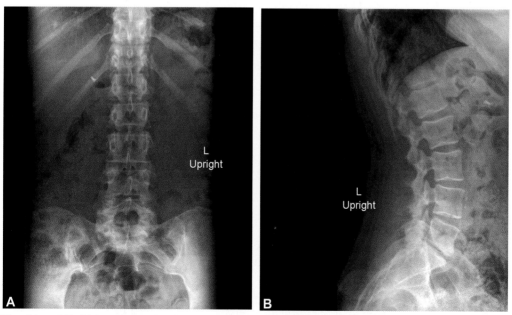

Figs 9A and B: Plain radiographs of the lumbar spine showing typical age-related degenerative changes at the level of L5-S1 including loss of disk space height, endplate sclerosis and osteophyte formation. (A) Anteroposterior view; (B) Lateral view

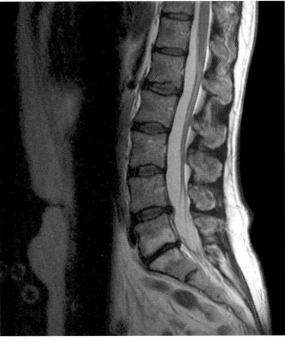

Fig. 10: Sagittal T2-weighted MRI of the lumbar spine showing loss of disk height, loss of fluid signal in the disk, osteophyte formation and endplate edema at the level of L5-S1. There are minor changes at the level of L4-L5 including minor disk bulging and loss of disk space height

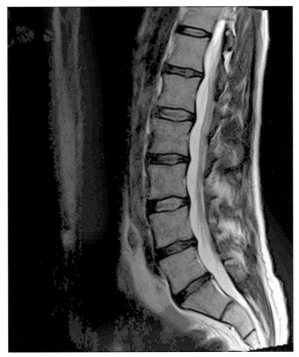

Fig. 11: The small increased signal intensity at the posterior aspect of L5-S1 disk on T2-weighted MRI showing a high intensity zone suggesting of annular tear

Table 1: Modic MRI vertebral endplate changes associated with age-related degeneration

Modic type	MRI findings
I	Decreased marrow signal on T1-weighted images Increased marrow signal on T2-weighted images
II	Increased marrow signal on T1-weighted images Isointense to slightly increased marrow signal on T2-weighted images
III	Decreased marrow signal on T1- and T2-weighted images

Table 2: Descriptive terms for disk herniation

Term	Description
Bulge	A small bump on edge of the disk without disruption of the annulus
Protrusion	Herniation of the disk with its base being at least as large as the herniated portion of the disk
Extrusion	The disk material is herniated out of the normal disk space with base of the herniation smaller than the herniated portion of the disk
Sequestration	A completely free fragment of disk separated from the remaining disk

be described according to the degree of disruption of the disk outside its normal confines as summarized in Table 2. Disk herniations can occur independently or in combination with other degenerative changes as shown in Figures 12A to C.

Stenosis can occur either centrally or in the foramen or in lateral recess. Central canal stenosis can occur due to disk herniation, congenitally short pedicles, osteophyte formation and facet or ligamentous hypertrophy. In the cervical and thoracic spine this can cause symptoms of myelopathy. In more severe cases spinal cord compression can occur that can lead to myelomalacia as shown in Figure 13. This is seen as increased signal intensity in the spinal cord on T2-weighted images with or without decreased signal intensity of the spinal cord on T1-weighted images. It is generally believed to be a poor prognostic factor associated with myelopathy.[10] Central stenosis in the lumbar spine can cause neurogenic claudication. Lateral recess stenosis can cause radicular symptoms similar to those of disk herniation and results from a lateral disk herniation, facet hypertrophy, facet cysts or lateral osteophyte formation.

Spinal Trauma

Plain radiographs are often the initial screening examination in the setting of spinal trauma. If the patient remains asymptomatic and has a reliable neurologic examination with negative plain imaging there is no need for further imaging studies. If the patient remains symptomatic with negative plain radiographs, additional imaging is needed to rule out a spinal injury. The details of the clinical algorithm are provided in Chapters 7 and 12 on Spinal Trauma.

Computed tomography scan of the spine has gained popularity in the setting of trauma due to its near universal availability in the hospital settings and the ability to visualize the entire spine quickly with improved bony detail.

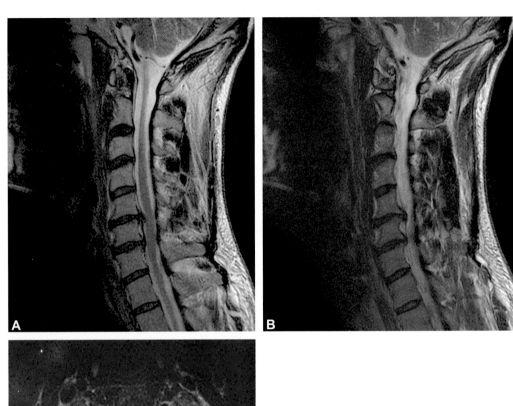

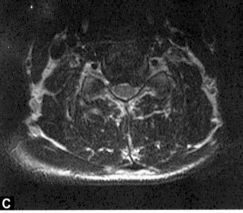

Figs 12A to C: Sagittal T2-weighted MRI. (A) Revealing degenerative disk disease at C5-C7 with disk herniation at C5-C6; (B) A more left-sided sagittal image revealing large osteophytes at C5-C6 and C6-C7 causing foraminal stenosis; (C) Axial T2-weighted image showing both the central and foraminal stenosis associated with disk herniation and osteophytes

In cases of neurologic deficit or suspected ligamentous injury MRI remains the gold standard imaging study. MRI can visualize the neurologic structures, assess for spinal canal compromise or neurologic compression, and assess for ligamentous disruption. Ligamentous disruption appears as increased signal intensity in soft tissues on T2-weighted images, and STIR images often provide a better view of this disruption as seen in Figures 14A and B. It is often possible to visualize a discrete interruption in the ligaments on MRI as well.

Neoplastic Disease

Tumors of the spine are most commonly the result of metastatic spread from remote areas, but primary spine tumors can occur as well. In some cases tumors of the spine can be identified on plain radiographs, but they are often initially missed until they become

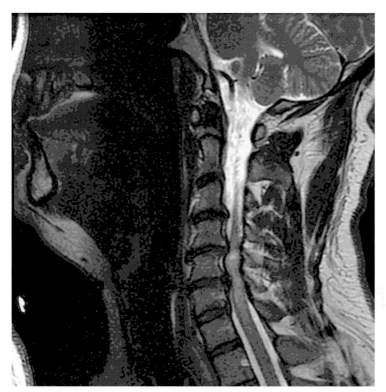

Fig. 13: Sagittal T2-weighted MRI revealing multiple level cervical spine stenosis with increased intensity signal in the spinal cord at the level of C4-C5 consistent with myelomalacia

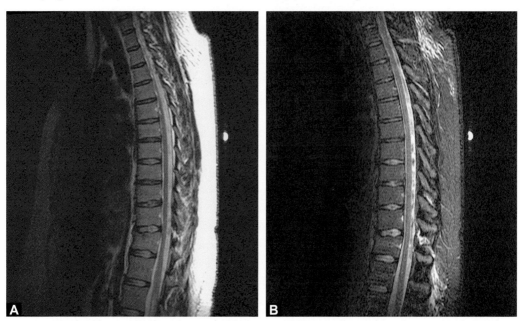

A

B

Figs 14A and B: MRI sequences. (A) Sagittal T2-weighted MRI revealing a traumatic disruption at the level of T11-T12 of ligamentum flavum and interspinous and supraspinous ligaments; (B) The short inversion-time inversion recovery (STIR) sequence providing a more obvious view of these ligamentous injuries

Table 3: Characteristics of spinal tumor versus infection based on MRI

Characteristics	Infection	Tumor
Disk space involvement	Involved	Spared
Vertebral endplate	Loss of definition	Spared
Contiguous vertebral involvement	More common	Less common
Soft tissue fat planes	Commonly diffusely obscured due to edema	Less commonly or more focally obscured

more advanced with greater bony destruction or pathologic fracture. As discussed earlier in this chapter, bone scans can be used to identify sites of metastatic spread of tumors throughout the body, but caution should be taken due to the high rates of false negative results with renal cell carcinoma and multiple myeloma. CT scans provide the best imaging for evaluation of bone involvement of tumors and assessment for potential signs of instability and canal compromise. MRI scans are often obtained as a gold standard, but in many cases can overestimate the degree of involvement due to surrounding soft tissue edema. In some cases it can be difficult to differentiate tumor from infection based on MRI findings. An et al. determined specific criteria to help differentiate between spinal infection and tumor using MRI as summarized in Table 3.[11] Specific characteristics of individual tumors have been discussed in more detail in Chapter 19.

Postoperative Imaging of the Spine

Imaging of the postoperative spine is commonly performed to assess for adequate healing, fusion status, proper placement of spinal instrumentation, adjacent level degeneration and continuation of preoperative symptoms. In many cases of spinal fusion, plain radiographs will be obtained to evaluate for the proper placement of spinal instrumentation and to assess for fusion. Either plain radiographs or fluoroscopic images are typically obtained to assess for placement of spinal instrumentation prior to leaving the operating room. Prior to leaving the hospital upright plain radiographs can be obtained to allow for better visualization than with intraoperative images. This allows for any necessary changes prior to the patient being discharged.

Evaluation for solid spinal fusion can be attempted with plain radiographs, dynamic radiographs or CT scans. Unfortunately, each of these has inherent limitations. Plain radiographs alone are the least reliable, but should be assessed for the appearance of bridging trabecular bone connecting the fused bony surfaces without the presence of radiolucent lines. The presence of lucency on either plain radiographs or CT scans surrounding screws is referred to as a Halo and suggests that there is continued motion due to a pseudoarthrosis as shown in Figure 15. The addition of dynamic radiographs provides further evidence of fusion, but can be limited by the presence of spinal instrumentation that can reduce the motion despite a potential pseudoarthrosis. CT scans provide the best imaging analysis for spinal fusion. They also have the ability to provide axial imaging of the vertebrae to evaluate proper

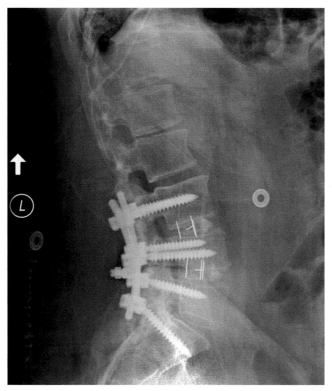

Fig. 15: Postoperative lateral plain radiograph of the lumbar spine showing previous spinal instrumentation from L3-S1. There is lucency surrounding the L3 pedicle screws (Halo sign) consistent with pseudoarthrosis at the level of L3-L4

placement of spinal instrumentation. MRI scans can be obtained postoperatively, even with the presence of spinal instrumentation, but are more limited by streak artifacts than CT scans.

In cases of continued or recurrent radicular symptoms postoperatively, an MRI should be obtained if possible to assess for stenosis or disk herniation. The risk of recurrent disk herniation following discectomy is approximately 6%. The addition of gadolinium to MRI can help differentiate a recurrent disk herniation from epidural fibrosis.[12] Postoperative MRI alone can show the presence of compressive epidural tissue, but the addition of contrast will result in the enhancement of scar tissue due to its blood supply, while recurrent disk herniation will not enhance with contrast as it does not have a blood supply.

☞ REFERENCES

1. Roberts FF, Kishore PR, Cunningham ME. Routine oblique radiography of the pediatric lumbar spine: is it necessary? AJR Am J Roentgenol. 1978;131(2):297-8.
2. Scavone JG, Latshaw RF, Weidner WA. Anteroposterior and lateral radiographs: an adequate lumbar spine examination. AJR Am J Roentgenol. 1981;136(4):715-7.
3. Kent DL, Haynor DR, Larson EB, et al. Diagnosis of lumbar spinal stenosis in adults: a meta-analysis of CT, MR, and myelography. AJR Am J Roentgenol. 1992;158(5):1135-44.

4. Coin CG. Cervical disk degeneration and herniation: diagnosis by computerized tomography. South Med J. 1984;77(8):385-90.

5. Modic MT, Ross JS, Masaryk TJ. Imaging of degenerative diseases of the cervical spine. Clin Orthop Rel Res. 1989;239:109-20.

6. Sobel DF, Barkovich AJ, Munderloh SH. Metrizamide myelography and postmyelographic computed tomography: comparative adequacy in the cervical spine. Am J Neuroradiol. 1984;5(4): 385-90.

7. Boden SD, McCowin PR, Davis DO, et al. Abnormal magnetic-resonance scans of the cervical spine in asymptomatic subjects. A prospective investigation. J Bone Joint Surg Am. 1990;72(8):1178-84.

8. Boden SD, Davis DO, Dina TS, et al. Abnormal magnetic-resonance scans of the lumbar spine in asymptomatic subjects. A prospective investigation. J Bone Joint Surg Am. 1990;72(3):403-8.

9. Modic MT, Steinberg PM, Ross JS, et al. Degenerative disk disease: assessment of changes in vertebral body marrow with MR imaging. Radiology. 1988;166(1 Pt 1):193-9.

10. Eck JC, Drew J, Currier BL. Effect of magnetic resonance imaging signal change in myelopathic patients: a meta-analysis. Spine. 2010;35(23):E1306-9.

11. An HS, Vaccaro AR, Dolinskas CA, et al. Differentiation between spinal tumors and infections with magnetic resonance imaging. Spine. 1991;16(8 Suppl):S334-8.

12. Haughton V, Schreibman K, De Smet A. Contrast between scar and recurrent herniated disk on contrast-enhanced MR images. AJNR Am J Neuroradiol. 2002;23(10):1652-6.

CHAPTER

3

Spinal Biomechanics

The spine is composed of a complex arrangement of tissues that allow it to perform its three basic functions: (1) transmit and withstand loads, (2) allow for segmental motion and (3) protect the spinal cord. The underlying mechanics that make these functions possible are very complex, but a basic comprehension of these principles is crucial in order to understand how the spine works, how it fails, and how it is affected by our interventions. The field of biomedical engineering was developed as a subdivision of mechanical engineering and deals with the understanding of mechanical properties related to the human body. While the basic principles of mechanical engineering can be applied to structures that make up the body, their complex interaction within the body and need for understanding of biology and physiology necessitated the need for this new field of study. An important subset of biomedical engineering that applies to the spine is termed spinal biomechanics. The purpose of this chapter is to provide an overview of the field of spinal biomechanics, focusing on the specific issues important to the spine surgeon.

☞ DEFINITIONS OF MECHANICAL AND MATERIAL PROPERTIES

The terms "force", "stress" and "strain" are purely mechanical terms, unrelated to a specific type of material. The term "force" is applied to any action that tends to change the state of rest or of motion of a body to which it is applied. It is known to be directly proportional to the acceleration of the object through Newton's famous equation $F = m \times a$, where F refers to the force, m is the mass of the object, and a is the acceleration of the object. There are different types of forces that can be applied to an object. A compressive force is one that tends to push the material together, a tensile force acts to elongate the material, and a torsional force applies a torque or twisting force to the object as shown in Figure 1. "Stress" is defined as the force per a unit of area using the equation $\sigma = F/A$, where σ refers to the stress, F is the force, and A is the area. "Strain" is the change in length of an object per unit length of the object subjected to a load using the equation $\varepsilon = (L_{final} - L_{initial})/L_{initial}$, where ε is the strain, L_{final} is the final length of the object, and $L_{initial}$ is the initial length of the object prior to the application of the load.

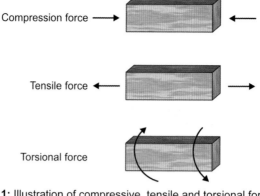

Fig. 1: Illustration of compressive, tensile and torsional forces

There are specific material properties that are intrinsic to the material based on its composition and are not dependent on geometry of the object. These properties include elasticity, plasticity and viscoelasticity. "Elasticity" refers to the property of a material that allows it to deform under an applied load and return to its original form or length after removal of a deforming load. A basic spring is a good example of this material property. The "elastic region" of a material is the range in which it remains elastic and retains its ability to return to its initial shape after removal of an applied force. If an object is subjected to a great enough load it will undergo a permanent change in its shape or length even after removal of the load. "Plasticity" refers to the permanent deformation of a material when it is loaded beyond its elastic range. The "plastic region" is the range in which a material has been loaded past the elastic range but still has an ability to partially recoil after removal of the applied load. The "yield point" defines the transition of a material between the elastic region and the plastic region. Once a material has been loaded beyond the yield point it is no longer able to return to its initial geometry due to a permanent deformation. The "elastic modulus" is the property of a given material that is commonly used to define its characteristics and is defined by the equation $E = \Delta\sigma/\Delta\varepsilon$, where E is the elastic modulus, $\Delta\sigma$ is the change in stress and $\Delta\varepsilon$ is the change in strain. The elastic modulus is an important concept when designing spinal instrumentation and has been previously defined for many commonly used materials and anatomic structures. The "strength" of a material is the point at which failure occurs and corresponds to the amount of force required to cause a structural failure to the material. These terms are illustrated in Figure 2 in a stress-strain curve. These curves can be created for any given material and vary significantly based on the intrinsic material properties.

"Viscoelasticity" of a material relates the time-dependent deformation of the material to the magnitude of the force applied on it. This means that when a force is applied to a viscoelastic material there will be an initial deformation of the object at a given rate until an equilibrium is reached. "Creep" refers to a state when the intrinsic resistance of the material is equal to the applied force. This causes an equilibrium where the applied force on the object can remain constant and there will be no further deformation of the object as illustrated in Figure 3. "Stress relaxation" refers to the state when a constant deformation occurs while the stress exponentially decays as shown in Figure 4. These viscoelastic properties of the

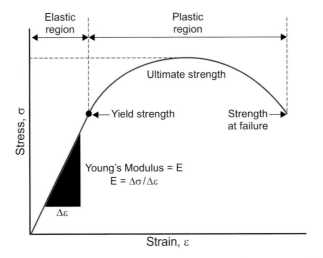

Fig. 2: The stress-strain curve for a given material defining intrinsic material properties and how the material reacts to applied load

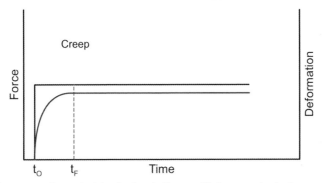

Fig. 3: The creep of a material referring to the equilibrium reached when a continued constant applied force no longer causes any deformation of the object

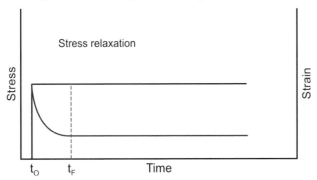

Fig. 4: The stress relaxation of a material occurring when the stress exponentially decays while a constant deformation continues

material help define their potential for failure. When viscoelastic materials are loaded more quickly they fail at higher forces and with less deformation than if loaded more slowly as shown in Figure 5.

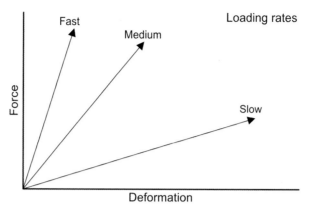

Fig. 5: Force-deformation graft showing the effects of viscoelasticity of a material. Faster loading rates allows for failure at higher forces but lower amounts of deformation

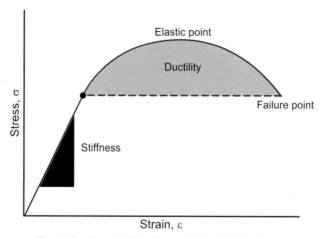

Fig. 6: Stress-strain curve illustrating the ductility of a material which is the amount of plastic deformation that a material can achieve beyond the elastic point but prior to failure

One of the most important determinations how well a material can withstand a given load without failure is its ductility. The "ductility" of a material is the amount of plastic deformation that can occur beyond the elastic point but prior to failure of the material as shown in Figure 6. Ductility is very important for contouring spinal rods to allow them to be countered in shape of the spine without breaking. "Fatigue failure" of a material refers to the concept where if a material is consistently loaded over time it will fail at loads of a lower magnitude than would induce failure if loaded with fewer cycles as shown in Figure 7. Repetitive bending of a paperclip illustrates this concept. If a paperclip is bent back and forth a small number of times it will not fail, but if this process is continued for many cycles the paperclip will eventually fail at a relatively low load. This is also an important concept for spinal instrumentation. These devices need be able to withstand millions of cycles of loading without failure over lifetime.

The "bending moment" is the product of applied force and length of the lever arm and is described by the equation $M = F \times d$, where M is the bending moment and d is the distance of the lever arm. This means that the further away from an object a force is applied, the

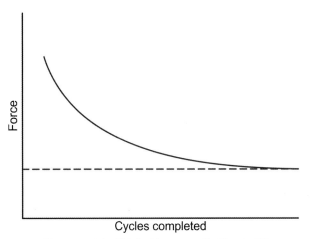

Fig. 7: Fatigue failure curve. The material will fail at lower applied loads if they are continuously applied for a high number of cycles. Failure at a lower number of cycles requires a higher applied load

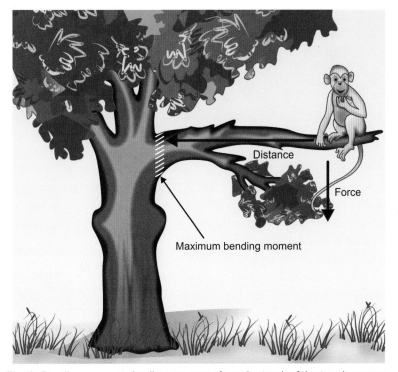

Fig. 8: Bending moment. As distance away from the trunk of the tree increases, the bending moment increases

larger the bending moment becomes as illustrated in Figure 8. This concept is important to consider in proper lifting mechanics. Carrying objects closer to the body places less bending moment on the spinal musculature and disks than carrying objects at arms reach as illustrated in Figure 9.

The "moment of inertia" of an object is related to its cross-sectional area and correlates to its ability to withstand bending moments. For cylindrical objects such as a spinal rod it

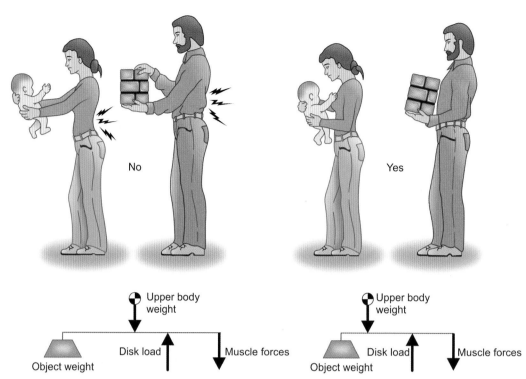

No

Yes

Upper body weight

Disk load

Muscle forces

Object weight

Upper body weight

Disk load

Muscle forces

Object weight

Fig. 9: Importance of proper lifting mechanics on the bending moment applied to the spine. Carrying objects as close to the body as possible reduces the bending moment to the spine

is described by the equation $I = \pi r^4/4$ where I is the moment of inertia and r is the radius of the object. As a result small increase in the diameter of a rod can greatly increase the structural properties of the rod. For rectangular objects such as a spinal plate the equation is $I = bh^3/12$, where I is the moment of inertia, b is the length of the plate and h is the thickness of the plate. Again, it is clear that increasing the thickness of the plate has a substantial impact on its mechanical properties.

The instantaneous axis of rotation is the point about which an object rotates. This is very important when considering vertebral motion and disk arthroplasty. In order to maintain normal motion and forces in the spine when performing disk arthroplasty it is crucial to recreate the normal axis of rotation of the vertebrae according to its instantaneous axis of rotation as shown in Figures 10A and B.

☛ FUNCTIONAL BIOMECHANICS OF THE DISK

The intervertebral disk is composed of the inner nucleus pulposus and the outer annulus fibrosus. The nucleus is composed predominantly of Type II collagen, proteoglycans and mucopolysaccharides. The annulus is composed of concentric layers of overlapping Type I collagen. The nucleus is predominately responsible for resisting compressive forces, while the annulus resists tensile forces. In the young healthy disk applied loads are distributed evenly through the nucleus and are transmitted to the annulus. As the disk ages the nucleus

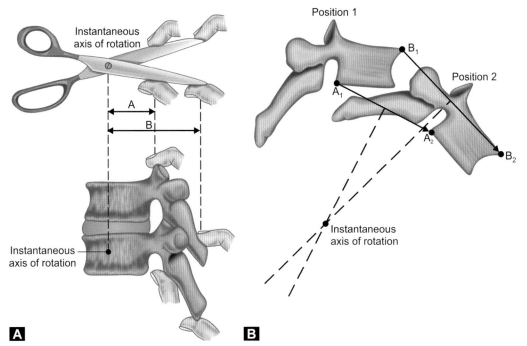

Figs 10A and B: The instantaneous axis of rotation. (A) The blades of the scissor rotate about a fixed point where they are connected; (B) The same is true of the vertebra that rotates about a central point

is less capable of resisting compressive forces and the loads are distributed asymmetrically to the annulus. This leads to higher tensile forces in the annulus and eventual disk degeneration, tears and disk herniation as shown in Figures 11A to C. Torsional loading of the disk is felt to be the most important in terms of injury and degeneration. When the disk is subjected to torsional loads it induces shear forces in both axial and horizontal planes, and the magnitude of these forces is directly proportional to the distance from the center of the disk as shown in Figure 12. The intradiscal pressures have been previously measured for different body positions.[1] It was determined that compared to standing, laying supine induces approximately 25% of the intradiscal pressure, sitting induces 140%, standing and bending forward induces 150%, and sitting, bending forward and holding weights induces 185% of the intradiscal pressure.

KINEMATICS OF THE SPINE

Segmental motion of the spine is often studied as a functional spinal unit consisting of the intervertebral disk and two neighboring vertebral bodies. This model consists of three joints: the disk and the two facet joints. The normal motion allowable in the spinal units is a function of anatomy. The unique anatomy of the upper cervical spine from the occiput to C2 allows for approximately half of the flexion/extension motion of the cervical spine to occur at the occipitocervical (occiput-C1) joint and half of the axial rotation of the cervical spine to occur at the atlantoaxial (C1-C2) joint. The remaining cervical spine motion is divided among the subaxial cervical spine segments. There is a gradual change in the orientation

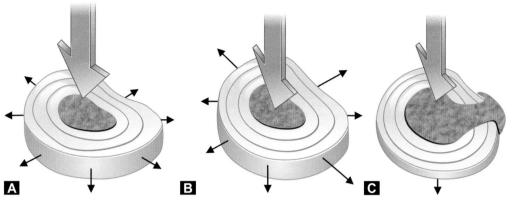

Figs 11A to C: Intervertebral disk showing applied loads. (A) Normal disk where compressive forces are resisted by the nucleus and are symmetrically transmitted to the annulus; (B) Degenerative disk showing asymmetric forces; (C) Herniated disk where asymmetric forces can lead to disk herniation

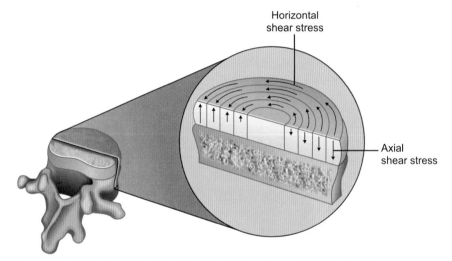

Fig. 12: Intervertebral disk showing torsional loading of the spine resulting in shear forces in both horizontal and axial planes, and these forces are directly proportional to the distance from the center of the disk

of facet joints from the cervical to the lumbar spine. In the cervical spine facet joints are oriented in the coronal plane, while in the lumbar spine they are oriented in the sagittal plane.

As disks undergo degeneration the kinematics also changes.[2] In moderate degrees of degeneration there is an increase in motion, while in cases of more severe disk degeneration the motion is decreased compared to normal. This is believed to be due to an initial laxity on restraints of the disk with moderate degeneration, followed by a decrease in motion due to osteophyte formation.

Another cause of alteration of spinal kinematics is the presence of previous spinal fusion. It is believed that the elimination of segmental motion through spinal fusion leads to an increased transmission of forces to the adjacent level. This has been measured by Eck et al. in the cervical spine.[3] A simulated anterior cervical fusion at C5-C6 led to an increase in adjacent level intradiscal pressure of 73.2% at C4-C5 and 45.3% at C6-C7 during flexion. Corresponding increases in segmental motion were also reported. These findings were in agreement of those of Hilibrand et al. who reported clinical risks of developing adjacent level degenerative changes following anterior cervical discectomy and fusion.[4] In a 2–21-year follow-up of 371 patients, they reported a 2.9% risk of developing new symptomatic adjacent level degenerative changes annually, and a 25.6% risk at 10 years. Two-thirds of those patients went on to additional surgery at the adjacent level. Similar risk of adjacent level degeneration following lumbar fusion was also present. It remains uncertain, however, how much of the adjacent level degeneration is the result of purely increased mechanical demand and how much of a role the natural history plays.

SPINAL STABILITY

The term spinal stability refers to ability of the spine under normal physiologic loads to limit patterns of displacement so as not to damage the neural structures and to prevent deformity or pain due to structural damage. There are some radiographic criteria for determining the presence of instability. In the cervical spine greater than 3.5 mm of translation or greater than 11° of angulation suggests possible instability. In the lumbar spine 4.5 mm of translation or greater than 22° of angulation suggests instability.[5] There are various classification systems for trauma and tumor cases of the spine that can be used for determining the presence of instability. These have been discussed in their respective chapters.

BIOMECHANICS OF SPINAL INSTRUMENTATION

A complete discussion of spinal instrumentation is beyond the scope of this chapter; however, there are several principles that are worthy of discussion. As discussed previously in this chapter different materials have different material properties. These differences can be used to select the most appropriate material for use in specific instrumentation systems. Three of the most commonly used metal materials for spinal implants are titanium, cobalt-chromium and stainless steel. Stainless steel has advantages of being strong, ductile and resistant to notch failure, but it is ferromagnetic, causes a high degree of postoperative image distortion and differs greatly from the elastic modulus of bone. Stainless steel is used in several of the metal-on-metal disk arthroplasty devices and in some cases of deformity correction, especially if there has been previous instrumentation failure. Titanium is currently widely used in spinal instrumentation as it has an elastic modulus more similar to bone, allows more load sharing and is more compatible with postoperative imaging studies. Cobalt-chromium is a newer option for spinal instrumentation with a profile between titanium and stainless steel. It is frequently used for deformity cases where there may be concern for failure of titanium rods.

Other nonmetallic materials include polyetheretherketone (PEEK) and bioresorbable materials. PEEK is a plastic material that has the advantage of being radiolucent, and provides for a better assessment of fusion radiographically. It also has an elastic modulus similar to bone. The place for bioresorbable materials in spinal instrumentation remains unclear. They have been shown to have an initial stability similar to titanium implants and allow for improved levels of load sharing; however, their use has not been well adopted.[6]

REFERENCES

1. Nachemson A, Morris JM. In vivo measurements of intradiscal pressure. Discometry, a method for the determination of pressure in the lower lumbar discs. J Bone Joint Surg Am. 1964;46:1077-92.
2. Miyazaki M, Hong SW, Yoon SH, et al. Kinematic analysis of the relationship between the grade of disc degeneration and motion unit of the cervical spine. Spine. 2008;33(2):187-93.
3. Eck JC, Humphreys SC, Lim TH, et al. Biomechanical study on the effect of cervical spine fusion on adjacent-level intradiscal pressure and segmental motion. Spine. 2002;27(22):2431-4.
4. Hilibrand AS, Carlson GD, Palumbo MA, et al. Radiculopathy and myelopathy at segments adjacent to the site of a previous anterior cervical arthrodesis. J Bone Joint Surg Am. 1999;81(4):519-28.
5. White AA, Johnson RM, Panjabi MM, et al. Biomechanical analysis of clinical stability of the cervical spine. Clin Orthop. 1975;109:85-96.
6. Vadapalli S, Sairyo K, Goel VK, et al. Biomechanical rationale for using polyetheretherketone (PEEK) spacers for lumbar interbody fusion–a finite element study. Spine. 2006;31(26):E992-8.

CHAPTER

4

History and Physical Examination of the Spine

One of the most important aspects to master in the care of the patient with a spinal disorder is the history and physical examination of the spine. It is during this initial evaluation of the patient that the clinician develops a differential diagnosis, indentifies potential emergent problems, initiates further testing if needed and begins to construct a potential treatment plan.

Despite the fact that spinal disorders are very common, an accurate diagnosis can remain challenging. There are certain clues that can be identified based on the patient's recent history, past medical history, age and physical examination findings that can lead the clinician to a differential diagnosis. The most important initial goal is to rule out the presence of any serious pathology that potentially needs emergent treatment. There are certain "red flags" that can lead the clinician to suspect the presence of more serious pathology as summarized in Table 1. These main categories of emergent problems include cancer, infection, fracture and cauda equina syndrome. Each of these needs to be identified early to initiate the appropriate treatment and decrease the associated complications. Cancer should be considered in the patient with a new onset or worsening pain that is not relieved with rest especially if the patient has a history of cancer or strong smoking. Infection of the spine can be difficult to diagnose initially, as spine infections do not typically present with the same constitutional symptoms as other systemic infections. Infection should be considered in patients who are immunocompromised or with a history of intravenous drug usage. Patients do not need to have fever, chills or elevated white blood cell count to have a spine infection. The most concerning infection is an epidural abscess that results in compression of the spinal cord and a progressive neurologic deficit. In many cases of spinal fracture a recent trauma has occurred. However, in patients with osteoporosis or inflammatory disorders including ankylosing spondylitis (AS) or diffuse idiopathic skeletal hyperostosis (DISH) fracture can occur with little or no trauma to the spine. Any patient with AS or DISH that has a change in the position of the spine or an increased range of motion should be considered to have a spinal fracture until proven otherwise. Cauda equina syndrome is the final category and is a surgical emergency. Patients present with saddle anesthesia, severe lower back and/or lower extremity pain and loss of bowel and/or bladder control. The loss of bowel control consists of bowel incontinence, while the bladder dysfunction consists of an initial inability to void followed by an overflow incontinence.

Table 1: List of "red flags" that may suggest more serious etiology of spinal disorders

Potential etiology	Finding or symptom
Cancer	Personal history of cancer
	History of smoking
	Unexplained weight loss
	Age > 50 years
	Pain at night or not relieved with rest
Infection	Fever
	Immunosuppression (from medications or illness)
	Intravenous drug use
	History of recent infection
Fracture	Age > 50 years
	Osteoporosis or osteopenia
	History of recent trauma
	Ankylosing spondylitis
	Diffuse idiopathic skeletal hyperostosis
	Use of corticosteroids
Cauda equina syndrome	Saddle anesthesia
	Loss of bowel or bladder control

PATIENT'S HISTORY

The first step in the patient evaluation is to obtain the chief complaint. This typically can be summarized in a single statement of why the patient is presenting to you. In most cases, this information can be obtained directly from the patient. However, in cases of trauma or dementia the chief complaint may need to be obtained from other sources. The chief complaint may be a simple statement of lower back or neck pain, while in other cases the patient may present with a presumptive diagnosis based on previous evaluation by other providers. Care should be taken to avoid being biased by the patient's presumptive diagnosis prior to your own history and physical examination.

Once the chief complaint has been established, further information regarding the patient's history can be determined with targeted questions. Key components that should be investigated include the duration of the patient's symptoms, whether or not there was any inciting event or trauma that was thought to cause these symptoms, what activities alleviate or exacerbate the symptoms, and whether or not the patient has had any prior history of similar symptoms in the past. Any prior treatment should be determined along with its degree of effectiveness.

The most common complaint of patients with spinal disorders is pain. The severity, character and specific location of the pain can help lead to a diagnosis. The severity of the pain can be rated on either a numeric rating scale (0–10) or a visual analog scale (the patient marks a point on a 10 cm line corresponding to the severity of pain). The character of the pain can be described as sharp, dull, burning, cramping, etc. It can either be isolated to the axial spine or radiate to the extremities. Axial pain is more commonly associated

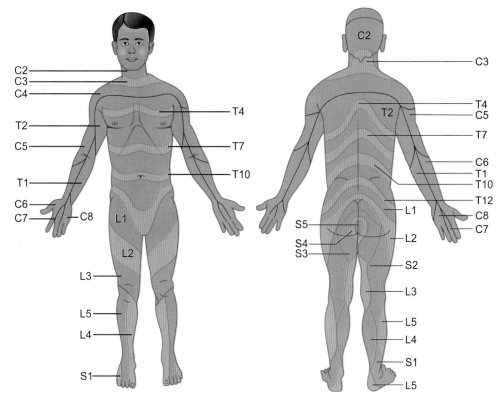

Fig. 1: Anterior and posterior location of spinal dermatomes

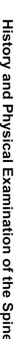

with degenerative disk disease, facet joint degeneration, and muscular and ligamentous structures. Radicular pain is more commonly caused by nerve root compression from disk herniations or stenosis. The location of radicular pain often follows a specific nerve root distribution that can assist in determining the location of the pathology (Fig. 1).

PAST MEDICAL HISTORY

In addition to information of the patient's current complaints, it is important to obtain a complete past medical history. This can help with the differential diagnosis as many spinal disorders can be associated with other medical conditions. The patient should be specifically questioned regarding the history of cancer, recent infection, immune suppression, current medications and previous surgeries. Conditions including vascular disorders, diabetes or herpes zoster can each result in peripheral pain complaints similar to radiculopathy from a spinal etiology. Patients with a history of osteopenia, osteoporosis or inflammatory disorders are more prone to fractures with minor trauma.

SOCIAL HISTORY

There are many factors related to the patient's lifestyle that can play a crucial role in both diagnosis and treatment of spinal disorders. The use of tobacco, alcohol or other drugs should be documented. Tobacco use can increase the level of pain and lead to further degeneration of the spinal structures. Additionally, nicotine is well-known to inhibit normal bone formation which can lead to failure of spinal fusion and chronic pain.[1,2] The use of illicit drugs can decrease the effectiveness of many pain medications. The use of intravenous drugs places the patient at increased risk for spinal infection including epidural abscess.

The patient's education and work status should be documented. Lack of satisfaction with work or poor perceived work environments can increase the incidence of chronic pain and disability and decrease the likelihood of treatment success.[3,4] Involvement of worker's compensation claim or litigation has also been reported to negatively affect patient outcomes.[5,6]

A history of psychological distress, anxiety or depression should also be determined. These conditions can negatively affect outcomes of treatment.[7,8] Additionally, medications for these comorbidities can potentially negatively interact with other medications used for spinal disorders.

☞ PHYSICAL EXAMINATION

After obtaining a complete history, the next step is to perform the physical examination. The examination is often targeted to the areas of complaints identified during the history. The components of the physical examination include inspection, palpation, neurological testing and special tests.

Inspection should begin with observing the patient ambulating into the examination room if possible. Abnormalities in the patient's gait pattern can provide clues to underlying spine pathology. The gait should be evaluated for overall balance, posture, stride length and steadiness. Poor balance could represent a sign of myelopathy, while a forward flexed posture could represent lumbar stenosis. Once in the examination room the patient should be undressed sufficiently to allow for adequate inspection of the entire spine and extremities. The skin should be inspected for any surgical or traumatic scars, rashes or pigment changes. Overall patient balance in the frontal and sagittal view can reveal the presence of scoliosis or increased kyphosis. The spine should be evaluated both in an upright stance as well as with the patient forward flexed to assess for changes in rib prominence. The level of the shoulders and iliac crest should be compared as well as identified as any asymmetric skin creases. Active range of motion testing should be performed of the cervical, thoracic and lumbar spine to assess flexibility and to identify any restrictions in motion or pain generators. The muscles should be inspected for signs of atrophy that could be the result of severe nerve root compression.

Palpation of the midline spinous processes should be performed to locate any area of tenderness or step-offs between the levels. The paraspinous muscles should be palpated to identify areas of localized or generalized tenderness. Any masses or muscles spasms should be noted. The greater trochanters should be palpated as trochanteric bursitis is commonly mistaken for a potential spinal disorder. Evaluation of peripheral pulses can identify potential vascular causes of pain.

The neurologic examination includes evaluation of the sensation, motor function and reflexes. The sensory examination assesses for areas of diminished sensation along specific dermatomes associated with specific nerve roots (Fig. 1). This can be performed for both

Table 2: Motor strength grading scale

Grade	Description
5	Full active motion against full resistance (normal strength)
4	Full active motion against some resistance
3	Active motion against gravity
2	Active motion without gravity
1	Muscle twitch only, no active motion
0	No muscular contraction

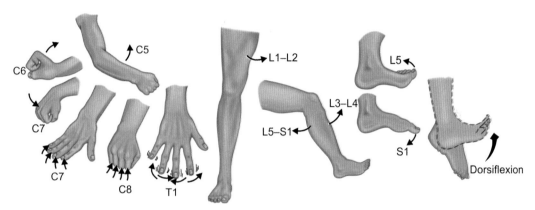

Fig. 2: Muscle strength testing associated with specific nerve roots

light touch and pin prick. More diffuse areas of sensory deficit including a "stocking" or "glove" distribution may suggest the presence of peripheral neuropathy or nonorganic pathology. The motor examination is performed to identify potential areas of muscle weakness that could be the result of specific nerve root dysfunction or a more global spinal cord injury. Muscle strength testing is graded on a five-point scale as described in Table 2. The specific nerve roots responsible for muscle function are illustrated in Figure 2. Testing for the presence of reflexes can also help identify spinal disorders. A reduction or absence of reflex is often associated with a lower motor neuron disorder, while an exaggerated reflex or hyperreflexia is associated with an upper motor neuron disorder. Figure 3 illustrates the reflexes associated with specific nerve roots.

After the history and physical examination have been completed, the clinician may start to form a differential diagnosis. Based on this list of potential diagnoses there are additional maneuvers and tests that can be performed to help confirm or eliminate some disorders from the differential diagnosis. A Spurling's maneuver is performed on patients with unilateral upper extremity radiculopathy. The patient's head is extended and bent toward the side of the symptoms. The clinician then gently pushes downward on the patient's head. A positive test causes an increase in the radiculopathy by causing additional compression of the exiting nerve roots in the cervical foramen. Lhermitte's sign is present if the patient experiences an electrical shock-like sensation radiating into the trunk and upper and lower extremities

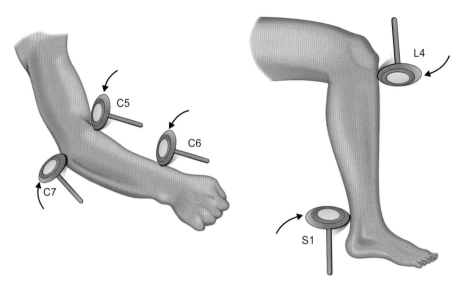

Fig. 3: Reflex testing associated with specific nerve roots

with flexion of the head and neck. This sign is present in some cervical spinal cord disorders and causes additional compression of the cervical spinal cord by reducing the spinal canal diameter. A Hoffman's sign is performed on patients with suspected myelopathy or upper motor neuron disorders. The patient relaxes the wrist, and the examiner places the wrist in slight extension. The distal aspect of the middle finger is flicked into flexion. A positive sign is when the patient's thumb or other fingers spontaneously flex. Beevor's sign is performed to evaluate for thoracic motor function. The patient performs a partial sit-up while the umbilicus is observed. If all thoracic nerve roots are functioning properly the umbilicus retracts proximally along the midline. If there is a dysfunction in the middle or lower thoracic nerve root the umbilicus would deviate to the contralateral side due to relative weakness in the abdominal musculature. The femoral nerve stretch test is performed for suspected upper lumbar (L2-L4) nerve root compression. The patient lies prone on the examination table while the examiner extends the knee and hip joint by lifting the knee off the bed. A positive test causes an increase in the radiculopathy by causing additional stretch or compression of the upper lumbar nerve root. The straight leg raise test is performed for suspected lower lumbar (L4-S1) nerve root compression. It can be performed with the patient seated and supine. The examiner gradually raises the patient's leg and evaluates for recreation or worsening of the radiculopathy. The test is positive if it causes radiating pain in the leg between 30° and 70° of elevation. The Valsalva maneuver can be performed on patients with a suspected lumbar disk herniation. The patient holds his or her breath while bearing down. A positive test causes an increase in the lower extremity radiculopathy by increasing the intradiscal pressure.

Table 3: Waddell's nonorganic physical signs in low back pain	
Sign	Description
Tenderness	
Superficial	Skin tender to light pinch over a wide area
Nonanatomic	Deep tenderness over a wide area
Simulation Test	
Axial loading	Low back pain elicited by vertical loading of the patient's head
Rotation	Low back pain with passive rotation of the shoulders and pelvis in the same plane
Distraction	
Straight leg raising	Variation in straight leg raising test results when the patient is otherwise distracted
Regional disturbances	
Weakness	Partial "giving way" of multiple muscles in a nonanatomic distribution
Sensory	Decreased sensation in a "stocking" or "glove" distribution as opposed to a dermatomal pattern
Overreaction	Presence of disproportionate response including verbalization, facial expression, tension, tremor or sweating

NONORGANIC SIGNS

If the clinician suspects the possibility of malingering or nonorganic causes of the patient's pain Waddell's signs can be tested[9] that are given in Table 3. These include five types of physical signs that could suggest the presence of a nonorganic component to the patient's complaints. If three or more of the five signs are found to be positive it is felt to be clinically significant. Caution should always be taken in evaluating for nonorganic causes of pain. All patients should be given the benefit of the doubt that their complaints are real. Inappropriately labeling a patient as malingering can lead to a potential delay in proper diagnosis.

KEY POINTS

- It is crucial to identify potential "red flags" that need more emergent treatment.
- A thorough history can help form a differential diagnosis.
- The physical examination can further confirm or eliminate an etiology from the differential diagnosis.
- The presence of nonorganic signs should be considered, but only as a diagnosis of exclusion.

REFERENCES

1. Andersen T, Christensen FB, Laursen M, et al. Smoking as a predictor of negative outcome in lumbar spinal fusion. Spine. 2001;26(23):2623-8.
2. Sanden B, Forsth P, Michaelsson K. Smokers show less improvement than nonsmokers two years after surgery for lumbar spinal stenosis: a study of 4555 patients from the Swedish spine register. Spine. 2001;36(13):1059-64.

3. Macfarlane GJ, Pallewatte N, Paudyal P, et al. Evaluation of work-related psychosocial factors and regional musculoskeletal pain: results from a EULAR Task Force. Ann Rheum Dis. 2009;68(6): 885-91.
4. Mielenz TJ, Garrett JM, Carey TS. Association of psychosocial work characteristics with low back pain outcomes. Spine. 2008;33(11):1270-5.
5. Carreon LY, Glassman SD, Kantamneni NR, et al. Clinical outcomes after posterolateral lumbar fusion in workers' compensation patients: a case-control study. Spine. 2010;35(19):1812-7.
6. Nguyen TH, Randolph DC, Talmage J, et al. Long-term outcomes of lumbar fusion among workers' compensation subjects: a historical cohort study. Spine. 2011;36(4):320-31.
7. Edmond SL, Werneke MW, Hart DL. Association between centralization, depression, somatization, and disability among patients with nonspecific low back pain. J Orthop Sports Phys Ther. 2010;40(12):801-10.
8. Kroenke K, Wu J, Bair MJ, et al. Reciprocal relationship between pain and depression: a 12-month longitudinal analysis in primary care. J Pain. 2011;12(9):964-73.
9. Waddell G, McCulloch JA, Kummel E, et al. Nonorganic physical signs in low-back pain. Spine. 1980;5(2):117-25.

CHAPTER

5

Cervical Disk Disease

☞ INTRODUCTION

Cervical spondylosis refers to normal age-related degenerative changes that occur in the cervical spine. These changes become much more prevalent as individuals age. Radiographic evidence of cervical disk disease is present in 25% of asymptomatic patients under age 40, and 85% of asymptomatic patients over 60 years of age.[1,2] Cervical disk disease can remain asymptomatic in many cases, but symptoms can include axial neck pain, cervical radiculopathy and cervical spondylotic myelopathy. The first two of these categories are the focus of the current chapter, while myelopathy has been discussed in Chapter 6.

The lifetime prevalence of clinically significant axial neck pain is 66%, with 5% reporting intractable pain at any time.[3] Cervical radiculopathy refers to pain, sensory findings, or neurologic deficits in a dermatomal distribution in the upper extremity, with or without neck pain. The incidence is 83 per 100,000 and is most common in individuals between 30 years and 55 years of age.[4] It occurs more frequently in males than females. Risk factors are known to include frequent lifting, driving, overhead work, athletics and smoking. Genetic factors also play an important role and can lead to a much earlier presentation of symptoms in those with a strong family history of disk disease.

Fortunately, in the majority of cases, the symptoms are self-limiting and respond well to a conservative treatment plan. For those patients who fail to respond to conservative treatment or have a neurologic deficit, various surgical interventions are available. This chapter discusses the etiology of these degenerative changes along with the patient presentation and the appropriate treatment options.

☞ PATHOPHYSIOLOGY

The intervertebral disk is composed of an inner nucleus pulposus and an outer annulus fibrosus. The nucleus consists of a mesh of Type II collagen and an extracellular matrix of proteoglycans that are hydrophilic, maintain a high water content, and resist compressive forces. The annulus is comprised of a concentric series of interwoven fibrous lamellae that provide tensile strength to the disk. They attach to the anterior and posterior longitudinal ligaments and the superior and inferior endplates. As individuals age there is a characteristic degenerative cascade that develops in the intervertebral disks. Typically, in the third decade there is a change in the proteoglycan content leading to reduced levels of chondroitin sulfate and increased levels of keratin sulfate.[5] These changes diminish the disk's ability to maintain its normal fluid concentration and leads to a decreased ability of the nucleus to resist normal compressive forces. This places additional stress on the outer annular fibers. The disk then looses a portion of its normal height. This causes buckling of the ligamentum flavum, facet joint capsules, and annulus into the spinal canal and neuroforamen. This increases the resultant loading of the facet joints and leads to facet joint degeneration. Additional bone spurs can form and cause further narrowing of the spinal canal and foramen.

One of the most common manifestations of cervical disk disease is a disk herniation. Disk herniations can be categorized as soft or hard. A soft disk herniation is the result of a disruption of the outer annular fibers with protrusion of the inner nucleus material causing compression of the exiting nerve roots. Soft disk herniations are most commonly seen in patient between 30 years and 50 years of age. A hard disk herniation is the result of osteophyte formation or calcification of disk material and typically causes chronic symptoms in patients greater than 55 years of age. Soft disk herniations can be further categorized as a bulge, protrusion, extrusion or sequestration (Figs 1A to D). A disk bulge is a caused by the nucleus pushing on the annulus but without any disruption of the

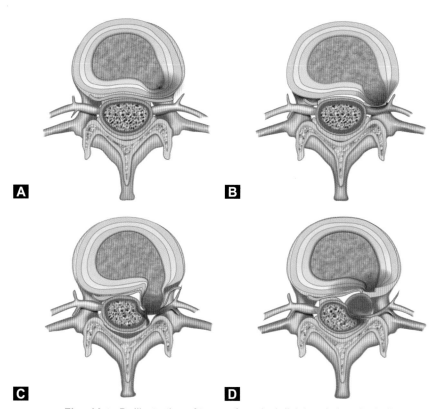

Figs 1A to D: Illustration of types of cervical disk herniations including
(A) Bulge; (B) Protrusion; (C) Extrusion; (D) Sequestration
Source: Eck JC, Voccaro A (Eds). Surgical Atlas of Spinal Operations. New York: Thieme Medical Publishers.

annular fibers. A protrusion is a small defect in the outer annular fibers with a portion of the nucleus displaced outside the annulus. The base of the protrusion is wider than the material displaced beyond the borders of the annulus. A disk extrusion consists of further displacement of the nucleus beyond the borders of the annulus where the diameter of the displaced material is greater than at the base. A sequestered disk herniation is a completely free piece of disk that has separated from the remainder of the disk.

In the cervical spine the nerve roots exit above the pedicle as compared to the lumbar spine where the nerve roots exit below the pedicle of the same number. For example the C6 nerve root will exit above the C6 pedicle at the C5-C6 disk space. The C8 nerve root exits at the C7-T1 disk space.

Axial neck pain can be caused by muscular or ligamentous deconditioning or injury. This can result from poor posture, fatigue, stress, and a poor ergonomic environment. Degenerative disk disease can also directly cause axial neck pain. The outer annular fibers are innervated by the sinuvertebral nerve, which is composed of fibers of the ventral nerve root and sympathetic plexus.[6] Studies have described a reproducible pattern of axial neck pain associated with provocative discography at each cervical disk level (Figs 2A to E).[7] The facet joints can also contribute to axial neck pain through their innervation from the medial branches of the dorsal rami.[8]

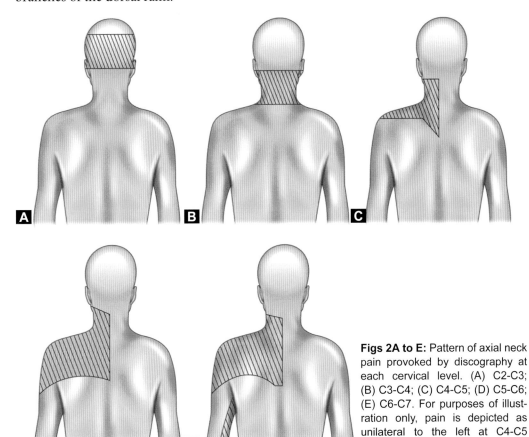

Figs 2A to E: Pattern of axial neck pain provoked by discography at each cervical level. (A) C2-C3; (B) C3-C4; (C) C4-C5; (D) C5-C6; (E) C6-C7. For purposes of illustration only, pain is depicted as unilateral to the left at C4-C5 through C6-C7

Cervical radiculopathy most commonly occurs due to direct compression of the exiting nerve root in the intervertebral foramen either due to disk herniation, osteophyte formation, or loss of disk height and subsequent foraminal height narrowing. Other known causes of cervical radiculopathy comprise of the normal blood supply to the nerve root and chemical radiculitis. A constriction of the venous blood flow from the nerve root can lead to edema and fibrosis of the nerve root.[9] Various neurogenic and non-neurogenic chemical pain mediators have also been reported to be released from the degenerative disk that can result in radicular symptoms. These include substance P, somatostatin, vasoactive intestinal peptide, calcitonin gene-related peptide, angiotensin II, bradykinin, serotonin, histamine, acetylcholine, and prostaglandin E1 and E2.

PATIENT PRESENTATION

Patients with cervical disk disease often present with a chief complaint of posterior neck pain. The pain is often located in the cervical paraspinous muscles with extension into the posterior shoulder girdles and trapezius muscles. Extension of the pain up to the occiput can frequently result in headaches. Patients may have "trigger points" deep in the muscles that are tender to palpation. Pain that worsens with neck flexion suggests a myofascial etiology, while exacerbation in neck extension suggests a discogenic origin.

Patients with cervical disk herniation or foraminal stenosis present with upper extremity complaints of pain, paresthesias or weakness with or without associated neck pain. In most cases of herniated disk the radiculopathy is unilateral, but in cases of a central disk herniation or foraminal stenosis, the symptoms can occur bilaterally. Patients may find a position of comfort when resting the affected arm over their head to relieve the pressure on the exiting nerve root, a finding known as the shoulder abduction sign. Extension and lateral bending toward the affected arm typically exacerbates the symptoms.

A complete neurologic examination can help identify cervical disk disease and locate the level of involvement. The location of the patient's axial neck pain can provide a reasonable estimation of the involved level as shown in Figures 2A to E. Similarly, the location of radicular symptoms including pain, motor and sensory deficits and altered reflexes can lead to the location of the pathology as summarized in Table 1.

Table 1: Neurologic findings associated with cervical radiculopathy			
Nerve root	Motor function	Sensory location	Reflex
C5	Deltoid, biceps	Lateral arm	Biceps
C6	Biceps, wrist extensors	Lateral forearm, thumb and index finger	Brachioradialis
C7	Triceps, wrist flexors, finger extensors	Middle finger	Triceps
C8	Finger flexors	Medial forearm, ring and small fingers	None
T1	Interossei muscles	Medial arm	None

The differential diagnosis of cervical disk disease includes cardiopulmonary disorders, angina, temporomandibular joint disease, inflammatory arthritis, peripheral nerve entrapment, rotator cuff pathology, brachial plexitis, herpes zoster, thoracic outlet syndrome, cervical epidural abscess, cervical stenosis, cervical spine fracture and cervical spine tumor.

IMAGING STUDIES

If cervical disk disease is suspected, imaging studies can be obtained to confirm the diagnosis. In cases without neurologic findings or the presence of "red flags" for more serious underlying pathology, imaging studies are typically not recommended during the first 6 weeks of symptoms. Plain radiographs can show a loss of disk space height, endplate sclerosis, and osteophyte formation (Figs 3A and B). Plain radiographs can also be used to identify other potential pathology including fracture or tumors. The Pavlov ratio can be calculated by dividing the anteroposterior diameter of the spinal canal by the anteroposterior diameter of the vertebral body. A normal value is 1.0 with a value less than 0.8 indicating spinal canal stenosis.[10] The presence of abnormal motion between the vertebral bodies can also be assessed with lateral flexion and extension radiographs to identify instability. Greater than 3.5 mm of translation or 11° of angulation in the subaxial cervical spine indicates the presence of instability or pathologic motion.[11]

Computed tomography (CT) scans can provide axial imaging of the cervical spine, evaluate for the presence of central or foraminal stenosis, ossification of the posterior longitudinal ligament and calcified disk fragments. It is useful in patients unable to obtain a magnetic resonance imaging (MRI) scan due to the presence of a pacemaker, certain

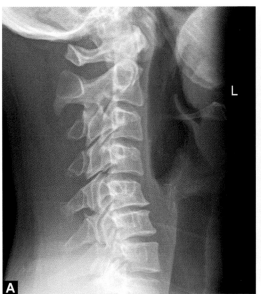
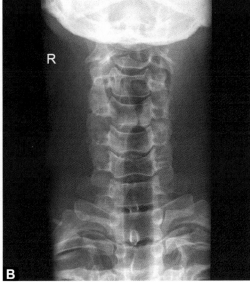

Figs 3A and B: (A) Plain lateral and (B) anteroposterior (AP) radiographs of the cervical spine of a 39-year-old male with neck and bilateral upper extremity pain and paresthesias. The radiographs reveal the presence of loss of disk space height, osteophyte formation and endplate sclerosis at C5-C6 and C6-C7 consistent with cervical disk disease. Additionally, the radiographs show a kyphotic sagittal plane alignment

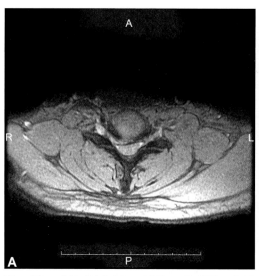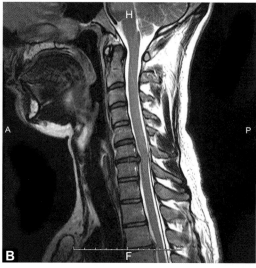

Figs 4A and B: (A) Axial and (B) sagittal T2-weighted MRI scans of a 37-year-old male with severe neck and right upper extremity pain. The MRI scan reveals loss of disk height and fluid signal, and osteophyte formation at C6-C7 with a C6-C7 right-sided disk herniation. This results in central and right-sided foraminal stenosis

metallic implants, or claustrophobia. CT scans can also provide better visualization in patients with deformity since the plane of the images can be adjusted along the curve of the deformity. CT can be combined with myelography for improved visualization of the neural structures. Drawbacks of this technique include being invasive and the exposure to increased levels of radiation.

Magnetic resonance imaging has become the gold standard for imaging evaluation of patients with suspected disk disease. It provides the most detailed view of the soft tissues including the spinal cord, nerve roots, intervertebral disk and ligaments. As with all imaging studies, any abnormalities identified must be closely correlated with the patient's history and physical examination findings. Asymptomatic MRI abnormalities have been reported to increase in frequency as individuals age.[12] MRI evidence of cervical disk disease can include loss of disk space height, osteophyte formation, loss of the normal fluid signal within the disk, endplate edema, disk herniation, and central and foraminal stenosis (Figs 4A and B).

☞ ELECTRODIAGNOSTIC STUDIES

Electrodiagnostic studies include electromyography (EMG) and nerve conduction studies (NCS). EMG involves the placement of intramuscular needle electrodes to evaluate for muscle function and is used to detect motor dysfunction due to nerve compression. NCS use surface electrodes to measure the amplitude and latency of peripheral nerves. These studies can be useful to help differentiate a nerve root compression associated with cervical disk disease from a peripheral nerve compression. EMG studies have a delay of approximately 4 weeks after nerve injury prior to revealing any abnormality. Additionally, there is a poor correlation between the results of electrodiagnostic studies and MRI findings.[13] As a result, electrodiagnostic studies can aid in refining a differential diagnosis but should not be relied upon without confirmation from other studies.

NONOPERATIVE TREATMENT

Fortunately, the majority of cases of axial neck pain or radiculopathy associated with cervical disk disease recover with a period of conservative treatment. This can include a short period of rest or activity modification, medications, injections, and manual techniques.

Long periods of bed rest or immobilization are discouraged as they lead to further muscle deconditioning and a prolonged recovery time. During an acute period of pain patients should be advised to avoid strenuous activities that exacerbate their symptoms. A soft cervical collar can be used for short periods to provide some pain relief, but patients should be warned again prolonged use to avoid muscle deconditioning.

Options for medication management include nonsteroidal anti-inflammatory drugs (NSAIDs), oral corticosteroids, narcotics, muscle relaxants, antidepressants and anticonvulsants. There are currently no specific guidelines for the pharmacologic management of neck pain and radiculopathy associated with cervical disk disease. General recommendations include the use of NSAIDs or acetaminophen as first-line options with patients without contraindications. Oral corticosteroids can be effective in relieving symptoms associated with inflammation, but their use should be limited due to potential adverse effects including weight gain and osteonecrosis. Caution should also be used in diabetic patients due to the risk of hyperglycemia. Opioids are the second-line option but should be used cautiously due to the increased risk for dependency and abuse. Muscle relaxants can be used for patients with severe muscle spasms, but patients should be cautioned on the potential for central nervous system side effects. Antidepressants should not be considered a primary treatment option for cervical disk disease, but there is anecdotal support for their use especially in patients with pre-existing symptoms of anxiety or depression that have been exacerbated by their pain complaints. Anticonvulsants including gabapentin and pregabalin have been shown to be effective in reducing symptoms of radiculopathy in patients with disk disease. These medications have numerous potential adverse effects that should be discussed with the patient prior to recommendation for use.

The use of steroid injections for cervical disk disease can provide short-term reduction in neck pain and radiculopathy in some patients. Patients with tender points in the muscles may benefit from the use of trigger point injections. These injections can be performed in the office setting without the use of fluoroscopy and are felt to be safe, but they provide only short-term benefits. Cervical epidural steroid injections (CESI) can provide some reduction in radicular symptoms in patients. In a systematic review from the Bone and Joint Decade Task Force on Neck Pain and its Associated Disorders Carragee et al. reported that there was evidence to support the short-term use of CESI for the symptomatic improvement of radicular symptoms in patients not involved in litigation (Table 2).[14] Clinicians should receive proper training in CESI prior to performing this procedure. There are several controversial issues related to CESI including the risks of particulate versus nonparticulate steroids and the use of an interlaminar (IL-CESI) versus transforaminal (TF-CESI) approach.

Table 2: Summary of findings from the Bone and Joint Decade Task Force on Neck Pain and its Associated Disorders

Evidence-based recommendations

- Cervical epidural steroid injections (CESI) can provide short-term symptomatic improvement of radicular symptoms in patients not involved in litigation
- No evidence that multiple injections (> 3) or repeated courses are beneficial
- No evidence that the use of CESI in seriously symptomatic patients can decrease the rate of open surgery
- CESI are associated with relatively frequent minor adverse events
- Serious adverse events are very uncommon (< 1%)

Source: Data from Carragee et al.[14]

Table 3: Recommendations to minimize risk associated with transforaminal cervical epidural steroid injections (TF-CESI)

Safety recommendations for TF-CESI

- Use real-time fluoroscopy with nonionic contrast and digital subtraction to minimize detection of intravascular uptake
- Use a test dose of local anesthetic prior to steroid injection
- Use microbore extension tubing to minimize needle manipulation
- Use minimal or no sedation to allow for neurologic monitoring
- Use shorter-acting local anesthetic to minimize high spinal anesthesia severity
- Use blunt needles
- Screen for arterial dissection risk factors
- Use nonparticulate steroids such as dexamethasone

Source: Data from Scanlon et al.[16]

Lee et al. performed a retrospective review of 185 TF-CESI in 159 patients to investigate the difference in short-term effectiveness of using triamcinolone versus dexamethasone.[15] When using the particulate steroid (triamcinolone) there was an 80.4% effectiveness for a mean period of 185 days, while with the nonparticulate steroid (dexamethasone) there was a 69.4% effectiveness for a mean period of 298 days. This difference was not statistically significant suggesting equivalent results regardless of the type of steroid utilized. Scanlon et al. reported on a survey study of 1,404 physicians that performed CESI regarding their associated risks.[16] When questioned on the type of steroid used the only steroid that was not associated with complications was dexamethasone, a nonparticulate steroid. Of those responding to the survey, 21.3% were aware of neurologic complications of TF-CESI, including 30 cases of spinal cord or brain infarct and 13 total fatalities. The recommendations based on this survey have been summarized in Table 3.

In another survey study of instructors from the International Spine Intervention Society, Derby et al. reported on results from 5,968 CESI (4,389 interlaminar and 1,579 transforaminal).[17] There was a total complication rate of 0.46% (0.52% for interlaminar injections vs 0.32% for transforaminal injections). There was no significant difference in complication rate based on the approach in this study of injections performed by expert instructors.

Based on the available evidence CESI are believed to be efficacious in the short-term treatment of neck pain and upper extremity radiculopathy, but they do not decrease the rates of surgery in patients with more severe symptoms. There is no difference in efficacy between particulate versus nonparticulate steroids, but nonparticulate steroids have a lower risk of associated adverse effects. Minor complications are relatively common but short-lived, while major complications are rare but can be devastating.

There are various manual therapy options available for the treatment of neck pain and upper extremity radiculopathy associated with cervical disk disease. These include physical therapy, spinal manipulation and traction. Physical therapy is typically felt to be a useful noninvasive treatment option for this patient population that can often provide improvement in symptoms. In addition to the traditional stretching and strengthening exercises it can include modalities including heat, ice, ultrasound, electrical stimulation, muscle energy and traction. In a randomized controlled trial Young et al. evaluated 81 patients with cervical radiculopathy undergoing treatment with physical therapy with or without traction twice a week for 4.2 weeks.[18] Both groups reported significant improvement in pain scale, neck disability index and functional capacity. The addition of cervical traction provided no additional benefit over a multimodal treatment program of physical therapy and exercises. The efficacy of these programs is highly dependent on patient participation both during and after the structured program. The more effort the patient exerts and the more the patient continues to implement these exercises into their normal routine for the long term, the better the associated results are likely to be.

The goals of spinal manipulation are to increase the range of motion of the functional spinal unit and to modulate the sensory input to the central nervous system. Systematic reviews of the literature have reported spinal manipulation to be effective for treatment of axial neck pain, but there are no randomized controlled trials comparing the efficacy of spinal manipulation for the treatment of cervical radiculopathy.[19] Small case series have reported positive benefits for both axial neck pain and cervical radiculopathy.[20] Caution should be exercised in the use of recommendations for cervical spine manipulation as serious complications including vascular injury, structural lesions and neurologic injury have been reported as detailed in Table 4.[21] Spinal manipulation should not be recommended for patient with cervical stenosis, spinal cord compression, fracture or instability, carotid artery stenosis, tumor, or severe osteoporosis.

OPERATIVE TREATMENT

For those patients with cervical disk disease who fail a period of nonoperative management and remain with intractable pain, surgery may be an option. Specific surgical techniques are available as options depending on the specific patient characteristics, imaging findings and physical examination. In general, options include anterior cervical discectomy and fusion (ACDF), cervical disk arthroplasty, posterior laminectomy with or without fusion, posterior laminoforaminotomy and laminoplasty.

Surgery for patients with axial neck pain without radicular symptoms remains somewhat controversial. There is a conception of many clinicians that surgery should be reserved for those patients with radicular or neurologic signs and avoided in patients with axial

Table 4: Serious complications associated with cervical spine manipulation

Category of complication	Reported complications
Vascular injury	Visual and hearing loss
	Vertebral artery and internal carotid dissection
	Cervical epidural hematoma
Structural lesions	Intradural cervical disk herniation
	Odontoid fracture
	Atlantoaxial injury
Neurologic injury	Brainstem trauma
	Diaphragmatic paralysis
	Quadriplegia
	Myelopathy
	Radiculopathy

Table 5: Summary of studies reporting on benefits of anterior cervical discectomy and fusion (ACDF) for axial neck pain

Author	Sample size	Outcomes
Dohn et al.[22]	34	62% good or excellent, 24% fair, 15% poor
Garvey et al.[23]	87	82% good or excellent, 16% fair, 2% poor
Riley et al.[24]	93	72% good or excellent, 18% fair, 10% poor
Robinson et al.[25]	56	73% good or excellent, 22% fair, 5% poor
Roth [26]	71	93% good or excellent, 1% fair, 6% poor
White et al.[27]	28	62% good or excellent, 23% fair, 23% poor
Zheng et al.[28]	55	76% good or excellent, 18% fair, 6% poor

neck pain alone. The main justification for this viewpoint is that it is difficult to accurately define the source of axial neck pain. As discussed previously, radiographic abnormalities in asymptomatic individuals are common and increase in frequency with advancing age. Based on this, it may not be possible to accurately isolate the source of axial neck pain based on radiographic abnormalities. Despite this, there are numerous clinical studies that have reported good results following surgery for axial neck pain (Table 5). In the majority of cases, when surgery is performed for axial neck pain, an ACDF is the procedure of choice. This allows for removal of the degenerative disk and elimination of motion at the segment perceived to be the pain generator. Whether the pain is related to degenerative disk disease or facet arthropathy, the ACDF acts to eliminate the potential source of pain. The obvious limitation of this lays in the accuracy of identifying the actual pain generator.

For patients with cervical radiculopathy, the procedure of choice of many surgeons is the ACDF. This technique allows for removal of herniated disks and osteophytes to relieve pressure on the exiting nerve roots while eliminating motion at that level to reduce pain from the degenerative disk or facet joint. The surgery can be performed on up to three levels through a small transverse incision. Often the incision can be placed in line with a skin crease for improved cosmesis. For more extensive cases an oblique or longitudinal incision is used. Many surgeons prefer a left-sided approach in an attempt to reduce the risk of injury to the

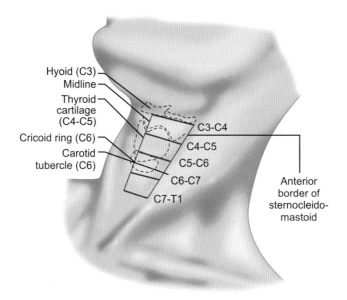

Hyoid (C3)
Midline
Thyroid cartilage (C4-C5)
Cricoid ring (C6)
Carotid tubercle (C6)

C3-C4
C4-C5
C5-C6
C6-C7
C7-T1

Anterior border of sternocleido-mastoid

Fig. 5: Illustration detailing the anatomic landmarks used to determine the location of skin incision for anterior cervical discectomy and fusion

recurrent laryngeal nerve. This nerve is believed to more predictably enter the thorax in the carotid sheath on the patient's left side, although others believe that the risk of injury is related to excessive retraction during surgery and is not side-dependent. Specific landmarks can be palpated to localize the skin incision (Fig. 5). The hyoid bone can be palpated at C3, the thyroid cartilage is palpated at C4-C5, and the cricoid is palpated at C6. After removal of the disk and osteophytes, a graft is placed in the disk space. The graft can be autologous iliac crest, allograft structural bone graft, or a cage packed with either autograft or allograft bone matrix. The perceived benefits of autograft include improved fusion rates, decreased cost, and lack of immune response. The perceived benefits of allograft include lack of donor site pain, unlimited supply, and decreased operative time due to lack of harvesting time. While initial studies reported improved fusion rates with autograft, the use of anterior cervical plates seems to have reduced this discrepancy. There is no universally accepted standard for graft material in ACDF. In an attempt to maximize fusion rates, the use of anterior cervical plates has become very common (Figs 6A and B). The plate helps to prevent graft dislodgement and also further reduces motion at the surgical level to enhance fusion. There are numerous designs for plates including various locking mechanisms, static and dynamic plates, and resorbable plates. Again, there is no universally accepted standard for use of a specific type of plating system.

While ACDF is a very commonly performed technique with good clinical results, there are potential complications. These include infection, injury to the surrounding vascular structures (internal carotid and vertebral arteries), spinal cord injury, nerve root injury, C5 nerve palsy, dysphasia, esophageal perforation, instrumentation failure, graft extrusion, pseudoarthrosis, and adjacent level degeneration. Fortunately, most of these risks are

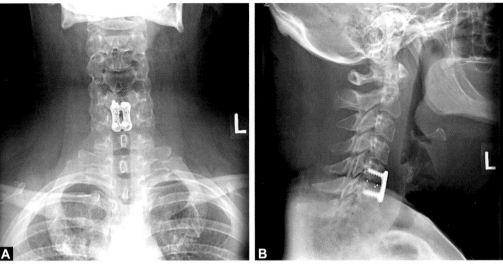

Figs 6A and B: (A) Plain lateral and (B) anteroposterior (AP) postoperative radiograph of 47-year-old female patient with C5-C6 disk herniation that underwent an anterior cervical discectomy and fusion with anterior plating, polyether-etherketone (PEEK) interbody spacer with allograft bone. These 1-year postoperative images reveal proper placement of the graft and plate with solid arthrodesis

uncommon, but they can be devastating. The most common of these complications is dysphasia which can occur in the majority of patients and is increased with multiple level surgeries and with revision surgery. The majority of these cases are short lived, but patients should be warned in advance of this common occurrence. The rate of C5 nerve palsy is approximately 5–8%. This can present as pain in the outer deltoid or weakness in the deltoid or biceps. In some patients the presentation can be delayed for several days after surgery, and in these cases it is believed to result for settling of the spinal cord causing a traction injury to the C5 nerve root. In the majority of these cases the symptoms completely resolve, but recovery may take up to 6 months.

Adjacent level degeneration is reported to occur in up to 25% of patients within 10 years of cervical fusion.[29] This is thought to be the result of increased biomechanical forces being placed across the adjacent level due to loss of motion at the fused segment. This has been supported by previous biomechanical studies showing an increase in adjacent level intradiscal pressure and segmental motion in levels adjacent to ACDF.[30] The position of the anterior plate has been reported to play a role in the development of adjacent level degeneration. Park et al. compared the development of adjacent level degenerative changes following ACDF with a plate within 5 mm of the adjacent disk versus those greater than 5 mm and reported 93% of cases with moderate to severe changes occurred with a plate within 5 mm of the disk space.[31] The incidence of cephalad adjacent level degeneration occurred in 67% of those with a plate within 5 mm of the disk versus 24% of those with the plate greater than 5 mm from the disk space.

In an attempt to reduce the risk of adjacent level degeneration following ACDF, disk arthroplasty techniques have been developed. The potential benefit of these devices is that the disk and osteophytes can be removed to address disk disease and radiculopathy, but

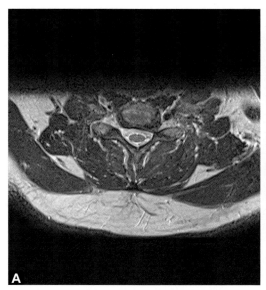
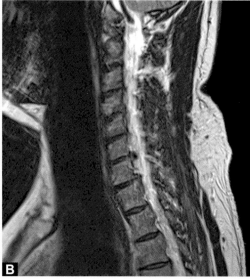

Figs 7A and B: (A) Axial and (B) sagittal MR images of 43-year-old male with left arm pain and paresthesias without axial neck pain. Images reveal a disk osteophyte complex on the left at C6-C7 causing foraminal stenosis and nerve root compression. The patient underwent a minimally invasive left C6-C7 laminoforaminotomy with good resolution of his radicular symptoms

normal kinematics at the surgical level are maintained. There are several devices available but they each share some common principles. A key technical difference compared to ACDF is the need for proper placement of the device in the disk space. For an ACDF, the exact location of the graft material or plate is less important as long as the patient goes on to a solid fusion. With disk arthroplasty, it is crucial to maintain as close to normal kinematics as possible to reduce the adverse effects on the adjacent level.[32] Since disk arthroplasty devices allow for continued motion, it is contraindicated in patients with moderate to severe facet arthrosis. Maintaining motion across the degenerative facets is likely potential source of postoperative pain. Care should be taken to avoid decorticating the endplates and anterior vertebral bodies as this increases the risk for heterotopic ossification and potential fusion across the disk space. Some surgeons recommend the use of prophylactic NSAIDs to reduce this risk.

For patients with isolated radiculopathy without axial neck pain from a cervical disk herniation a posterior laminoforaminotomy provides a useful treatment alternative to ACDF (Figs 7A and B). In this technique the exiting nerve root is decompressed through a laminotomy, and a partial discectomy can be performed through a posterior approach (Figs 8A to D). The discectomy is limited to cases of a lateral disk herniation. Due to the inability to retract the spinal cord, central disk herniations cannot be removed through this technique. The major benefit of this technique is the ability to relieve the compression of the exiting nerve root while avoiding the need for fusion. This reduces the risk of adjacent level degeneration, and it allows for a quicker return to activities as the patient is not restricted while waiting for the fusion to heal. This technique can be performed through either an open approach or a minimally invasive approach through tube dilators.

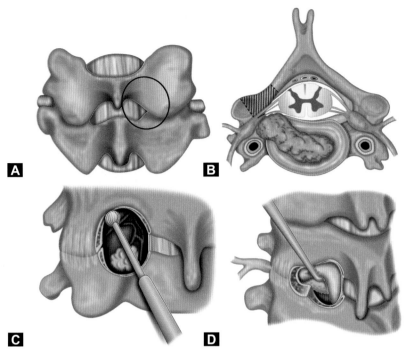

Figs 8A to D: (A) Illustration showing the location of bone resection for the laminoforaminotomy; (B) Illustration showing the foraminal stenosis resulting from the disk and osteophyte formation with nerve root compression; (C) Illustration showing the burr creating the laminoforaminotomy; (D) Gentle retraction of the exiting nerve root can be performed to reveal the underlying herniated disk

In cases of multiple level cervical disk disease, a posterior approach may provide a better surgical alternative. This approach allows for decompression of the neural elements and fusion of multiple levels. This technique is frequently performed for patients with multiple level spinal stenosis and signs of myelopathy, and it has been discussed in detail in Chapter 6.

☞ REFERENCES

1. Lehto IJ, Tertti MO, Komu ME, et al. Age-related MRI changes at 0.1T in cervical discs in asymptomatic subjects. Neuroradiology. 1994;36(1):49-53.
2. Matsumoto M, Fujimura Y, Suzuki N, et al. MRI of cervical intervertebral discs in asymptomatic subjects. J Bone Joint Surg Br. 1998;80(1):19-24.
3. Cote P, Cassidy JD, Carroll LJ, et al. The annual incidence and course of neck pain in the general population: a population-based cohort study. Pain. 2004;112(3):267-73.
4. Radhakrishnan K, Litchy WJ, O'Fallon WM, et al. Epidemiology of cervical radiculopathy. A population-based study from Rochester, Minnesota, 1976 through 1990. Brain. 1994;117:325-35.
5. Shedid D, Benzel EC. Cervical spondylosis anatomy: pathophysiology and biomechanics. Neurosurgery. 2007;60:S7-13.
6. Bogduk N, Windsor M, Inglis A. The innervation of the cervical intervertebral discs. Spine. 1988;13(1):2-8.

7. Grubb SA, Kelly CK. Cervical discography: clinical implications from 12 years of experience. Spine. 2000;25(11):1382-9.

8. Bogduk N, Marsland A. The cervical zygapophysial joints as a source of neck pain. Spine. 1988;13(6):610-7.

9. Cooper RG, Freemont AJ, Hoyland JA, et al. Herniated intervertebral disc-associated periradicular fibrosis and vascular abnormalities occur without inflammatory cell infiltration. Spine. 1995;20(5):591-8.

10. Pavlov H, Torg JS, Robie B, et al. Cervical spinal stenosis: determination with vertebral body ratio method. Radiology. 1987;164(3):771-5.

11. White AA, Panjabi MM. Update on the evaluation of instability of the lower cervical spine. Instr Course Lect. 1987;36:513-20.

12. Boden SD, McCowin PR, Davis DO, et al. Abnormal magnetic-resonance scans of the cervical spine in asymptomatic subjects. A prospective investigation. J Bone Joint Surg Am. 1990;72(8):1178-84.

13. Nardin RA, Patel MR, Gudas TF, et al. Electromyography and magnetic resonance imaging in the evaluation of radiculopathy. Muscle Nerve. 1999;22(2):151-5.

14. Carragee EJ, Hurwitz EL, Cheng I, et al. Treatment of Neck Pain. Injection and surgical interventions: Results of the Bone and Joint Decade 2000-2011 Task Force on Neck Pain and Its Associated Disorders. Spine. 2008;33(4 Suppl):S153-69.

15. Lee JW, Park KW, Chung SK, et al. Cervical transforaminal epidural steroid injection for the management of cervical radiculopathy: a comparative study of particulate versus nonparticulate steroids. Skeletal Radiol. 2009;38(11):1077-82.

16. Scanlon GC, Moeller-Bertram T, Romanowsky SM, et al Cervical transforaminal epidural steroid injections. More dangerous than we think? Spine. 2007;32(11):1249-56.

17. Derby R, Lee SH, Kim BJ, et al. Complications following cervical epidural steroid injections by expert interventionalists in 2003. Pain Physician. 2004;7(44):45-9.

18. Young IA, Michener LA, Cleland JA, et al. Manual therapy, exercise, and traction for patients with cervical radiculopathy: a randomized clinical trial. Phys Ther. 2009;89(7):632-42.

19. Hurwitx EL, Aker PD, Adams AH, et al. Manipulation and mobilization of the cervical spine. A systematic review of the literature. Spine. 1996;21(15):1746-59.

20. Dougherty P, Bajwa S, Burke J, et al. Spinal manipulation postedpidural injection for lumbar and cervical radiculopathy: a retrospective case series. J Manipulative Physiol Ther. 2004;27(7):449-56.

21. Malone DG, Baldwin NG, Tomecek FJ, et al. Complications of cervical spine manipulation therapy: 5-year retrospective study in a single-group practice. Neurosurg Focus. 2002;13:1.

22. Dohn DF. Anterior interbody fusion for treatment of cervical disk conditions. JAMA. 1966;197(11):897-900.

23. Garvey T, Transfeldt E, Malcolm J, et al. Outcome of anterior cervical discectomy and fusion as perceived by patients treated for dominant axial-mechanical cervical spine pain. Spine. 2002;27(17):1887-95.

24. Riley L, Robinson R, Johnson K, et al. The results of anterior interbody fusion of the cervical spine. J Neurosurg. 1969;30:127-33.

25. Robinson R, Walker E, Ferlic D, et al. The results of anterior interbody fusion of the cervical spine. J Bone Joint Surg Am. 1962;44:1569-87.

26. Roth DA. A new test for definitive diagnosis of the painful-disk syndrome. JAMA. 1976;235(16):1713-4.

27. White A, Southwick W, Panjabi M. Clinical instability in the lower cervical spine. Spine. 1976;1:15-27.

28. Zheng Y, Liew S, Simmons E. Value of magnetic resonance imaging and discography in determining the level of cervical discectomy and fusion. Spine. 2004;29(19):2140-5.

29. Hilibrand AS, Carlson GD, Palumbo MA, et al. Radiculopathy and myelopathy at segments adjacent to the site of a previous anterior cervical arthrodesis. J Bone Joint Surg Am. 1999;81(4):519-28.

30. Eck JC, Humphreys SC, Lim TH, et al. Biomechanical study on the effect of cervical fusion on adjacent level intradiscal pressure and segmental motion. Spine. 2002;27(22):2431-4.

31. Park JB, Cho YS, Riew KD. Development of adjacent-level ossification with an anterior cervical plate. J Bone Joint Surg Am. 2005;87(3):558-63.

32. Dmitriey AE, Cunningham BW, Hu N, et al. Adjacent level intradiscal pressure and segmental kinematics following a cervical total disc arthroplasty: an in vitro human cadaveric model. Spine. 2005;30(10):1165-72.

CHAPTER

6

Cervical Spine Stenosis

👉 INTRODUCTION

Cervical spine stenosis refers to a condition that is often age-related that leads to a progressive narrowing of the spinal canal and compression of the spinal cord. It is part of the category of cervical disorders known as cervical spondylosis or cervical degenerative disease, initially discussed in Chapter 5. It can occur either as part of the broader category with axial neck pain and cervical radiculopathy or in isolation.

When it becomes symptomatic it causes cervical spondylotic myelopathy. While this is a relatively common disorder with the potential for severe neurologic consequences, it is frequently misdiagnosed or ignored in its early stages. Due to the high rate of misdiagnosis of this disorder, the actual prevalence is unknown. It is important for the clinician to be able to recognize the early subtle findings of cervical myelopathy, council patients on the progressive natural history of the disorder, and provide reasonable treatment options.

This chapter provides an overview of the pathophysiology of cervical spine stenosis, and guides for the evaluation and treatment of the patient with cervical spondylotic myelopathy.

👉 PATHOPHYSIOLOGY

The normal anteroposterior diameter of the subaxial cervical spinal canal is 17–18 mm and the diameter of the spinal cord is approximately 10 mm.[1] A spinal canal diameter of 13 mm or less is considered to be stenotic.[2] The anteroposterior and transverse diameters of the spinal cord have been reported to vary from 8.8 mm × 12.4 mm at C2 to 8.7 mm × 14 mm at C4 to 7.4 mm × 11.4 mm at C7. The mean cross-sectional area of the spinal cord is 110 mm² at C2, 121.9 mm² at C4 and 84.6 mm² at C7.[3]

With advancing degenerative changes of the cervical spinal canal, there is less space available for the spinal cord and subsequent spinal cord compression. The symptoms of cervical spondylotic myelopathy are believed to occur from a combination of the extrinsic compressive forces on the spinal cord as well as the alteration of the normal spinal cord blood supply. The cross-sectional area of the spinal cord at the most involved level has been found to be the most accurate predictor of neurologic recovery in patients with cervical spondylotic myelopathy.[4]

The compression ratio of the spinal cord refers to the ratio between the anteroposterior and transverse diameter of the spinal cord. The value of this ratio at the site of greatest compression has been reported to predict clinical function. Bucciero et al. found that patients with a ratio of 40% or greater had improved neurologic function as compared to patients with a ratio of 38% or less. Additionally, patients with a compression ratio of 10% or less had worse neurologic function than those with a ratio of 15% or more. In this study, patients with a ratio of less than 10% did not improve following decompression surgery, while those with a ratio of 15% or more did achieve some neurologic improvement postoperatively.[5]

The prognostic effects of the compression ratio has been validated by Ogino et al. who reported that improving the compression ratio to 40% or more or increasing the cross-sectional area of the spinal cord to greater than 40 mm^2 was a strong predictor of neurologic improvement following decompression surgery.[6]

There are normal changes in the canal dimensions during range of motion of the neck that can result in dynamic cord compression. The change in canal diameter is linearly related to the amount of flexion or extension motion in the neck.[7] In addition to altering the canal diameter, flexion and extension of the neck lead to morphologic changes in the spinal cord. The spinal cord is stretched during neck flexion, and shortens and thickens with neck extension.[8] Thickening of the spinal cord can increase the risk of pressure from the infolded ligamentum flavum or lamina. During flexion there is increased risk of extrinsic pressure anteriorly on the spinal cord from bulging disks or osteophytes from the vertebral body.

Additionally, instability of a motion segment adjacent to an area of stenosis can lead to further spinal cord compression. Wang et al. reported that radiographic evidence of segmental instability was present in 71.4% of patients with severe disk degeneration versus only 22.7% of patients without severe disk degeneration.[9] Segmental instability can also compromise the spinal cord's intrinsic blood supply leading to further potential damage.[10,11]

Autopsy studies have been performed on the spinal cords of patients with myelopathy to document the intrinsic damage to the spinal cord. Ito et al. reported that there is a common pattern of lesion progression associated with progressive cervical myelopathy.[12] The initial findings include atrophy and neuronal loss in the anterior horn and intermediate zone. This is followed by degeneration of the lateral and posterior funiculi.

PATIENT PRESENTATION

As discussed previously, patients with cervical spondylotic myelopathy can present with a wide variety of vague symptoms that can often lead to a misdiagnosis or delay in diagnosis. The most common symptoms include clumsiness, altered gait, or loss of fine motor skills in the hands. These symptoms are often attributed to other causes including aging, poor vision, clumsiness and arthritis. Patients or their family members may notice a worsening gait pattern or more frequent falls. Axial neck pain or upper extremity radiculopathy are commonly present due to cervical spondylosis, but do not have to be present. In more severe cases, patients may complain of motor weakness or muscle atrophy in the upper or lower extremities. Loss or alteration of bowel and bladder function is also possible in more advanced cases. There are several grading scales for myelopathy including the Nurick classification (Table 1) and the Japanese Orthopaedic Association score (Table 2).

Table 1: Nurick disability classification for cervical spondylotic myelopathy

Grade	Description
0	Root signs or symptoms, nor cord involvement
I	Signs of cord involvement, normal gait
II	Mild gait involvement, able to be employed
III	Gait abnormality prevents employment
IV	Able to ambulate only with assistance
V	Chairbound or bedridden

Table 2: Japanese Orthopaedic Association myelopathy score

Involved area	Score	Description
Upper extremity	0	Impossible to eat with chopsticks or spoon
	1	Possible to eat with spoon but not with chopsticks
	2	Possible to eat with chopsticks, but inadequately
	3	Possible to eat with chopsticks, but awkwardly
	4	Normal
Lower extremity	0	Impossible to walk
	1	Need cane or air on flat ground
	2	Need cane or aid on stairs
	3	Possible to walk without cane or aid, but slowly
	4	Normal
Upper extremity sensation	0	Apparent sensory loss
	1	Minimal sensory loss
	2	Normal
Lower extremity sensation	0	Apparent sensory loss
	1	Minimal sensory loss
	2	Normal
Trunk sensation	0	Apparent sensory loss
	1	Minimal sensory loss
	2	Normal
Bladder function	0	Complete retention
	1	Severe disturbance: Inadequate evacuation, straining, dribbling of urine
	2	Mild disturbance: Urinary frequency, hesitancy
	3	Normal

The medical history should include questions regarding the patient's gait and balance, loss of strength or sensation, and loss of fine motor skills. Patients can be asked if they have difficulty picking up small objects such as change or buttoning the buttons on their shirt. While degenerative changes are the most common reasons for developing cervical stenosis and myelopathy, patients should be questioned to rule out other potential pathologic causes

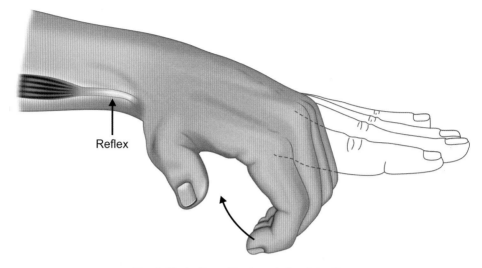

Fig. 1: Illustration of the inverted radial reflex

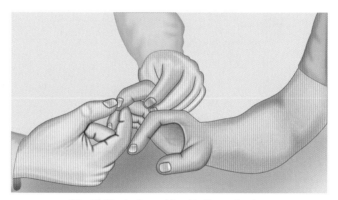

Fig. 2: Illustration of the Hoffmann's sign

of spinal cord compression such as fracture, infection or neoplasm. It is often helpful if a family member or spouse is present as they are often able to identify subtle changes prior to the patient noticing a change.

The physical examination should include testing for sensation and motor strength of the upper and lower extremities. Pain, temperature, proprioception and vibratory sensations may all be affected. There are several abnormal reflexes associated with myelopathy that should be evaluated. Patients with spinal cord compression often have hyperreflexia in the upper and lower extremities. Pathologic reflexes include the inverted radial reflex, Hoffmann's sign and the extensor plantar response (Babinski sign).

The inverted radial reflex tests for spinal cord compression at C5-C6. The brachioradialis tendon is tapped at the distal radius. A pathologic response is a lack of the normal extensor response with a hyperactive finger flexion (Fig. 1). The Hoffmann's sign is elicited by rapidly snapping the distal phalanx of the long finger and watching for a spontaneous flexion of the index finger and thumb (Fig. 2). This reflex is present in approximately 5% of the

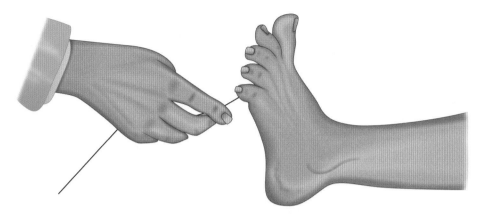

Fig. 3: Illustration of the Babinski sign

normal population. It can occur either unilaterally or bilaterally and can be accentuated by relaxing and passively extending the wrist during testing. The extensor plantar response, or Babinski, sign is present when the toes extend when the sole of the foot is stimulated (Fig. 3). It is present in approximately 50% of myelopathic patients.

There are numerous pathologic signs that can be tested in the hands of patients with suspected myelopathy. This constellation of findings known as myelopathy hand includes loss of dexterity, diffuse numbness, wasting of the intrinsic muscles, poor grip and release, and the finger escape sign. The rapid grip and release test requires the patient to open and close the hand quickly and firmly. A positive test occurs if the patient can perform less than 20 cycles in 10 seconds. The finger escape sign results from a deficiency of adduction or extension of the ring and small fingers. It is the earliest sign of intrinsic muscle weakness. The test is positive if the patient is unable to hold the hands forward and pronated with the small finger adducted for greater than 30 seconds. The larger more powerful extrinsic muscles overpower the intrinsic muscles. It progresses from the small to the ring to the long finger. It represents damage to the central pyramidal tracts of the spinal cord. It is important to rule out any ulnar nerve palsy or peripheral nerve neuropathy.

The scapulohumeral reflex is present in approximately 95% of myelopathic patients with spinal cord compression above the level of C3. It is performed by tapping the spine of the scapula or acromion and eliciting elevation of the scapula or abduction of the humerus.

IMAGING STUDIES

Imaging studies of patients with suspected cervical stenosis begin with plain radiographs in an upright position. The images should be assessed for degenerative changes including disk space narrowing, facet arthrosis, osteophyte formation and endplate sclerosis. The sagittal plane alignment is an important factor to consider in these patients. The plain radiograph is the best method to evaluate this as other more advanced imaging studies are typically performed with the patient in a supine position. The amount of cervical lordosis can play a role in surgical planning.

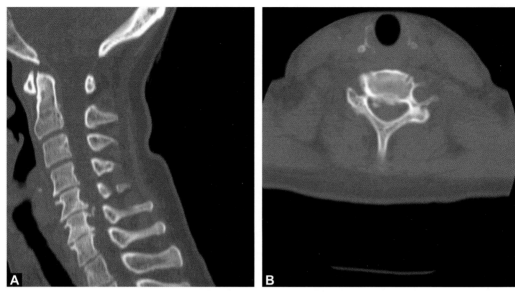

Figs 4A and B: (A) Sagittal and (B) axial CT scan of patient with progressive myelopathy from stenosis related to a large calcified disk

The Pavlov ratio is determined by dividing the anteroposterior diameter of the spinal canal by the anteroposterior diameter of the vertebral body. A normal value is 1.0, and a value of less than 0.8 suggests stenosis. However, it has not been shown to correlate well with the space available for the spinal cord. Flexion and extension radiographs can be obtained to evaluate for any abnormal motion or instability. Measurement of greater than 3.5 mm of translation or 11° of angulation are considered unstable.[13]

Computed tomography (CT) scans provide an improved visualization of the bony details (Figs 4A and B). It is useful for distinguishing osseous from soft tissue compressive structures and evaluating for the presence of ossification of the posterior longitudinal ligament. CT scans are often preferred in patients with spinal deformity, pacemaker or with a history of previous spinal instrumentation. It can be combined with myelography for improved imaging of the neural structures, but this is an invasive test.

The gold standard for imaging of patients with cervical spondylotic myelopathy is magnetic resonance imaging (MRI). MRI scans can show the degree of spinal cord and nerve root compression from disk, osteophytes and ligamentous structures (Figs 5 and 6). It is important to correlate all imaging findings with the clinical examination finding as imaging findings are frequently found in asymptomatic individuals.[14,15]

Magnetic resonance imaging scans can also identify intramedullary changes within the substance of the spinal cord. There is ongoing debate over the relevance of the signal changes in the spinal cord of myelopathic patients. Ohsio et al. found a direct correlation between histopathological features and intramedullary signal change on MRI.[16] It is generally believed that increased signal intensity of T2-weighted MRI scans represent edema which may resolve and has less clinical significance. A combination of high signals on T2-weighted images and low signals on T1-weighted images may represent more severe lesions including necrosis, myelomalacia or spongiform changes.

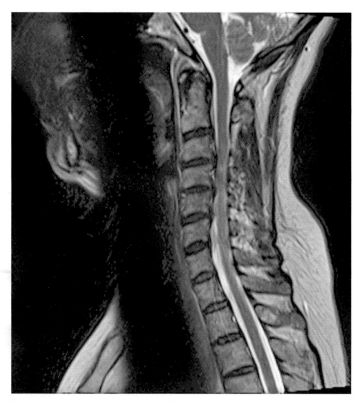

Fig. 5: Sagittal T2-weight MRI scan of patient with myelopathy revealing cervical spine stenosis from multiple level disk and osteophyte compression. The image also reveals increased signal intensity within the spinal cord

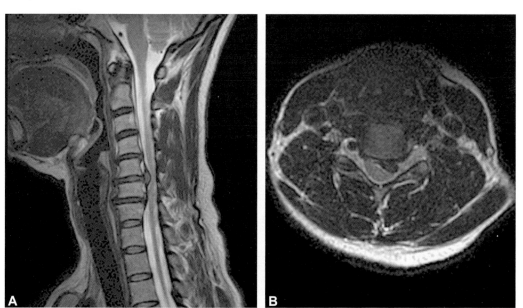

Figs 6A and B: (A) Sagittal and (B) axial MRI of patient with focal stenosis from large extruded disk herniation causing myelopathy

Previous investigators have investigated the importance of differences among these signal changes in myelopathic patients. Well-demarcated signal changes are felt to be a worse prognostic factor than a signal change with a fuzzy border.[17] In a meta-analysis of the literature Eck et al. reported that myelopathic patients without MRI signal changes had statistically better preoperative and postoperative the Japanese Orthopaedic Association scores and recovery rates following surgery compared to those with signal changes.[18]

The cross-sectional area and shape of the spinal cord at the level of the greatest compression have also been reported to be predictors of outcomes. An area less than 45 mm^2 correlates with a poor clinical outcome.[19] Spinal cords with a boomerang or teardrop shape have better outcomes than those with a triangular shape.[20]

ELECTRODIAGNOSTIC STUDIES

Electrodiagnostic studies can provide useful clinical information for patients with known or suspected cervical myelopathy. This includes the use of somatosensory evoked potential (SEP) and motor evoked potential (MEP) studies from the upper and lower extremities. Both SEP and MEP signals can be abnormal in patients with MRI evidence of spinal cord compression without clinical signs of myelopathy.[21,22] Bednarik et al. performed a prospective study of 30 patients with asymptomatic cervical stenosis with spinal cord compression and obtained SEP and MEP studies over 2 years.[22] They identified neurophysiologic abnormalities in half of the patients at the beginning of the study. Clinical signs of myelopathy developed in 5 of these 15 patients, but in none of the patients with normal electrodiagnostic studies. It was believed that there is a significant association between abnormal electrophysiological studies and the development of cervical myelopathy in patients with cervical spine stenosis.

Other studies have reported on potential predictive factors for surgical outcomes. Patients who have normal preoperative SEP have improved postoperative recovery rates.[23] Additionally, a 50% decrease in MEP correlates well with a postoperative motor deficit.[24]

NONOPERATIVE TREATMENT

Nonoperative management of patients with cervical spine stenosis should be limited to those without progressive cervical spondylotic myelopathy. If patients have axial neck pain or upper extremity radiculopathy they can often be effectively managed with anti-inflammatory medications, physical therapy, chiropractic and activity modification. Modalities including heat, ultrasound and electrical stimulation can be effective in some patients.

The use of epidural steroid injections can be beneficial in some patients with cervical radiculopathy. In most cases interlaminar injections or nonparticulate steroids are the preferred method.

Patients with symptomatic myelopathy should be cautioned against higher risk activities that could increase their risk of a spinal cord injury. These patients should avoid all contact sports and make changes in their home environment to decrease the risks of falls including removing loose rugs and cords and avoiding climbing on step ladders. In most cases patients with progressive symptomatic myelopathy are recommended for surgery.

OPERATIVE TREATMENT

Patients with cervical spine stenosis causing myelopathy generally experience a gradual, stepwise deterioration of neurologic function. The rate of neurologic decline varies among patients, but improvement without surgery is uncommon. The goals of surgery are to decompress the spinal cord and stabilize the spine. There are several methods available to achieve this goal. The decision of the optimal treatment depends on imaging findings and surgeon experience. Both anterior and posterior approaches are available.

The anterior approach to cervical myelopathy consists of anterior cervical discectomy and fusion (ACDF), corpectomy and fusion, and disk arthroplasty. Each of these utilizes a well-known anterior cervical approach. The ACDF can be performed at single or multiple levels depending on the pathology. Disk arthroplasty is currently only approved for use in a single level. The corpectomy and fusion is useful in cases of either extruded disk material that had migrated posterior to the vertebral body, large vertebral body osteophyte formation or multiple level ventral compression (Figs 7A and B). Both the ACDF and corpectomy procedures can be beneficial in cases of cervical kyphosis where there is a need to restore more normal lordosis. Each of the anterior procedures can be used in patients with concomitant axial neck pain and cervical radiculopathy.

The posterior surgical approach is utilized for either laminectomy and fusion or laminoplasty. Laminectomy alone without fusion is less commonly performed due to the potential for developing postlaminectomy kyphosis. Laminectomy and fusion is recommended for patients with multiple level cervical spine stenosis (Figs 8A and B). It can also be beneficial for the patient with axial neck pain or radiculopathy. It can help restore

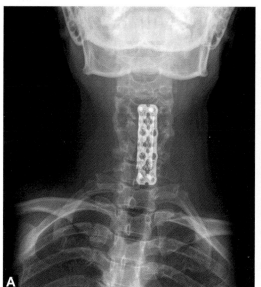
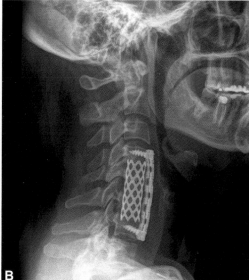

A **B**

Figs 7A and B: (A) Postoperative anteroposterior and (B) lateral radiographs of patient following C5-C6 corpectomy and C4-C7 anterior cervical fusion. Preoperative images are shown in Figure 6

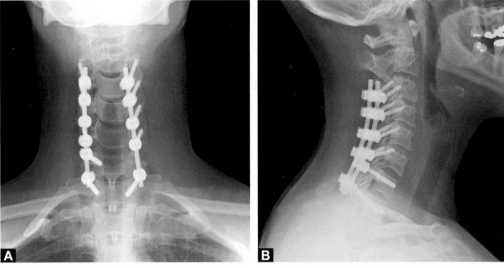

Figs 8A and B: (A) Postoperative anteroposterior and (B) lateral radiographs of patient following C3-T1 posterior decompression and instrumented fusion. Preoperative images are shown in Figure 5

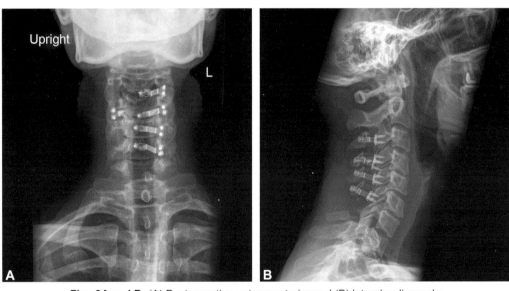

Figs 9A and B: (A) Postoperative anteroposterior and (B) lateral radiographs of a patient following C3-C6 laminoplasty

some cervical lordosis by compressing the screws together prior to their final attachment to the rods. It is also often utilized in patients with ossification of the posterior longitudinal ligament in an attempt to avoid the risk of dural tear from the anterior approach.

Laminoplasty can be performed through the posterior approach for the patient with multiple level stenosis that has limited axial neck pain, and some remaining cervical lordosis (Figs 9A and B). It can be combined with unilateral foraminotomies to address concomitant unilateral cervical radiculopathy. Laminoplasty has the benefit of maintaining approximately 50% of preoperative motion at the operative levels compared to complete loss of motion at the operative levels associated with a fusion. If upright radiographs reveal cervical kyphosis, laminoplasty is typically contraindicated as this would prevent the spinal cord from being able to shift posteriorly postoperative, and the cord would remain stretched over the posterior aspect of the vertebral bodies.

REFERENCES

1. Matsunaga S, Sakou T, Taketomi E, et al. The natural course of myelopathy caused by ossification of the posterior longitudinal ligament in the cervical spine. Clin Orthop. 1994;305:168-77.
2. Bohlman H. Cervical spondylosis and myelopathy. Inst Course Lect. 1995;44:81-97.
3. Sherman JL, Nassaux PY, Citrin CM. Measurements of normal cervical cord on MR imaging. Am J Neuroradiol. 1990;11:369-72.
4. Koyanagi T, Hirabayashi K, Satomi K, et al. Predictability of surgical results of cervical compression myelopathy based on presurgical computed tomographic myelography. Spine. 1993;18:1958-63.
5. Bucciero A, Vizioli L, Tedeschi G. Cord diameters and their significance in prognostication and decisions about management of cervical spondylotic myelopathy. J Neurosurg Sci. 1993;37(4): 223-8.
6. Ogino H, Ikata T, Okada K, et al. Canal diameter, anteroposterior compression ratio, and spondylotic myelopathy of the cervical spine. Spine. 1983;8:1-15.
7. Holmes A, Han ZH, Dang GT, et al. Changes in cervical canal volume during in vitro flexion-extension. Spine. 1996;21(11):1313-9.
8. Breig A, Turnbull I, Hassler O. Effects of mechanical stresses on the spinal cord in cervical spondylosis. A study on fresh cadaver material. J Neurosug. 1966;25:45-56.
9. Wang B, Liu H, Wang H, et al. Segmental instability in cervical spondylotic myelopathy with severe disc degeneration. Spine. 2006;31(12):1327-31.
10. Gooding MR, Wilson CB, Hoff JT. Experimental cervical myelopathy. Effects of ischemia and compression of the canine cervical spinal cord. J Neurosurg. 1975;43:9-17.
11. Gooding MR. Pathogenesis of myelopathy in cervical spondylosis. Lancet. 1074;2:1180-1.
12. Ito T, Oyanagi K, Takahashi H, et al. Cervical spondylotic myelopathy: Clinicopathologic study on the progression pattern and thin myelinated fibers of the lesions of seven patients examined during complete autopsy. Spine. 1996;21:827-33.
13. White AA 3rd, Panjabi MM. Update on the evaluation of instability of the lower cervical spine. Instr Course Lect. 1987;36:513-20.
14. Boden SD, McCowin PR, Davis DO, et al. Abnormal magnetic-resonance scans of the cervical spine in asymptomatic subjects. A prospective investigation. J Bone Joint Surg Am. 1990;72: 1178-84.
15. Teresi LM, Lifkin RB, Reicher MA, et al. Asymptomatic degenerative disk disease and spondylosis of the cervical spine: MR imaging. Radiol. 1987;164:83-8.
16. Ohsio I, Hatayama A, Kaneda K, et al. Correlation between histopathologic features and magnetic resonance images of spinal cord lesions. Spine. 1993;18:1140-9.
17. Wada E, Ohmura M, Yonenobu K. Intramedullary changes of the spinal cord in cervical spondylotic myelopathy. Spine. 1995;20:2226-32.
18. Eck JC, Drew J, Currier BL. Effects of magnetic resonance imaging signal change in mylopathic patients. A meta-analysis. Spine. 2010;35(23):E1306-9.
19. Fukushima T, Ikata T, Taoka Y, et al. Magnetic resonance imaging study on spinal cord plasticity in patients with cervical compression myelopathy. Spine. 1991;16(10 Suppl):S534-8.

20. Matsuyama Y, Kawakami N, Yanase M, et al. Cervical myelopathy due to OPLL: clinical evaluation by MRI and intraoperative spinal sonography. J Spinal Disord Tech. 2004;17:401-4.
21. Simo M, Szirmai I, Aranyi Z. Superior sensitivity of motor over somatosensory evoked potentials in the diagnosis of cervical spondylotic myelopathy. Eur J Neurol. 2004;11:621-6.
22. Bednarik J, Kadanka Z, Vohanka S, et al. The value of somatosensory and motor evoked potentials in preclinical spondylotic cervical cord compression. Eur Spine J. 1988;7:493-500.
23. Liu RK, Tang LM, Chen CJ, et al. The use of evoked potentials for clinical correlation and surgical outcome in cervical spondylotic myelopathy with intramedullary high signal intensity on MRI. J Neurol Neurosurg Psychiatry. 2004;75:256-61.
24. Nakagawa Y, Tamaki T, Yamada H, et al. Discrepancy between decreases in the amplitude of compound muscle action potential and loss of motor function caused by ischemic and compressive insults to the spinal cord. J Orthop Sci. 2002;7:102-10.

7

Cervical Spine Trauma

INTRODUCTION

Cervical spine injuries occur in up to 3% of all blunt traumas.[1] The potential for instability and catastrophic neurologic injury makes it imperative that a high index of suspicion should be maintained along with early precautions and aggressive evaluation and management when necessary. The consequences of missed cervical injuries can be catastrophic neurologically.[2] In the evaluation and management of cervical spine trauma, three key factors should always be considered: (1) spinal stability, (2) neurology and (3) patient factors. These factors guide the surgeon's formulation of a treatment plan and shape the goals of treatment. Spinal stability is one of the most important considerations in the definitive management of cervical spine trauma. Spinal stability is defined by White and Panjabi as the "ability of the spine under physiologic loads to limit patterns of displacement so as not to damage or irritate the spinal cord or nerve roots and, in addition, to prevent incapacitating deformity or pain due to structural changes".[3-5] The patient's presenting neurology and observation of its evolution (i.e. deterioration or improvement) provides the surgeon with essential information to guide treatment. The presence, extent and evolution of neurologic injury can especially shape the timing and type of interventions as well as the patient's prognosis. The role of patient factors such as medical comorbidities, other organ system injuries and underlying spine diagnoses, i.e. ankylosing spondylitis (AS) cannot be overemphasized.

The cervical spine is comprised of two anatomically distinct zones: (1) the atlantoaxial (AA) spine and (2) subaxial spine. There are also two "junctional zones" that are often addressed as separately: (1) the occipitocervical (OC) and (2) cervical-thoracic spine. The AA spine comprises C1 and C2, and the subaxial cervical spine comprises C3-C7. C7 also behaves as a junctional portion of the cervical spine as it comprises the cervical-thoracic junction. For the purposes of this chapter, distinctions have been made based on the distinct anatomic zones with some attention also placed on the junctional regions.

PATHOPHYSIOLOGY

The pathophysiology of cervical fractures is best understood by first understanding the distinct anatomical features and functions of the zones of the cervical spine. Understanding the pathoanatomy of cervical injury has guided surgeons in the development of injury

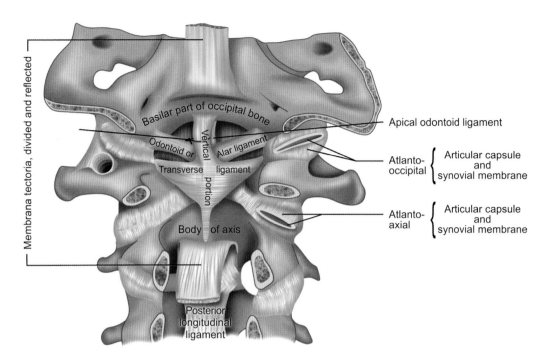

Fig. 1: Ligamentous anatomy of the occipitocervical and atlantoaxial region

classification systems. These classification systems become the language that surgeons use to describe injuries, communicate, guide treatment and prognosticate on specific injuries. Most injury classification systems attempt to describe an injury either morphologically, mechanistically and neurologically, or a combination of the three can be employed. Ultimately, they are meant to help the surgeon assess cervical stability and thus the need for treatment.

Establishing the stability of a particular cervical spine injury is not a binary (yes-or-no) issue but rather a matter of assessing and determining the extent of instability along a continuum.[6] White and Panjabi developed a checklist that takes into consideration the competence of the anterior and posterior spinal elements, the extent of static and dynamic displacement (including the stretch test), the presence of neurologic injury, and the anticipated physiologic loads to which the spine subsequently would be subjected.[3,4] This assessment of stability is based largely on a static radiographic assessment of the bone anatomy. It is now recognized that much of the stability of the cervical spine, particularly its ability to resist kyphosis, is attributable to the posterior capsule-ligamentous structures, which cannot be directly visualized with X-ray or computed tomography (CT) and has inconsistent reliability even with magnetic resonance imaging (MRI).[6,7]

Occipitocervical Injury

The OC articulation is made up of the junction of the occipital condyles to the "atlas" (C1). Occipitocervical injuries typically occur via blunt mechanism. The OC articulation is quite robust and is maintained by a network of complex ligaments (Fig. 1). In order

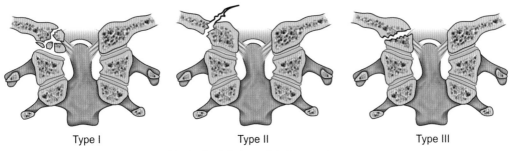

| Type I | Type II | Type III |

Fig. 2: Occipital condyle fracture types

to cause instability, injuries must typically be high energy and cause rupture of multiple ligamentous structures. Typically, a combination of major hyperextension, hyperflexion and lateral deviation or axial dissociation needs to occur in order for an OC injury to take place. The injuries are often fatal due to brainstem injury and polytrauma. A high index of suspicion should be maintained to detect these injuries. Symptoms are often impossible to attribute specifically to OC injury but may include facial and occipitocervical swelling, shortness of breath [diminished respiratory drive (pentaplegia)], cranial nerve injury and cruciate paralysis. Occipital condyle fractures are typically classified by the Anderson and Montesano method.[8] Type I injuries have comminution of the condyle and are usually stable. Type II injuries consist of a skull base fracture extending through one of the condyles. These are also typically considered stable. Type III injuries consist of bony avulsion of the occipital condyle through its alar ligament attachment (Fig. 2). These injuries tend to be associated with cranial cervical dissociation and should be suspicious for instability.[8] Also patients with bilateral occipital condyle fracture should be assumed to have an unstable cranio-cervical dissociation until proven otherwise.

Craniocervical dissociation is typically associated with blunt injury such as motor vehicle crashes or falls. Major deceleration trauma is common. The tensile load capacity to failure of each alar ligament has been described as being about half of an anterior cruciate ligament. There are very few specific physical examination findings or clinical signs to hint at the presence of craniocervical dissociation. There may be significant swelling of the head and neck and associated skull injury. Neurologic injuries are common but can vary widely. The overall combination and arrangement of the craniocervical ligaments offer significant protection against minor trauma. Major trauma involving likely hyperextension with disruption of the tectorial membrane and lateral hyperflexion with disruption of the alar ligaments is likely necessary to produce craniocervical dissociation. Atlanto-occipital dissociation or dislocation is most typical in the anterior direction or the vertical (axial) direction. Posterior displacement is the rarest type. The Harborview atlanto-occipital dissociation classification emphasizes craniocervical injury severity.[9] Type I injuries consist of incomplete ligament injuries such as unilateral alar ligament tear. Type II injuries consist of complete craniocervical dissociation with initial lateral radiographs showing borderline screening measurement abnormalities. Type III injuries demonstrate obvious major craniocervical displacement on plane imaging and Type IIID injury identifies death from craniocervical dissociation in the first 24 hours following injury.[9]

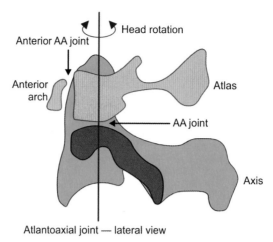

Atlantoaxial joint — lateral view

Fig. 3: Atlantoaxial (AA) articulation

Atlantoaxial Cervical Spine

The AA region of the spine is distinct in its anatomic and functional differences from the subaxial cervical spine due to the shape and relationship of the C1-C2 articulation. It is composed of the C1 (atlas) and C2 (axis). The C1-C2 articulation is a "biconcave joint" (Fig. 3). The odontoid (dens) acts as the "axis" or post around which the C1 vertebra rotates. Approximately 50% of cervical rotation motion comes from the AA articulation. The transverse ligament, which inserts upon the medial C1 lateral masses, resists anteroposterior translation of C1 on C2.

Besides contributing about 50% of the cervical rotation, the AA spine contributes about 20° of flexion and extension to overall cervical range of motion. C1 fractures contribute to about 10% of all cervical spinal fractures. They have a high association with other spine fractures.[10] Fractures of the atlas are classified based upon fracture location. The atlas is composed of two lateral masses, an anterior arch and a posterior arch. Lateral mass fractures typically occur from a lateral compression type injury or mechanism. They are usually unilateral and stable. If they have associated ligamentous injury, they may have a higher degree of instability.

A Jefferson fracture is a burst fracture of the atlas. It typically results from an axial load mechanism. Fracturing of the anterior and posterior arches of the atlas can lead to spreading of the lateral masses. If the lateral masses of C1 overhang the lateral masses of C2 by a combined distance of 6.9 mm then disruption of the transverse ligament is likely (Fig. 4).[11] This is based on open-mouth odontoid plain X-ray examination. If utilizing a CT scan, 8.1 mm of lateral mass overhang is considered a critical value of instability. The transverse ligament is the main restraining structure to prevent anterior and posterior translation of the atlas over the axis.

Atlantoaxial rotatory instability is an uncommon injury in adults. It is more common in children. If it does occur in adults, it is most likely associated with traumatic injuries and upper cervical spine fractures. The normal constraints to excessive AA instability

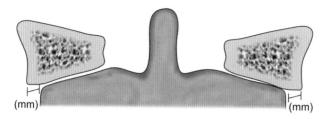

Fig. 4: "Rule of Spence" identifying the overhang of C1 lateral masses to identify transverse ligament disruption

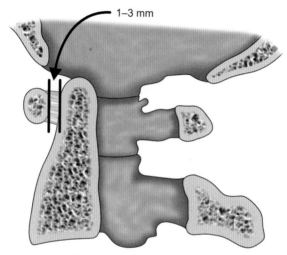

1–3 mm

Fig. 5: Atlanto-dens interval

are provided by the alar and transverse ligaments. These injuries may be missed in the initial evaluation. They may present late with pain, torticollis and limited head rotation. Fielding and Hawkins devised a classification for AA rotatory instability.[12] Type I: rotatory fixation without anterior displacement of the atlas. Type II: rotatory fixation with anterior displacement of the atlas of 3–5 mm. Type III: rotatory fixation with anterior displacement greater than 5 mm. Type IV: rotatory fixation with posterior displacement. Type I injuries do not have associated ligamentous injuries. By definition, rupture of one or more of the ligaments including the transverse and/or alar ligaments will be disrupted with type II-IV injuries.[12] When these types of injuries are suspected, CT scan is the optimal diagnostic modality. Dynamic CT scanning may help increase the diagnostic information.

Anteroposterior AA instability occurs when the transverse ligament or its attachments are disrupted. Occasionally, the alar ligaments may be ruptured as well. This typically occurs from a flexion mechanism. The presence of traumatic AA instability can be determined by measuring the anterior atlanto-dens interval (AADI). In adults, a 3 mm AADI is considered within normal limits (Fig. 5). In children, an AADI of 4 mm or less is considered normal. When this injury is suspected, a CT scan will allow identification of subluxation of the AA region as well as identification of associated fractures.

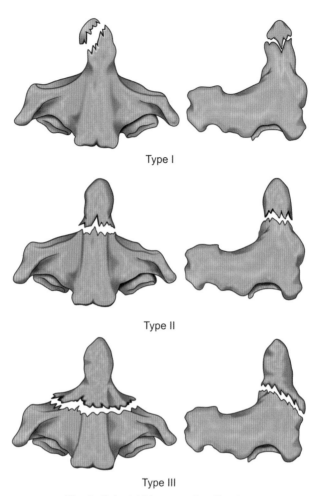

Type I

Type II

Type III

Fig. 6: Odontoid fracture classification

Odontoid Fractures

Odontoid fractures are common. They may occur in upwards of 20% of all cervical spine fractures. They tend to occur in a bimodal distribution (young adults who have experienced high-energy trauma and in older adults due to low-energy mechanisms such as fall). The classification of odontoid fractures is based upon the morphology and location of the fracture line.[13] Type I fractures are the least common. They result in an avulsion of the odontoid tip. They are considered stable injuries. These may be associated with OC injuries and thus should arouse suspicion of other injuries. Type II fractures occur at the base of the odontoid. They occur through the junction of the dens and C2 vertebral body. Type III fractures occur through cancellous bone portion of the C2 vertebral body (Fig. 6).

Traumatic Spondylolisthesis of the Axis

Traumatic spondylolisthesis of the axis is also referred to as a Hangman's fracture. This fracture typically occurs in young adults who sustain high-energy trauma. The most

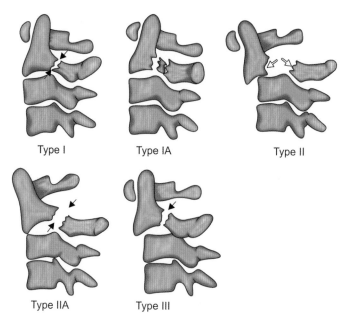

Type I   Type IA   Type II

Type IIA   Type III

Fig. 7: Hangman's fracture classification

common mechanism is hyperextension. It is rarely associated with neurological deficits. The classification has four primary subtypes with one-fifth addition as an atypical pattern.[14] (1) Type I: bilateral pars fracture with less than 3 mm displacement and no angulation. (2) Type II: vertical fracture line through the pars with displacement of greater than 3 mm and significant angulation. (3) Type IIA fractures differ from type II fractures in that they have an oblique fracture of the pars with no displacement of the fracture but significant angulation. The angulation is typically greater than 15°. It is thought that the injury mechanism for this type of fracture is due to flexion distraction with resultant disk disruption at C2-C3 and rupture of the posterior longitudinal ligament (PLL). It is important to distinguish between type II and type IIA. Type IIA fractures should not have attempts at reduction with traction due to the disruption of the PLL and C2-C3 disk. (4) A type III fracture is similar to a type I fracture, but it also has bilateral C2-C3 facet dislocation (Fig. 7).

Starr and Eismont also identified an atypical fracture pattern Hangman's variant.[15] In this case, the fracture is similar to a type I, but instead of the fracture lines both propagating through the pars the fracture propagates through the posterior body of C2. This has been labeled a type IA. Displacement of this fracture type may result in neurologic injury due to a retained hook of bone in the posterior wall of C2 (Fig. 8). Typically, a Hangman's fracture opens the spinal canal. However, in the case of IA fracture type, a displacement of C2 could theoretically increase the risk of neurologic compression.

Subaxial Cervical Spine

The vertebrae of the subaxial cervical spine share similar anatomy with regard to the anterior and posterior bony elements, intervertebral disks, joint capsules, ligaments and surrounding neurovascular structures. The transverse process contains the transverse foramen, through

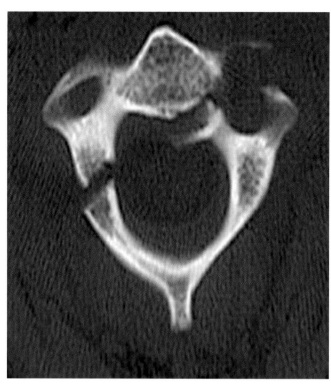

Fig. 8: Hangman's Type IA variant with one fracture line extending into the posterior vertebral body wall

which the vertebral artery passes (between C3 and C6); the vertebral artery may be injured in the setting of subaxial cervical spine fracture or dislocation. Important soft-tissue structures in the posterior aspect of the cervical spine include the facet capsules, ligamentum flavum, interspinous ligaments and supraspinous ligaments. They play a crucial role in providing tensile stability to the cervical spine in flexion as is demonstrated by the kyphosis that can develop when they are disrupted by force transmission during traumatic injury.[6]

The design of any fracture classification system is challenged by large variability in fracture mechanisms, morphology and clinical presentations. A fracture classification system ought to capture the essence of the most important factors while not being so cumbersome as to make communication difficult. Allen and Ferguson reviewed 165 subaxial cervical spine injuries.[16] Based solely on static radiographs and the documented and/or inferred mechanisms of injury, they devised a classification that grouped injuries into phylogenies according to their radiographic appearance, then arranged them along a spectrum of anatomic disruption.[16] Six general categories include: (1) flexion-compression, (2) vertical compression, (3) flexion-distraction, (4) extension-compression, (5) extension-distraction and (6) lateral flexion. Within each phylogeny is a series of stages based on the severity of anatomic disruption.[16] The flexion-distraction category is the most widely identifiable and subcategorized group. It progresses in severity from facet subluxation to unilateral facet dislocation to bilateral facet dislocation. This scheme, though descriptive, does not guide the surgeon's treatment plan.

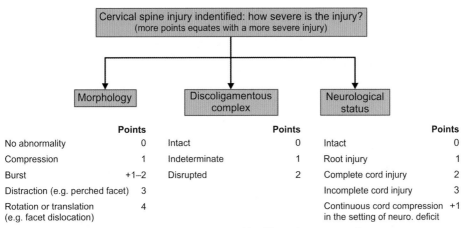

Fig. 9: Outline of subaxial injury classification system (SLIC) scoring system. It encompasses scores for injury morphology, neurology and discoligamentous complex

Mechanistic classification systems attempt to predict the primary injury vector from pattern seen on radiographs. Many of the mechanisms that have been classified have been accepted as common nomenclature to describe specific injuries. In some cases, the mechanistic nomenclature has also come to imply a specific morphologic pattern of injury such as compression fracture or flexion-distraction injury. Unfortunately, mechanistic classifications do not account for the multiple force vectors that tend to occur in traumatic cervical spine injury. For example, a flexion moment may occur at one level and an extension moment may occur at another.[17]

Most mechanistic classifications fall short in that they do not account for instability. White and Panjabi have defined stability as the ability of the spine under physiologic loads to maintain an association between vertebral segments in such a way that there is neither damage nor subsequent irritation of the spinal cord or nerve roots and in addition there is no development of incapacitating deformity or pain due to structural changes. This definition has been well accepted from a biomechanical standpoint but the scoring system that has been developed by those authors has not been clinically validated.[18,19]

The most recently constructed and validated classification system for the subaxial region is called the subaxial injury classification (SLIC) system.[7] No subaxial cervical injury classification to date has been universally validated except the SLIC system. All prior systems were based on one of three factors: (1) mechanism of injury, (2) morphologic features, or (3) degree of instability. The SLIC system was designed to be a simple, reliable system that allows easy communication and helps guide treatment. It is comprised of three main components: (1) injury morphology (2) patient neurology and (3) integrity of the discoligamentous complex (DLC). For each category, a score is assigned based on severity of the morphology, neurology or discoligamentous injury (Fig. 9). The morphology component can be scored from 0 (no abnormality) to 4 (rotation or translation instability). A score of 1 corresponds to a compression fracture. A burst fracture adds an additional point to score 2. A distraction injury such as a facet perch or hyperextension is assigned a score of 3. The most severe morphology score of 4 may include facet dislocations, translation injuries or advanced flexion-compression injuries.

The neurologic component is scored from 0 to 3 with a +1 modifier for ongoing spinal cord compression. No neurologic injury scores a 0. Nerve root injury is assigned a score of 1. Complete spinal cord injury is assigned a score of 2, and incomplete spinal cord injury is assigned a score of 3. Injuries with a score of 5 or greater tend to be treated surgically, and injuries with a score of 3 or less tend to be treated nonoperatively. Injuries that score 4 are indeterminate and can typically be treated either way.[20]

☞ PATIENT PRESENTATION

When missed at initial evaluation, unstable cervical spine fractures and/or dislocations have the potential to lead to sudden, catastrophic and permanent disability. Thus, the importance of a careful, thorough clinical and radiographic evaluation cannot be overstated. Physical examination of the patient with a suspected cervical spine injury should begin with the standard trauma resuscitation as outlined by the Advanced Trauma Life Support (ATLS) protocol.[21] Life-threatening compromise to the airway, breathing and circulation should be promptly addressed. Specifically for the cervical spine, the collar should be carefully removed and the posterior cervical spine palpated for tenderness along the midline or paraspinal tissues.[22] The examiner should note how the patient holds his or her head, looking specifically for angular or rotational deformities that may, for example, point to a unilateral facet dislocation. The face and scalp should be examined for evidence of direct trauma, which may not only suggest a closed head injury but also provide insight about the forces during the accident that were imparted to the head and neck.[22]

Physical examination or presenting mechanisms do not necessarily lend themselves to make the presence of occipital condyle injuries or OC dissociation injuries obvious. A high degree of suspicion should be maintained for any patient involved in a high-energy trauma, especially those with head or facial injuries. Certain aspects of the history should also be accounted for because they may provide important clues. The physician should review the available details of the accident, the energy and mechanism of injury, the general condition of the patient at the scene, and the presence or absence of neurologic deficits. A history of a high-energy trauma or transient neurologic symptoms should raise the level of suspicion for injuries that may not be readily evident at first glance.[22] Associated injuries such as facial bruising or laceration may indicate hyperextension injury in patients who have fallen and hit their head. These mechanisms are common in patients who suffer odontoid fractures. It is also important to identify other associated conditions and comorbidities that might influence either the nature of the injury or the means by which it is managed. Associated conditions that are particularly relevant for patients with suspected cervical spine injury include AS, diffuse idiopathic skeletal hyperostosis (DISH), previous cervical spine fusion (congenital or acquired), and connective tissue disorders leading to ligamentous laxity.[22] Negative plain radiographs alone should not be used as the rationale for discharging the patient home. More definitive imaging (e.g. CT, MRI) is mandatory. The typical guidelines used to determine the stability of spinal injuries are inapplicable to the patient with an ankylosed spine. To rationalize that the injury is relatively stable because of the lack of displacement can be a catastrophic error because the ankylosis and the altered biomechanics make these injuries much more likely to be unstable.[22]

Paramount to the evaluation of the cervical spine injured patient is full neurologic assessment. The chapter on spinal cord injury goes into an in-depth review of internationally standardized methods for assessment and documentation of neurologic examinations.[23] The ability to perform a proper comprehensive baseline neurologic examination and subsequently recognize changes of that examination in a timely fashion is one of the most important skills a clinician can develop in the management of cervical spine trauma.

🖝 IMAGING

The goal of clearing the cervical spine in the evaluation of trauma is to efficiently and safely rule out an injury that might, if missed, lead to neurologic injury or late instability.[22] Clinical protocols exist that allow clearance of the cervical spine in asymptomatic patients without imaging. The National Emergency X-Radiography Utilization Study (NEXUS) and Canadian C-spine rules are highly sensitive in ruling out clinically significant cervical injuries without radiographs.[24-28] Patients do not typically need X-rays if they are fully alert and oriented, has been involved in a low-energy trauma, is devoid of neurologic signs or symptoms, has no midline tenderness, can actively rotate the head 45° in both directions, and lacks distracting injuries that might divert his or her attention away from a severe neck injury, the Canadian cervical spine imaging protocol was developed and studied so as to limit the number of unnecessary cervical radiographs in patients presenting to the emergency department. It is typical for these criteria to be used in other countries (especially the United States) to determine whether a patient may have their cervical orthosis removed, once radiographs have been performed and are normal. Considerable care and judgment should always be exercised on a case by case basis when cervical injury is suspected. It has been shown that despite being both "clinically and radiographically cleared" late cervical instability can still develop after injury.[2] Plain X-rays, CT and MRI are not universally flawless, and most studies are unlikely to observe the proper number of patients to capture the very low frequency event of delayed cervical instability with normal radiographs.

It should also be emphasized that utilization of a rigid cervical collar to protect the "uncleared" cervical spine does not eliminate all cervical motion or need for diligent protection. Transporting patients, log-rolling or manipulating them in bed may still lead to unwanted motion in a collared, injured spine that could potentially cause neurologic deterioration.[29]

Patients with neck pain, tenderness, neurologic symptoms, appropriate mechanism for spine injury and obtunded patients require radiologic evaluation. Patients with distracting injuries or short-term cognitive dysfunction can either be protected with spinal precautions until management of these issues is completed and definitive clinical examination possible, or if urgency dictates, can be examined under the same criteria as the obtunded patient.[22]

In patients who do require radiographic investigation, the optimal choice of imaging modality is evolving. Clinicians are less reliant on plain X-ray imaging and are utilizing CT scans in comprehensive trauma screening protocols more frequently. Modern helical CT has been found to be more sensitive, specific and efficient than conventional radiography.[22]

The increased utilization of CT scan has made detection of OC injuries much more reliable. The basion-dens interval (BDI) and the basion posterior atlantal interval (BAI) are two measurements devised by Harris et al. to aid in the detection of OC

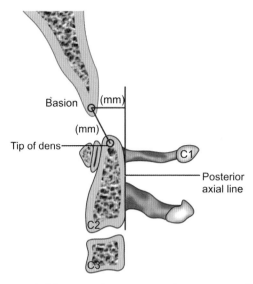

Fig. 10: The basion-dens interval (BDI) and basion posterior atlantal interval (BAI) are illustrated. The BDI is drawn from the basion to the tip of the dens. The BAI is a horizontal line drawn from the basion to the posterior axial line. Both measurements should be 12 mm or less.

dislocation (Fig. 10).[30] When the BDI and BAI are greater than 12 mm, OC dissociations are highly likely. The Harris line is believed to be the most useful, sensitive, and reproducible of radiographic parameters for detecting and characterizing OC dissociation and dislocations.

Bono et al., in conjunction with the Spine Trauma Study Group, developed a consensus paper on subaxial cervical imaging measurements.[31] Their premise was that optimal measurement methods need to be standardized so that important injury characteristics can be communicated clearly and consistently. They felt that standardization of injury measurement techniques would be both beneficial for clinical trials and diagnostic and therapeutic decision making.[31] Two methods have been described for defining cervical kyphosis. The first method utilizes the Cobb measurement. The measurement is taken from the cephalad endplate of the vertebral body above the injury that is unaffected and the inferior endplate of the caudal unaffected vertebral body. An alternative method is to utilize the vertebral body tangent lines (Fig. 11). Lines can be drawn along the posterior vertebral body of the two affected levels, and kyphosis angulation can be measured from their intersection.

Measurement of vertebral body translation should be performed by drawing a line along the posterior vertebral body of the two affected levels. The distance between these two lines indicates translation of one vertebral body over the other. The amount of facet overlap in cervical spine injuries has been considered an important variable to identify extent of facet subluxation. By utilizing reformatted CT images or lateral X-rays, the observer should measure the amount of intact overlapping facet articular surface. The length of the superior articular process is measured and is considered the numerator. The length of the inferior articular surface is also measured and is considered the denominator. A ratio is developed to identify the percentage of facet overlap.[32]

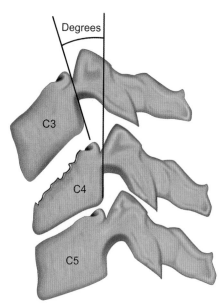

Fig. 11: Posterior vertebral body tangential line measurement to assess kyphosis

Utilization of MRI is typically recommended in the setting of neurologic deficit either transient, stable or progressive. It is especially useful if the patient's neurologic examination/ deficit does not match with the level of bony injury found on CT or X-ray. MRI in the setting of spinal cord injury can provide information about the neurologic structures including regions of edema, hemorrhage, compression or even transection. MRI findings in the setting of spinal cord injury have been found to be prognostic of recovery.[33] MRI is also useful in helping to define discoligamentous injury. In the setting of facet dislocation, the presence of disk herniation may be a guiding factor in whether a clinician decides to utilize closed reduction traction maneuvers or proceeds directly to open anterior discectomy and reduction. Investigators have studied the utility of MRI in assessing the integrity of the posterior ligamentous complex. The interpretation of traumatic MRI can be very sensitive and accurate regardless of years of training of the observer. However, the attending-level spine surgeon has been shown to be statistically more specific in the evaluation of injury on MRIs.[34] The fluid-weighted STIR sagittal sequences are most useful in determining injury to the supraspinous and interspinous ligaments, ligamentum flavum and cervical facets capsules.[34] However, studies such as this are often difficult to generalize due to small numbers of patients and observers. Also MRI has a tendency to overestimate posterior ligamentous injuries.

Not all abnormal findings on MRI are necessarily clinically significant. Some studies correlating MRI findings with direct surgical inspection illustrate the tendency of MRI to overestimate injury to the cervical and thoracolumbar posterior ligamentous complex.[35,36] How MRI should be incorporated into the evaluation of the obtunded patient remains a contentious issue. Some suggest that a negative helical CT alone can clear an unexaminable patient of clinically meaningful injuries while others state that both CT and MRI are necessary for definitive clearance.[22] Despite having excellent access and ability to utilize advanced three-dimensional imaging, there are still reports of patients who have had late spine instability and/or neurologic deficit when all imaging of the cervical spine was deemed negative.[2]

Associated vascular injury in the setting of cervical spine fractures is relatively common (especially those that involve significant displacement or disruption of the transverse foramen).[37-39] Magnetic resonance and CT angiography are becoming popular as relatively easy methods of evaluating the vertebral artery in the setting of cervical trauma. Their ability to demonstrate injury of the vertebral artery is not questioned. The optimal management of such injuries, however, remains controversial, because most are asymptomatic, and prophylactic anticoagulation poses potential risk of epidural hematoma and neurologic deterioration.[37-39]

NONOPERATIVE TREATMENT

Occipitocervical Injury

Nonoperative treatment for OC dissociation revolves around ATLS principles. Ensuring life-saving measures is the most important initial treatment. If possible, closed reduction maneuvers and temporary stabilization with Halo bracing or skeletal traction should be utilized. Since there is a propensity toward distraction of the OC region, care should be taken to limit the weight that is utilized. Halo vest immobilization is the preferable initial stabilization method when operative treatment cannot be undertaken right away. In adults, gross instability at the OC junction definitively requires surgical stabilization when the patient's medical condition allows. In children, there is less conviction about the requirement of surgical stabilization for definitive stabilization.

Jefferson Fractures

Most Jefferson fractures can be treated nonoperatively. Soft or rigid collars are appropriate for "stable" fractures. Fractures that meet Spence's rule or clearly have evidence of transverse ligament injury should be treated with halo vest immobilization. Surgical fixation can also be performed. In the setting of multiple cervical injuries, the surgical plan is typically dictated by the other fractures. Most Jefferson fractures can be treated with collar or halo immobilization. If nonunion or delayed instability occurs, surgical treatment can be undertaken.

Traumatic Spondylolisthesis of the Axis (Hangman's Fractures)

Type I and type IA fractures typically can be treated with rigid cervical collar immobilization. Consideration for halo vest for the first 4 weeks and then transfer to rigid collar is also a reasonable option. Type IA injuries should be watched closely for any translation. These types of fractures may have increased risk of neurologic injury due to the maintenance of a partially closed spinal canal. The posterior wall spike of bone may become an impinging factor.

Type II and type IIA fractures typically require reduction before immobilization with a halo. Again transition to rigid collar may occur after 4–6 weeks if the fracture maintains alignment with initial aggressive immobilization. Type II fractures can be reduced with traction followed by halo vest application. It has traditionally been advocated that reduction of type II fractures should be followed by 4–6 weeks of bed rest and traction prior to mobilization. However, mobilizing the patient in a halo acutely is typically safe. The fracture can be monitored with sequential imaging to identify its behavior pattern.

Odontoid Fractures

Type I odontoid fractures do not pose risk for neurologic impairment. Treatment for these fractures is symptomatic. Bracing is not typically required. Type II and type III odontoid fractures have been studied extensively. A plethora of scientific articles over the past several decades have discussed treatment methods for these fractures. Despite such an extensive body of literature, the indications for selection of specific treatment modality for these fractures have not been firmly established.[40-42]

There appears to be a significant role for separating fracture scenarios by age. Younger patients tend to be involved in much higher-energy injuries, and these fractures behave in a more unstable fashion. The choice of optimum external brace immobilization for odontoid fractures is based on surgeon choice, but age and energy of injury are important factors to consider. Young patients tend to tolerate halo vest immobilization better than elderly patients, whereas elderly patients have a much higher rate of complications including mortality. For younger patients, halo vest immobilization or cervical bracing are both viable options for the treatment of type II and type III odontoid fractures. The benefits of utilizing halo immobilization for the elderly typically do not outweigh the risk.

Multiple studies have shown the high rate of healing with type III odontoid fractures. Type II odontoid fractures have a higher rate of nonunion. For these fractures, factors that affect healing include degree and direction of displacement, angulation, age, delay in diagnosis and definitive treatment. Angulation greater than 10°, translation greater than 5 mm, age greater than 65 years, posterior displacement and comminution at the base of the odontoid are all risk factors for nonunion.

Unfortunately, treatment objectives that constitute acceptable outcome for odontoid fractures have not been firmly established. For instance, anatomical alignment and bony union are typically treatment goals of spinal fractures. However, fibrous nonunion in elderly patients may be an acceptable outcome given the very low rate of delayed neurologic consequences.[43] It has been shown in the elderly population that treatment with a cervical collar for 12 weeks generates a high rate of fibrous nonunion. However, the functional outcomes are not significantly different from age-matched controls.[43-45]

Subaxial Cervical Spine Fractures

There is a wide variety of subaxial fractures that can safely be treated with a rigid cervical collar. The SLIC classification helps guide this assessment. Some isolated injuries such as C7 spinous process fractures (clay shoveler's fracture) or isolated lamina fractures do not typically require any bracing at all for stability. Bracing may be chosen for comfort. Most isolated facet or lateral mass fractures can be treated with a collar alone and will not require surgery. Halliday et al. utilized MRI to help predict stability of unilateral facet fractures. They stated that plain radiographs of the cervical spine lack sensitivity to detect the presence of lateral mass/facet fractures. And the appearance of the fracture on CT does not indicate instability. The degree of ligamentous injury at the level of the fracture demonstrated on MRI correlates with instability for unilateral lateral mass fractures that present with a subluxation or that have injury to at least three of the following ligaments: the facet region, the interspinous ligament, the anterior longitudinal ligament and the PLL.[46] However, they admit that further validation is required due to the small study size. The authors recommend that bracing is safe in most unilateral non- or minimally displaced facet fractures without neurologic deficit. Close observation and judicious use of follow-up X-ray should be utilized to monitor for progression of spinal deformity when nonoperative treatment is employed. This is typically safe and may allow avoidance of unnecessary surgery.

The utilization of traction and closed reduction plays a significant role in subaxial facet dislocation injuries. It should be noted that extension-distraction type cervical injuries should not be treated with traction as this tends to exaggerate the deformity. Most subaxial cervical spine injuries that benefit from traction are flexion-distraction type injuries. These injuries tend to lead to the facet subluxation or dislocation. Traction and closed reduction can be a first-line treatment for neurologic decompression and temporary stabilization. Most facet dislocations can be reduced by closed means. Prompt reduction can lead to significant neurologic recovery. Closed reduction may be achieved by traction when the patient is awake and able to be examined. This can be a very safe method of monitoring the neurologic examination. MRI studies have demonstrated the ability of in-line traction to reduce neurologic compression in cervical flexion-distraction injuries, even in the setting of cervical disk herniation.[47] Some authors also advocate the use of reduction maneuvers under general anesthesia with intraoperative neurologic monitoring if traction fails.[48]

There is a very limited role for bracing alone for flexion-distraction injuries of the cervical spine. Only those with minimal displacement and mostly bony injury should be considered for bracing. These injuries need to be monitored very closely for progression of deformity or occurrence of neurologic deficit. Surgical treatment with internal fixation provides reliable stability.

☞ OPERATIVE TREATMENT

Occipitocervical Injury

The basic concepts of surgical treatment include obtaining rigid stabilization and neurologic decompression as well as spinal realignment. Instability of the OC junction has been defined as clear evidence of mobile subluxation of more than 1 mm in any direction of the osseous components under fluoroscopic manipulation.

The choice of specific fixation and fusion levels depends upon the injury variables such as the amount and direction of displacement, fracture locations, presence of noncontiguous injuries and bone quality. Most methods for fixation of the OC junction utilize plates or rods with various types of attachments to fix the occiput to the cervical spine. The occiput fixation devices usually utilize plate and screw constructs. These attach typically two rods which in turn attach to screws fixed in the cervical spine either in the pedicles, lamina or lateral masses. Sublaminar cables can also be utilized. Typically, the strongest bone for screw purchase in the occiput is just distal to the external occipital protuberance. Midline or parasagittal anchors can be placed.

Jefferson Fractures

Isolated C1 fractures generally do not require surgical stabilization. C1 burst fractures are typically considered "unstable" if the combined lateral mass overhang is greater than 6.9 mm on plain X-ray. Operative treatment (fixation of C1-C2 or OC fixation) can also be considered, especially if the patient develops a painful nonunion after attempted brace/halo immobilization. Late deformity can effectively be treated with OC fusion.[49]

Traumatic Atlantoaxial Instability

Treatment of traumatic AA instability typically requires internal fixation. This is especially true when the injury is primarily ligamentous. Halo immobilization alone does not appear to provide reliable long-term stability. C1-C2 posterior fixation and fusion is typically the treatment of choice. This allows reduction and rigid stabilization. C1 is typically anchored with lateral mass screws but may also be fixed with sublaminar wires or cables. C2 can be fixed with transpedicular screws, pars screws or intralaminar screws or sublaminar wires/cables.

Traumatic Spondylolisthesis of the Axis (Hangman's Fractures)

Type II fractures may be treated nonoperatively or surgically fixed. The surgeon may use a period of mobilization to assess the behavior of the fracture. If unacceptable displacement occurs then surgical fixation may be chosen. Repair of the pars fracture may be performed by inserting transpedicular lag screws. Fusion may also be chosen either through an anterior approach at C2-C3 or via posterior approach at C2-C3. Given the extent of comminution or presence of other injuries, the surgeon may choose to extend fixation to C1. Type III fractures require open posterior reduction and internal fixation. Traction is unlikely to achieve closed reduction due to the discontinuity of the pars and concomitant dislocation of the C2-C3 facet.

Odontoid Fractures

Due to the presence of significant clinical equipoise in the outcome of type II odontoid fractures in those patients that are neurologically intact, there is little agreement on whether operative or nonoperative treatment is optimal.[40,42,50] Operative treatment may lead to moderately higher morbidity.[44] The most commonly reported major complications after odontoid fracture surgery in the elderly include cardiac failure (6.8%), deep vein thrombosis (3.2%), stroke (3.2%), pneumonia (9.9%), respiratory failure (7.7%), liver failure (6.7%)

and severe infection (3.2%). The overall mortality rate after surgery is 10.1% (in-hospital, 6.2%; postdischarge, 8.8%). Similar mortality rates were found following anterior surgery (7% in-hospital, 9% overall) and posterior surgery (8% in-hospital, 9% overall); there were no differences in the rate of major airway complications between these groups (anterior: 17%; posterior: 18%). There was, however, a higher rate of site-specific complications, including nonunion, technical failure and the need for revision surgery, following anterior surgery as compared with posterior surgery.[51]

Treatment for odontoid fractures in octogenarians has been comparatively studied.[41] In the octogenarian population, operative treatment typically leads to higher length of hospital stay, and greater than 20% may have respiratory complications requiring tracheostomy.[41] Short-term mortality rate for either group is over 10%. This is very sobering information.

Surgical treatment for odontoid fractures can be performed by a number of different methods. Posteriorly, C1 can be fixed to C2 with sublaminar cabling or wiring. C1 lateral mass screws can be used to fix C1 to C2 pedicle screws or translaminar screws. Anterior fixation of odontoid fractures can be achieved with a single lag screw fixation technique. A number of series have been published to support acceptable clinical outcomes for each method. The authors encourage surgeons to recognize the importance of bone quality (often inferred from age, imaging and fracture mechanism), fracture pattern and anatomic considerations prior to choosing a fixation strategy. Anterior odontoid screw placement should not be attempted in fracture patterns anterior-inferior to posterior-superior because a lag screw will not effectively cross and compress this fracture.

Subaxial Cervical Spine Fractures

Dvorak et al., in conjunction with the Spine Trauma Study Group, performed a systematic review and developed an expert opinion consensus on surgical approaches to subaxial cervical injuries. They utilized the SLIC system to guide classification. The goal was to identify well-accepted surgical protocols to treat subaxial cervical injuries.

Subaxial spine injuries where the primary injury is an axial load can cause either endplate compression or burst fractures without disruption of the DLC. The neurology and presence of residual compression of the spinal cord are therefore the strongest determinants of treatment. With complete or incomplete neurologic injury, the SLIC system will add two, three or four points to the two morphology points leading to a score of 4 to 6, and thus favoring surgery with scores of 5 or greater. In the presence of intact posterior elements, the use of an anterior locking plate and strut graft provides adequate stability. Caution should be taken to avoid a solitary anterior reconstruction if there is endplate compromise upon which a graft will be situated. Otherwise, posterior fixation is rarely required for these injuries.[20]

Distraction injuries occur in two general patterns: (1) hyperextension, often occurring in the stiff, ankylosed or spondylotic spine and (2) hyperflexion leading to facet subluxations or perched facets.[20] Classically, hyperextension injuries occur in elderly individuals with spondylotic or stiff spines. Anterior retropharyngeal soft tissue swelling, widening of the disk space, high fluid signal in an otherwise degenerative disk space along with avulsion fractures of anterior osteophytes, or the anteroinferior corner of a vertebral body all point to this pattern of injury. Assessing this injury in terms of its morphology and DLC status, these injuries score 3 for morphology and 2 for DLC with the addition of any score resulting from neurologic impairment. Most of these injuries require surgical stabilization. The surgical approach is informed by the pattern of DLC disruption (primarily anterior), and thus most commonly an anterior cervical discectomy and fusion with plating is acceptable. This injury seems to occur most commonly in the elderly where the spine is spondylotic. If the spondylosis is severe or in the case of DISH or AS, the stiffness of adjacent segments creates long lever arms that may best be neutralized with the addition of posterior fixation.[20]

Flexion-distraction injuries can lead to fractured or perched facets. When the disk is essentially intact or merely disrupted without frank herniation, the surgeon can choose anterior or posterior fixation. Variables that may influence this decision include the available equipment and the training and familiarity of the surgeon with each approach. From the patients' perspective, anterior issues such as neck scar, the risk of temporary dysphagia or hoarse voice, and injury to visceral structures (esophagus) may be compared with the additional muscle dissection and local wound infection risk found with posterior approaches.[20] Anterior approaches are typically less painful and lead to a shorter hospital stay and yield slightly better radiographic results. But anterior alone approaches should be avoided if an endplate compression fracture exists along with a facet fracture. This has a high rate of graft subsidence and early failure. It is also important to take into consideration whether there is a loose piece of disk in the canal causing neurologic compression.

Vertebral burst fractures with dislocation or severe translation are the result of failure of the posterior ligamentous complex and anterior structures. Often the anterior vertebral bone causes neurologic compression. Surgical treatment is geared toward neurologic decompression, spinal reconstruction and stabilization. It is recommended that the majority of these injuries should be treated with a combined anterior and posterior surgery.[20] The most severe injuries of the cervical spine involve translation and/or rotation of one vertebral body over another. Surgical treatment should be planned based on presence and location of fractures and area of residual neurologic compression.

REFERENCES

1. Lowery DW, Wald MM, Browne BJ, et al. Epidemiology of cervical spine injury victims. Ann Emerg Med. 2001;38:12-6.
2. Brandenstein D, Molinari RW, Rubery PT, et al. Unstable subaxial cervical spine injury with normal computed tomography and magnetic resonance initial imaging studies: a report of four cases and review of the literature. Spine (Phila Pa 1976). 2009;34:E743-50.
3. Panjabi MM, Hausfeld JN, White AA 3rd. A biomechanical study of the ligamentous stability of the thoracic spine in man. Acta Orthop Scand. 1981;52:315-26.
4. Panjabi MM, White AA 3rd, Keller D, et al. Stability of the cervical spine under tension. J Biomech. 1978;11:189-97.
5. White AA 3rd, Johnson RM, Panjabi MM, et al. Biomechanical analysis of clinical stability in the cervical spine. Clin Orthop Relat Res. 1975;(109):85-96.
6. Kwon BK, Vaccaro AR, Grauer JN, et al. Subaxial cervical spine trauma. J Am Acad Orthop Surg. 2006;14:78-89.

7. Vaccaro AR, Hulbert RJ, Patel AA, et al. The subaxial cervical spine injury classification system: a novel approach to recognize the importance of morphology, neurology, and integrity of the disco-ligamentous complex. Spine (Phila Pa 1976). 2007;32:2365-74.

8. Anderson PA, Montesano PX. Morphology and treatment of occipital condyle fractures. Spine (Phila Pa 1976). 1988;13:731-6.

9. Bellabarba C, Mirza SK, West GA, et al. Diagnosis and treatment of craniocervical dislocation in a series of 17 consecutive survivors during an 8-year period. J Neurosurg Spine. 2006;4:429-40.

10. Torretti JA, Sengupta DK. Cervical spine trauma. Indian J Orthop. 2007;41:255-67.

11. Spence KF Jr, Decker S, Sell KW. Bursting atlantal fracture associated with rupture of the transverse ligament. J Bone Joint Surg Am. 1970;52:543-9.

12. Fielding JW, Hawkins RJ. Atlanto-axial rotatory fixation. (Fixed rotatory subluxation of the atlanto-axial joint). J Bone Joint Surg Am. 1977;59:37-44.

13. Anderson LD, D'Alonzo RT. Fractures of the odontoid process of the axis. J Bone Joint Surg Am. 1974;56:1663-74.

14. Levine AM, Edwards CC. The management of traumatic spondylolisthesis of the axis. J Bone Joint Surg Am. 1985;67:217-26.

15. Starr JK, Eismont FJ. Atypical hangman's fractures. Spine (Phila Pa 1976). 1993;18:1954-7.

16. Allen BL Jr, Ferguson RL, Lehmann TR, et al. A mechanistic classification of closed, indirect fractures and dislocations of the lower cervical spine. Spine (Phila Pa 1976). 1982;7:1-27.

17. Moore TA, Vaccaro AR, Anderson PA. Classification of lower cervical spine injuries. Spine (Phila Pa 1976). 2006;31:S37-43; discussion S61.

18. Panjabi M, Abumi K, Duranceau J, et al. Spinal stability and intersegmental muscle forces. A biomechanical model. Spine (Phila Pa 1976). 1989;14:194-200.

19. White AA 3rd, Panjabi MM, Posner I, et al. Spinal stability: evaluation and treatment. Instr Course Lect. 1981;30:457-83.

20. Dvorak MF, Fisher CG, Fehlings MG, et al. The surgical approach to subaxial cervical spine injuries: an evidence-based algorithm based on the SLIC classification system. Spine (Phila Pa 1976). 2007;32:2620-9.

21. Ali J, Adam R, Stedman M, et al. Advanced trauma life support program increases emergency room application of trauma resuscitative procedures in a developing country. J Trauma. 1994;36:391-4.

22. Schouten R, Albert T, Kwon BK. The spine-injured patient: initial assessment and emergency treatment. J Am Acad Orthop Surg. 2012;20:336-46.

23. Chafetz RS, Gaughan JP, Vogel LC, et al. The international standards for neurological classification of spinal cord injury: intra-rater agreement of total motor and sensory scores in the pediatric population. J Spinal Cord Med. 2009;32:157-61.

24. Dickinson G, Stiell IG, Schull M, et al. Retrospective application of the NEXUS low-risk criteria for cervical spine radiography in Canadian emergency departments. Ann Emerg Med. 2004;43:507-14.

25. Hoffman JR, Wolfson AB, Todd K, et al. Selective cervical spine radiography in blunt trauma: methodology of the National Emergency X-Radiography Utilization Study (NEXUS). Ann Emerg Med. 1998;32:461-9.

26. Knopp R. Comparing NEXUS and Canadian C-Spine decision rules for determining the need for cervical spine radiography. Ann Emerg Med. 2004;43:518-20.

27. Michaleff ZA, Maher CG, Verhagen AP, et al. Accuracy of the Canadian C-spine rule and NEXUS to screen for clinically important cervical spine injury in patients following blunt trauma: a systematic review. CMAJ. 2012;184:E867-76.

28. Mower WR, Hoffman J. Comparison of the Canadian C-Spine rule and NEXUS decision instrument in evaluating blunt trauma patients for cervical spine injury. Ann Emerg Med. 2004;43:515-7.

29. Horodyski M, DiPaola CP, Conrad BP, et al. Cervical collars are insufficient for immobilizing an unstable cervical spine injury. J Emerg Med. 2011;41:513-9.

30. Harris JH Jr, Carson GC, Wagner LK. Radiologic diagnosis of traumatic occipitovertebral dissociation: 1. Normal occipitovertebral relationships on lateral radiographs of supine subjects. AJR Am J Roentgenol. 1994;162:881-6.

31. Bono CM, Vaccaro AR, Hurlbert RJ, et al. Validating a newly proposed classification system for thoracolumbar spine trauma: looking to the future of the thoracolumbar injury classification and severity score. J Orthop Trauma. 2006;20:567-72.

32. Bono CM, Vaccaro AR, Fehlings M, et al. Measurement techniques for lower cervical spine injuries: consensus statement of the Spine Trauma Study Group. Spine (Phila Pa 1976). 2006;31:603-9.

33. Bozzo A, Goulet B, Marcoux J, et al. The role of magnetic resonance imaging in the management of acute spinal cord injury. J Neurotrauma 2011;28:1401-11.

34. Crosby CG, Even JL, Song Y, et al. Diagnostic abilities of magnetic resonance imaging in traumatic injury to the posterior ligamentous complex: the effect of years in training. Spine J 2011;11: 747-53.

35. Rihn JA, Fisher C, Harrop J, et al. Assessment of the posterior ligamentous complex following acute cervical spine trauma. J Bone Joint Surg Am. 2010;92:583-9.

36. Rihn JA, Yang N, Fisher C, et al. Using magnetic resonance imaging to accurately assess injury to the posterior ligamentous complex of the spine: a prospective comparison of the surgeon and radiologist. J Neurosurg Spine. 2010;12:391-6.

37. Biffl WL, Moore EE, Offner PJ, et al. Blunt carotid and vertebral arterial injuries. World J Surg 2001;25:1036-43.

38. Biffl WL, Ray CE Jr, Moore EE, et al. Treatment-related outcomes from blunt cerebrovascular injuries: importance of routine follow-up arteriography. Ann Surg. 2002;235:699-706; discussion-7.

39. Biffl WL, Ray CE Jr, Moore EE, et al. Noninvasive diagnosis of blunt cerebrovascular injuries: a preliminary report. J Trauma. 2002;53:850-6.

40. Smith HE, Kerr SM, Fehlings MG, et al. Trends in epidemiology and management of type II odontoid fractures: 20-year experience at a model system spine injury tertiary referral center. J Spinal Disord Tech. 2010;23:501-5.

41. Smith HE, Kerr SM, Maltenfort M, et al. Early complications of surgical versus conservative treatment of isolated type II odontoid fractures in octogenarians: a retrospective cohort study. J Spinal Disord Tech. 2008;21:535-9.

42. Smith HE, Vaccaro AR, Maltenfort M, et al. Trends in surgical management for type II odontoid fracture: 20 years of experience at a regional spinal cord injury center. Orthopedics. 2008;31:650.

43. Molinari RW, Khera OA, Gruhn WL, et al. Rigid cervical collar treatment for geriatric type II odontoid fractures. Eur Spine J. 2012;21:855-62.

44. Molinari RW, Dahl J, Gruhn WL, et al. Functional outcomes, morbidity, mortality, and fracture healing in 26 consecutive geriatric odontoid fracture patients treated with posterior fusion. J Spinal Disord Tech. 2013;26:119-26.

45. Molinari W, Khera O, Gruhn W, et al. Functional outcomes, morbidity, mortality and fracture healing rates in 58 consecutive geriatric odontoid fracture patients treated with cervical collar or posterior fusion. Evid Based Spine Care J. 2011;2:55-6.

46. Halliday AL, Henderson BR, Hart BL, et al. The management of unilateral lateral mass/facet fractures of the subaxial cervical spine: the use of magnetic resonance imaging to predict instability. Spine (Phila Pa 1976). 1997;22:2614-21.

47. Darsaut TE, Ashforth R, Bhargava R, et al. A pilot study of magnetic resonance imaging-guided closed reduction of cervical spine fractures. Spine (Phila Pa 1976). 2006;31:2085-90.

48. Vital JM, Gille O, Senegas J, et al. Reduction technique for uni- and biarticular dislocations of the lower cervical spine. Spine (Phila Pa 1976). 1998;23:949-54; discussion 55.
49. Bransford R, Falicov A, Nguyen Q, et al. Unilateral C-1 lateral mass sagittal split fracture: an unstable Jefferson fracture variant. J Neurosurg Spine. 2009;10:466-73.
50. Chapman J, Smith JS, Kopjar B, et al. The AOSpine North America Geriatric Odontoid Fracture Mortality Study: A Retrospective Review of Mortality Outcomes for Operative versus Non-Operative Treatment in 322 Patients with Long-Term Follow-Up. Spine (Phila Pa 1976) 2013.
51. White AP, Hashimoto R, Norvell DC, et al. Morbidity and mortality related to odontoid fracture surgery in the elderly population. Spine (Phila Pa 1976). 2010;35:S146-57.

CHAPTER

8

Spinal Cord Injury

🖝 INTRODUCTION

Spinal cord injury (SCI) is rare in frequency but has devastating effects on patients and families, and puts large stresses on health systems and communities.[1] The national rate of SCI is about 40 per million people in the United States. It typically occurs in a bimodal age distribution with young men being the most common patient population. As our population ages and remains more active we are seeing a greater number of older patients with SCI as a trend.[1] The management of SCI patients requires a multidisciplinary approach. Adherence to basic advanced trauma life support (ATLS) principles and attention to multisystem injuries in the initial management of SCI typically make the difference between life and death.

The role of the spine surgeon in the management of SCI involves assessment of patient neurology, spinal stability and ultimately to generate a treatment plan that will optimize these patient needs.

🖝 PATHOPHYSIOLOGY

Acute SCI involves both primary and secondary mechanisms of injury.[2] The primary mechanism, usually caused by rapid spinal cord compression from bone displacement of fracture-dislocation or burst fracture, is irreversible. It may occur from a number of different mechanisms. In the aging population that may have a higher prevalence of pre-existing stenosis, lower energy injuries with hyperextension, and minimal or no bony injury for example, may be all that is required to compress and mechanically deform the spinal cord. The common theme is that traumatic SCI results from primarily mechanical injury to the spinal cord. This then initiates a cascade of secondary injury mechanisms, including ischemia, electrolyte derangements and lipid peroxidation. Secondary injury is preventable and may be reversible.[2] It is not within the scope of this chapter to provide a comprehensive description of the pathophysiology and pathology of acute SCI, but a brief discussion is warranted. The acute traumatic forces imparted on the spinal cord at the moment of injury cause significant primary damage to the neural tissue, and this is rapidly followed by an interrelated series of pathophysiologic processes, which includes ischemia, excitotoxicity, inflammation and oxidative stress.[3] Calcium channel blockers, such as nimodipine, have been investigated to inhibit vasospasm and promote improved blood supply to the cord.[3] The importance of excitotoxicity in many forms of neural trauma has led to interest in N-methyl-D-aspartate (NMDA) receptor antagonists as neuroprotective agents; such was attempted in human SCI with the clinical evaluation of gacyclidine.[3] The contribution of lipid peroxidation and inflammation to secondary damage rationalized the human investigation of steroids such as methylprednisolone and tirilazad mesylate in the National Acute Spinal Cord Injury Study (NASCIS) trials.[3]

Animal studies have shown that acute SCI results in systemic and disrupted local and vascular autoregulation.[4-6] Human studies have all shown that after SCI, bradycardia, hypotension, decreased systemic vascular resistance and cardiac output are all common.[5,7-10] Respiratory insufficiency is also an equally serious life-threatening complication. The physiologic sequelae and resultant hypoxia may lead to further secondary SCI.[11] Respiratory insufficiency is an independent risk factor for mortality and a major source of post SCI morbidity that is also related to level of injury.[12-14] Cardiovascular and respiratory complications can be transient and episodic and may occur after periods of relative stability. Early detection and aggressive treatment reduces morbidity and mortality of cardiac and respiratory dysfunction that is common with acute SCI.[11]

PATIENT PRESENTATION

By adopting a high level of suspicion, a systematic evaluation and judicious care, the physicians and team involved in initial evaluation of the SCI patient can play a significant role in protecting the patient from the devastating morbidity of SCI. Once appropriate immobilization is secured, a structured initial assessment, including a thorough neurologic examination, can identify individuals at risk.[15]

The initial care of the SCI patient centers on life-saving measures and provisional spinal stabilization. Definitive treatment is rendered based on a number of factors including patient health, other injuries and neurologic injury.[1,2,16,17] Evaluation is initially guided by ATLS principles. The standard assessment and order of evaluation and management of airway, breathing, circulation, neurologic disability and bodily exposure/inspection hold true. A full review of these concepts have been discussed by Harris et al.[18]

The authors would like to emphasize the importance of the secondary survey and neurologic examination to the spine practitioner. The ability to effectively evaluate the patient's level and severity of neurologic injury is one of the most important skills that he/she can have. There is perhaps no more important factor than the ability for the clinician to recognize a neurologic deterioration is perhaps the most important factor in determining the timing of surgical intervention.

NEUROLOGIC ASSESSMENT

A careful neurologic examination is critical to the spinal evaluation. However, such an examination is often not possible in a multi-traumatized patient or one who is intoxicated,

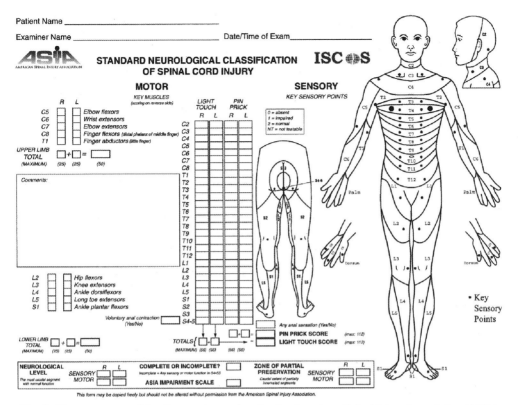

Fig. 1: Diagram summarizing the scoring system for the American Spinal Injury Association (ASIA) impairment evaluation for patients with spinal cord injury

sedated, or intubated and pharmacologically paralyzed. Within the context of acute spinal trauma, the neurologic examination is performed in accordance with the International Standards for the Neurologic Classification of Spinal Cord Injury (ISNCSCI), formerly the American Spinal Injury Association (ASIA) standards.[15,19] The authors have found it very useful to standardize communication by adopting the ASIA standardized neurologic assessment form into chart documentation (Fig. 1). This helps to ensure a standard of communication and reminds clinicians of the importance of every key element necessary for a thorough examination. This also facilitates scientific and clinical follow-up.

The motor examination measures the strength of five key upper and five lower extremity myotomes according to the grading scheme of 0 to 5 (Table 1). In the upper extremity, these include C5, elbow flexion; C6, wrist extension; C7, elbow extension; C8, long finger flexion; and T1, finger abductors. In the lower extremity, these include L2, hip flexion; L3, knee extension; L4, ankle dorsiflexion; L5, long toe extension; S1, ankle plantar flexion. The documentation of motor and sensory function, and determination of the severity of paralysis is critical for patients with spinal cord injuries. The ISNCSCI motor score is comprised of the strength in 10 key muscle groups, while the sensory score for light touch and pinprick is comprised of sensation within 28 dermatomes.[19] The sensation is documented as either absent, impaired, or normal and is scored 0, 1 or 2 respectively.

Table 1: Summary of the American Spinal Injury Association (ASIA) muscle grading scale	
ASIA muscle grading	
0	Total paralysis
1	Palpable or visible contraction
2	Active movement, full range of motion, gravity eliminated
3	Active movement, full range of motion, against gravity
4	Active movement, full range of motion, against gravity and provides some resistance
5	Active movement, full range of motion, against gravity and provides normal resistance
5*	Muscle able to exert, in examiner's judgment, sufficient resistance to be considered normal if identifiable inhibiting factors were not present

Table 2: Summary of the American Spinal Injury Association (ASIA) level of impairment scale	
ASIA grade	Level of impairment
A	No motor or sensory function preserved in the lowest sacral segments (S4 and S5)
B	Sensory but no motor function preserved, including the lowest sacral segments (S4-S5)
C	Motor function present below the injury, but the strengths of more than half of the key muscles are graded less than 3 of 5
D	Motor function present below the injury, but the strengths of more than half of the key muscles are graded more than or equal to 3 of 5
E	Motor and sensory functions in key muscles and dermatomes are normal

It is critical to test the perianal sensation and anal contraction to determine whether any function has been preserved in the lowest sacral segments, S4-S5. Testing of the S4-S5 dermatome is performed at the anal mucocutaneous junction.[15] Assignment of an ASIA grade is based on these neurologic findings (Table 2). The final but most important motor function to be tested is voluntary anal contraction, which should be documented as being present or absent.

Reflexes change over time in patients with spinal cord injuries. Acutely, the deep tendon reflexes are typically absent, and the limbs are flaccid; later in the course of SCI, they become hyperreflexic. The pathologic Babinski response, which is associated with upper motor neuron impairment, is elicited by stroking the lateral planter surface of the foot with a rigid, semi-sharp object. It manifests as an extension of the great toe, with flexion and spreading of the lateral toes. The bulbocavernosus reflex is elicited by digitally stimulating the glans or clitoris or by gently tugging on the bladder catheter and determining whether reflex anal contraction exists.

The ASIA impairment scale (AIS) is the most universally accepted scoring system for broadly categorizing the neurologic function of spinal injured patients. The patients in whom no motor or sensory function is preserved in the lowest sacral segments (S4-S5) are deemed to be AIS A, which is now the preferred method of describing what had previously been deemed "ASIA A." Those with sensory sparing in the lowest sacral segments with no motor function are AIS B. Those with preserved motor function below the neurologic level, with the majority of myotomes having a muscle grade of 2 or less, are AIS C, whereas those with a muscle grade of 3 or more are AIS D. Patients with normal motor and sensory function are considered to be AIS E. The AIS highlights the importance of the rectal and perianal examination to confirm the presence or absence of sacral sparing. If light touch or pinprick sensation is at all present at the S4-S5 dermatome (whether intact or impaired), or if any anal sensation or voluntary anal contraction is found on digital rectal examination, then the patient is deemed to have an incomplete SCI. The neurologic level describes the remaining sensory and motor functions on each side of the body. The sensory level is defined as the most caudal dermatome in which both pinprick and light touch sensation are normal. The motor level is defined as the most caudal myotome with intact innervation, below which motor deficits exist. Because of muscle polyinnervation, the most caudal muscle to have at least grade 3 power is considered to be fully innervated.

In patients with complete spinal cord injuries, the "zone of partial preservation" refers to the most caudal dermatome, and myotome beyond the motor and sensory level that has some limited preserved function.[15]

The ability of some patients to recover function following SCI remains poorly understood. Previous studies have reported on predictors of functional recovery and found that the initial AIS is one of the most reliable factors.[20] The more severe the neurologic injury, the less potential there appears to be recovery.[21] Region of spinal injury has been shown to correlate with prognosis with thoracic SCI having a poorer chance of recovery.[20-22] Energy of injury has been linked to recovery, with low-energy injuries having a 5.5 times greater recovery rate compared to high-energy injuries.[21,22] It has been shown that the characteristics of injury on magnetic resonance imaging (MRI) can have prognostic value.[17,23] Bozzo et al. described four patterns of MRI signal from normal, to single level cord signal, multilevel edema to cord hemorrhage. Multilevel cord hemorrhage has the worst prognosis.[23] Also, specific management options have been reported to improve functional outcomes including maximizing blood flow to the spinal cord through elevation of mean arterial pressure (MAP) to more than 85 mm Hg for the first week after injury, early transfer to a specialty SCI center, and early surgical decompression within 24 hours when medically feasible.[24-26]

For the traumatic SCI patient hypotension should first be assumed to be of a hemorrhagic etiology, and a detailed search for injuries with the potential for extensive bleeding should be initiated. A trauma survey should include all major body systems to rule out concomitant injury to other common regions such as the abdomen or thorax.

Hypovolemic shock should clearly be differentiated from neurogenic shock. Neurogenic shock typically occurs due to SCI rostral to T4 and upon presentation to emergency department can be seen in 20% of cases.[27] A distinct physiologic condition exists in which the heart rate is typically less than 80 beats per minute and the systolic blood pressure is less than 100 mm Hg. This occurs because of an over-powering of vagal output combined with a physiologic loss of sympathetic function. Once a patient is adequately volume resuscitated, neurogenic shock should be managed with pressor support and occasionally cardiac pacing is required.

The concept of spinal shock (though likely mechanistically related to neurogenic shock) is an entity which dates back over 150 years in description.[28] It is still not fully fundamentally understood, and it is currently considered an evolution of return of a series of spinal reflexes.[28,29] The presence of spinal shock has typically been thought to "mask" the true neurologic state of a patient due to the predilection for flaccid areflexic paralysis. Spinal shock, which is distinct from neurogenic shock, is a controversial topic. Conceptually, spinal shock is the temporary physiologic state of the acutely traumatized spinal cord, manifested by the transient absence of reflexive function caudal to SCI. Its end is heralded by the gradual return of reflex activity, such as the bulbocavernosus reflex, typically within 24–48 hours after injury.[15] In principle, the diagnosis of a "complete" SCI cannot be made until this neural "shock" resolves. It is unusual to witness an individual with complete paralysis in the presence of a severely displaced fracture-dislocation revert to being drastically improved once the bulbocavernosus reflex returns.[15] Ditunno and colleagues have sought to revise the understanding of spinal shock through an in-depth review and have attempted to link molecular mechanisms and neuroanatomic pathways to the clinical persistence or return of standard clinical reflex findings.[28,29] They describe four phases of spinal shock which is seen as a continuum of reflex return and persistence throughout multiple months. An extensive series of molecular mechanisms and neuroanatomic rationales are proposed, but the clinical and prognostic implications are still being investigated.[28] Ko et al. studied the subject of spinal shock with Ditunno's group and concluded that the prognosis for ambulation based on reflexes early after SCI should not be linked to current descriptions of spinal shock. In fact, the view of spinal shock, based on the absence of reflexes and the recovery of reflexes in a caudal to rostral sequence, is of limited clinical utility and should be discarded. The evolution of reflexes over several days following injury may be more relevant to prognosis than the use of the term spinal shock and the presence or absence of reflexes on the day of injury. They found that the delayed plantar response (DPR), a pathologic reflex, was the first reflex to recover most often, followed by the bulbocavernosus (BC) and cremasteric (CRM) in the first few days and later followed by the deep tendon reflexes (ankle and knee jerk) by 1–2 weeks respectively. Less than 8% of subjects had no reflexes on the day of injury, and the reflexes did not follow a caudal-rostral pattern of recovery.[28]

🖝 IMAGING

Imaging to assess spinal trauma is covered in the chapters on cervical and thoracolumbar spine trauma. The same principles apply to SCI evaluation. Some key points to consider about SCI are outlined below.

The choice of initial spinal survey imaging is evolving. Over the last decade the use of thin slice CT scans have dramatically increased. In addition to providing better resolution of the bony elements, CT overcomes the difficulties that often arise in adequately visualizing the occipitocervical and cervicothoracic junctions.[15] CT is also gaining utilization as CT angiogram screening for blunt vertebral artery injury is becoming more prevalent.[30,31]

Magnetic resonance imaging has become the gold standard for imaging neurologic tissues including the spinal cord. MRI is strongly recommended when a patient presents with spinal column injury that does not correlate with neurologic level of injury. It is also recommended to aid the clinician in assessing the prognostication of acute SCI. The sagittal T2 sequence is particularly valuable. Presently, four signal patterns based on sagittal T2-weighted sequences are commonly identified. Pattern 1 shows a normal MRI signal in the cord; pattern 2 represents single-level edema; pattern 3 is multilevel edema; and pattern 4 is mixed hemorrhage and edema. Neither T1 sequences nor T2 axial images have been shown to have prognostic value.[23] More recent sequences, such as gradient echo images (GRE), which are the best for visualizing hemorrhage, have not yet been incorporated into classification systems.[23] It is recommended that MRI should be used to direct clinical decision making. MRI has a role in clearance, the ruling out of injury, of the cervical spine in the obtunded patient only if there is abnormality of the neurological examination.[23] It has been shown that neurologic recovery tends to be correlated with the severity (magnitude) of signal pattern. For example, signal pattern 4 (hemorrhage) has the worst prognosis for neurologic recovery.

Magnetic resonance imaging is unequivocally superior in identifying ligamentous injury, intervertebral disk extrusions, and neural element trauma and compression. MRI may be the only modality able to detect this pathology in cases of transient dislocation-subluxation followed by spontaneous reduction and bony realignment.[15]

Persons with ankylosing spondylitis (AS) or diffuse idiopathic skeletal hyperostosis (DISH) can suffer catastrophic neurologic injuries from spinal injuries caused by low-energy trauma that may be missed in the initial emergency evaluation. Upwards of 80% of patients with ankylosing spinal disorders and delayed diagnosis can suffer abrupt neurologic deterioration.[32,33] Recognizing that the spine is ankylosed is a frank warning sign: such a patient who presents with neck or back pain should be assumed to have an unstable fracture with the potential to cause serious neurologic deficit until proven otherwise.[15] CT scan and/or MRI are highly recommended in the patient with AS or DISH, who presents with neck pain even after minor trauma. These patients typically have poor bone quality (especially AS) and are more prone to low-energy fragility fractures.

NONOPERATIVE TREATMENT

Patients with traumatic SCI derive considerable benefit (often lifesaving) from nonoperative care. Whether definitive treatment for the spinal injury is operative or not, care of the SCI patient requires a well-co-ordinated multidisciplinary approach. Nonoperative SCI care fits three general categories:

Vale et al. performed a prospective case series which claims that neurologic recovery in the setting of ICU care must have been attributed to ICU care as all of the other factors such as selection for surgery and timing did not have a significant effect. The frequency and severity of life-threatening complications after SCI are common enough and the benefits of ICU care are great enough to justify that all SCI patients initially (within 7–14 days of injury) should receive ICU level care.[34]

1. Neuroprotective measures: Neuroprotective strategies can take many forms including physiologic optimization to pharmacologic intervention to help prevent further secondary SCI. The scientific interest in pharmacologic intervention for the prevention of secondary

SCI is exploding. Multiple clinical trials are ongoing. We plan to give a concise overview, but currently there are no accepted standard pharmacologic treatments to enhance SCI recovery or prevent secondary injury. The initial insult in spinal cord trauma is mechanical. This leads to secondary injury resulting from vascular compromise, ischemia, inflammation, edema, complex biochemical dysregulation and ultimately neuronal cell death.[7-11,35] Maintenance of optimized cardiac output, blood pressure and tissue oxygenation may also protect from secondary SCI.[5,7-10,35] Many studies set a goal for MAP for a minimum of 85–90 mm Hg. These studies often employ the analogy of SCI to traumatic brain injury (TBI). In TBI, hypoxia and hypotension worsens secondary neuronal injury and hinders optimal recovery.[10,36] Studies of TBI suggest that MAP less than 90 or hypoxia ($paO_2 < 60$ mm Hg) has been shown to significantly increase morbidity and mortality.[8,10,35,36]

Animal studies suggest that avoidance of hypotension has a protective effect on the spinal cord and a beneficial effect on spinal cord recovery.[4-6] No study in human patients directly compares systemic hypotension and SCI outcome. Despite a lack of strong human clinical trial evidence, general principles of physiology management are to correct hypotension with volume replacement (crystalloid first followed by colloid as necessary).[11] Vasopressors may also be needed and can safely be used.[11] Occasionally patients may necessitate cardiac pacing to maintain cardiac output. Current standard of care management includes support of arterial oxygenation and spinal cord perfusion pressure. Maintenance of MAP for SCI patients more than or equal to 85–90 mm Hg is a safe clinical practice.[11]

While many advances in the basic science of SCI provide optimism for future treatments, clinical science lags. At present, there are no pharmacologic strategies of proven benefit. Although steroids continue to be given to patients with SCI in many institutions, evidence of deleterious effects continues to accumulate.[37] The routine use of steroids in patients with spinal cord injuries has been largely abandoned and has been even considered a harmful standard of care.[38] At best, the use of methylprednisolone in patients with acute SCI should be regarded as a treatment option only and not a standard of care. Central to the criticism of methylprednisolone is the fact that the neurologic benefit reported in NASCIS II and III was extremely modest, whereas the complications associated with prolonged infusion (e.g. sepsis, pneumonia and prolonged stay in the ICU) were substantial.[39-43] Many centers have subsequently abandoned the use of methylprednisolone for acute SCI, although the medicolegal climate in the United States compels many physicians into continuing to administer it. Individual institutions are encouraged to meet by committee to reach consensus and to formalize a treatment protocol.[15] The authors do not recommend the use of corticosteroid pharmacologic treatment in the setting of traumatic SCI.

2. Indirect reduction and spinal immobilization: Besides life-saving measures the main priority of SCI treatment is to prevent neurologic deterioration, regain spinal stability and possibly gain back neurologic function. Once a patient is brought under the care of medical personnel, there is still a real risk of neurologic deterioration of 6–10%.[44] The spinal cord injured patient deserves special attention due to the need for "controlled mobilization". Initial immobilization for the patient with SCI often involves bed rest with "spine precautions". A

rigid cervical orthosis is maintained until cervical spine injury can be ruled out. Studies on the unstable cervical spine in cadavers have shown that rigid collars allow similar amounts of motion compared to cadavers with no collars, in a stretcher to bed, or bed to bed transfer situation.[45] The cervical collar thus may not protect against transfer induced C-spine motion. The utmost in care must be taken when transferring patients, despite the presence of a collar.

Previous studies have shown that the spine injured patient who is subjected to bed rest (which is the initial form of spine immobilization in the trauma bay or ICU) is at risk for pulmonary complications, skin breakdown, deep vein thrombosis (DVT) and muscle atrophy.[46-50] Frequent patient repositioning has been shown to decrease morbidity of bed rest.[47,49,51] A mechanized version of patient repositioning has been developed by creating a laterally rotating bed which generates "kinetic therapy" (KT). We have found KT to be useful as a preoperative measure of spine immobilization.

The goal for the patients with spinal instability is to mobilize them effectively throughout their hospital care whether it is for imaging, ICU care or operative positioning, while also maintaining strict spinal immobilization. Patient transfers and positioning have the potential to confer dangerous amounts of motion to the unstable spine, which may lead to neurologic deterioration.[44] Thus, we consider spine immobilization as a paramount goal of nonoperative treatment whether in the ICU or not.

Rechtine et al. performed a study on embalmed cadavers that compared logroll to kinetic therapy treatment (KTT). They looked specifically at patient mobilization as might occur in an ICU setting. Embalmed cadavers with cervical and thoracolumbar instability were used. They found that KTT generated significantly less cervical and thoracolumbar spine motion, when compared to logroll.[52] Conrad et al. found similar results when fresh cadavers were studied.[53] When Rechtine et al. studied hospital bed transfers in cadavers they found that the act of transferring a patient from stretcher to bed may impart potentially dangerous amounts of cervical spine motion in the unstable spine whether a rigid collar is used or not.[45] They emphasized that patients with true cervical instability should be handled with inline manual cervical stabilization whenever a patient transfer is performed. The presence of a rigid collar should not be a sign that one can be less attentive to the head and neck, but rather the converse is true. The collar will not protect against transfer induced cervical motion.

Following that same theme, the cervical collar is not adequate enough to optimally immobilize the cervical spine in operating room supine to prone positioning. This has been demonstrated in multiple cadaver studies for C1-C2 and C5-C6 instability.[54-56] In these scenarios, the Jackson table turning technique immobilizes the cervical spine to a significantly greater degree in the majority of motion parameters for angular displacement (axial rotation, lateral bending and flexion-extension) and linear displacement (anteroposterior, axial and medial-lateral) whether a rigid collar is used or not.[57] The Jackson table prone positioning technique involves positioning a patient supine on the flat Jackson table and then applying the carbon frame, with pads over the ventral surface of the patient. The patient is held in place with tension in the system created by the locking T-pins and safety straps are applied around the whole setup. The patient is flipped prone by unlocking the manual lock at the head and foot of the bed, and then rotating the whole system. The Jackson table turning method has also been proven to provide better spine immobilization in the setting of thoracolumbar instability, when compared to a standard logroll, for supine to prone positioning.[54-56]

Based on the data presented, we recommend that KTT should be used for initial immobilization of patients with cervical, thoracic or lumbar instability. KTT appears to allow adequate controlled mobilization of the patient, while also providing optimum spine immobilization. The biomechanical data also supports the use of the Jackson table turn in the preoperative supine to prone patient transfer. In all scenarios (whether in the ICU or operating room) the logroll maneuver is vastly inferior when it comes to optimally immobilizing the unstable spine.

☞ OPERATIVE TREATMENT

The trend in definitive treatment for traumatic SCI has dramatically favored surgical treatment over the last decade.[1] It has become widely accepted that surgical stabilization of spinal injuries in the setting of neurologic deficit allows the patient to mobilize earlier, and decreases medical complications as well as ICU length of stay.[24,38] It has also been shown that early surgical decompression and stabilization for traumatic SCI can be safe and does not pose an increased morbidity or mortality risk to patients as was once believed.[58] It is beyond the scope of this chapter to review specific surgical techniques for the entire spectrum of spinal cord injuries. However, the subject of timing of surgical (or indirect) decompression performed for traumatic SCI is an evolving subject. Although a plethora of animal studies and anecdotal examples exist supporting the concept that early decompression after acute SCI improves long-term neurologic outcomes, only recently has this been supported by a well-designed human clinical study.[15] The objective difficulties in designing and conducting large prospective randomized studies and, at the same time, the urgent necessity to clarify the role of surgery has spurred a reanalysis of the enormous quantity of data produced in the past decades regarding SCI. Fehlings et al.[59,60] reviewed the literature using the modern criteria of evidence-based medicine. They provided a qualitative evaluation of the available data, concluding that there are Class III data suggesting a role for urgent decompression in the setting of bilateral facet dislocation, and in incomplete injuries in patients with neurological deterioration. The authors considered those observations as options since derived from retrospective data. A multicenter prospective trial, the Surgical Treatment of Acute Spinal Cord Injury Study recently reported that following cervical injuries, patients who received surgical or closed decompression within 24 hours had a higher rate of significant neurologic recovery (defined as at least a two grade AIS improvement) at 6-month follow-up, compared with those receiving delayed (> 24 hours) decompression (19.8% versus 8.8%).[61]

☞ REFERENCES

1. Fisher CG, Noonan VK, Dvorak MF. Changing face of spine trauma care in North America. Spine (Phila Pa 1976). 2006;31:S2-8.

2.   Fehlings MG, Perrin RG. The timing of surgical intervention in the treatment of spinal cord injury: a systematic review of recent clinical evidence. Spine (Phila Pa 1976). 2006;31:S28-35.

3.   Kwon BK, Sekhon LH, Fehlings MG. Emerging repair, regeneration, and translational research advances for spinal cord injury. Spine (Phila Pa 1976). 2010;35:S263-70.

4.   Amar AP, Levy ML. Pathogenesis and pharmacological strategies for mitigating secondary damage in acute spinal cord injury. Neurosurgery. 1999;44:1027-39.

5.   Dolan EJ, Tator CH. The effect of blood transfusion, dopamine, and gamma hydroxybutyrate on posttraumatic ischemia of the spinal cord. J Neurosurg. 1982;56:350-8.

6.   Ducker TB, Kindt GW, Kempf LG. Pathological findings in acute experimental spinal cord trauma. J Neurosurg. 1971;35:700-8.

7.   Osterholm JL. The pathophysiological response to spinal cord injury. The current status of related research. J Neurosurg. 1974;40:5-33.

8.   Tator CH. Vascular effects and blood flow in acute spinal cord injuries. J Neurosurg Sci. 1984;28:115-9.

9.   Tator CH. Review of experimental spinal cord injury with emphasis on the local and systemic circulatory effects. Neurochirurgie. 1991;37:291-302.

10. Tator CH, Fehlings MG. Review of the secondary injury theory of acute spinal cord trauma with emphasis on vascular mechanisms. J Neurosurg. 1991;75:15-26.

11. Blood pressure management after acute spinal cord injury. Neurosurgery. 2002;50:S58-62.

12. Claxton AR, Wong DT, Chung F, et al. Predictors of hospital mortality and mechanical ventilation in patients with cervical spinal cord injury. Can J Anaesth. 1998;45:144-9.

13. Jackson AB, Groomes TE. Incidence of respiratory complications following spinal cord injury. Arch Phys Med Rehabil. 1994;75:270-5.

14. Lemons VR, Wagner FC, Jr. Respiratory complications after cervical spinal cord injury. Spine. 1994;19:2315-20.

15. Schouten R, Albert T, Kwon BK. The spine-injured patient: initial assessment and emergency treatment. J Am Acad Orthop Surg. 2012;20:336-46.

16. Farmer J, Vaccaro A, Albert TJ, et al. Neurologic deterioration after cervical spinal cord injury. J Spinal Disord. 1998;11:192-6.

17. Fehlings MG, Cadotte DW, Fehlings LN. A series of systematic reviews on the treatment of acute spinal cord injury: a foundation for best medical practice. J Neurotrauma. 2011;28:1329-33.

18. Harris MB, Sethi RK. The initial assessment and management of the multiple-trauma patient with an associated spine injury. Spine (Phila Pa 1976). 2006;31:S9-15.

19. Chafetz RS, Gaughan JP, Vogel LC, et al. The international standards for neurological classification of spinal cord injury: intra-rater agreement of total motor and sensory scores in the pediatric population. J Spinal Cord Med. 2009;32:157-61.

20. Harrop JS, Naroji S, Maltenfort MG, et al. Neurologic improvement after thoracic, thoracolumbar, and lumbar spinal cord (conus medullaris) injuries. Spine (Phila Pa 1976). 2011;36:21-5.

21. Al-Habib AF, Attabib N, Ball J, et al. Clinical predictors of recovery after blunt spinal cord trauma: systematic review. J Neurotrauma. 2011;28:1431-43.

22. Fisher CG, Noonan VK, Smith DE, et al. Motor recovery, functional status, and health-related quality of life in patients with complete spinal cord injuries. Spine. 2005;30:2200-7.

23. Bozzo A, Goulet B, Marcoux J, et al. The role of magnetic resonance imaging in the management of acute spinal cord injury. J Neurotrauma. 2011;28:1401-11.

24. Furlan JC, Noonan V, Cadotte DW, et al. Timing of decompressive surgery of spinal cord after traumatic spinal cord injury: an evidence-based examination of pre-clinical and clinical studies. J Neurotrauma. 2011;28:1371-99.

25. Furlan JC, Noonan V, Singh A, et al. Assessment of disability in patients with acute traumatic spinal cord injury: a systematic review of the literature. J Neurotrauma. 2011;28:1413-30.

26. Parent S, Barchi S, LeBreton M, et al. The impact of specialized centers of care for spinal cord injury on length of stay, complications, and mortality: a systematic review of the literature. J Neurotrauma. 2011;28:1363-70.

27. Guly HR, Bouamra O, Lecky FE. The incidence of neurogenic shock in patients with isolated spinal cord injury in the emergency department. Resuscitation. 2008;76:57-62.

28. Ditunno JF, Little JW, Tessler A, et al. Spinal shock revisited: a four-phase model. Spinal Cord. 2004;42:383-95.

29. Ko HY, Ditunno JF Jr, Graziani V, et al. The pattern of reflex recovery during spinal shock. Spinal Cord. 1999;37:402-9.

30. Biffl WL. Computed tomographic angiography for blunt cerebrovascular injuries: is it good enough? J Trauma. 2010;68:508-9.

31. Biffl WL, Moore EE. Computed tomographic angiography for blunt cerebrovascular injuries: don't throw out the baby with the bathwater. Ann Surg. 2011;253:451-2.

32. Caron T, Bransford R, Nguyen Q, et al. Spine fractures in patients with ankylosing spinal disorders. Spine (Phila Pa 1976). 2010;35:E458-64.

33. Westerveld LA, Verlaan JJ, Oner FC. Spinal fractures in patients with ankylosing spinal disorders: a systematic review of the literature on treatment, neurological status and complications. Eur Spine J. 2009;18:145-56.

34. Management of acute spinal cord injuries in an intensive care unit or other monitored setting. Neurosurgery. 2002;50:S51-7.

35. King BS, Gupta R, Narayan RK. The early assessment and intensive care unit management of patients with severe traumatic brain and spinal cord injuries. Surg Clin North Am. 2000;80: 855-70.

36. Chesnut RM. The management of severe traumatic brain injury. Emerg Med Clin North Am. 1997;15:581-604.

37. Hurlbert RJ. Strategies of medical intervention in the management of acute spinal cord injury. Spine (Phila Pa 1976). 2006;31:S16-21.

38. Stahel PF, VanderHeiden T, Finn MA. Management strategies for acute spinal cord injury: current options and future perspectives. Curr Opin Crit Care. 2012;18:651-60.

39. Bracken MB, Shepard MJ, Holford TR, et al. Administration of methylprednisolone for 24 or 48 hours or tirilazad mesylate for 48 hours in the treatment of acute spinal cord injury. Results of the third national acute spinal cord injury randomized controlled trial. National acute spinal cord injury study. JAMA. 1997;277:1597-604.

40. Hugenholtz H, Cass DE, Dvorak MF, et al. High-dose methylprednisolone for acute closed spinal cord injury--only a treatment option. Can J Neurol Sci. 2002;29:227-35.

41. Lee HC, Cho DY, Lee WY, et al. Pitfalls in treatment of acute cervical spinal cord injury using high-dose methylprednisolone: a retrospect audit of 111 patients. Surg Neurol. 2007;68 (Suppl 1):S37-41.

42. Matsumoto T, Tamaki T, Kawakami M, et al. Early complications of high-dose methylprednisolone sodium succinate treatment in the follow-up of acute cervical spinal cord injury. Spine (Phila Pa 1976). 2001;26:426-30.

43. Sayer FT, Kronvall E, Nilsson OG. Methylprednisolone treatment in acute spinal cord injury: the myth challenged through a structured analysis of published literature. Spine J. 2006;6:335-43.

44. Harrop JS, Sharan AD, Vaccaro AR, et al. The cause of neurologic deterioration after acute cervical spinal cord injury. Spine. 2001;26:340-6.

45. Rechtine GR, Del Rossi G, Conrad BP, et al. Motion generated in the unstable spine during hospital bed transfers. J Trauma. 2004;57:609-11.

46. Chulay M, Brown J, Summer W. Effect of postoperative immobilization after coronary artery bypass surgery. Crit Care Med. 1982;10:176-9.

47. Convertino VA, Bloomfield SA, Greenleaf JE. An overview of the issues: physiological effects of bed rest and restricted physical activity. Med Sci Sports Exerc. 1997;29:187-90.

48. Curry K, Casady L. The relationship between extended periods of immobility and decubitus ulcer formation in the acutely spinal cord-injured individual. J Neurosci Nurs. 1992;24:185-9.

49. Dittmer DK, Teasell R. Complications of immobilization and bed rest. Part 1: Musculoskeletal and cardiovascular complications. Can Fam Physician. 1993;39:1428-32, 35-7.

50. Krishnagopalan S, Johnson EW, Low LL, et al. Body positioning of intensive care patients: clinical practice versus standards. Crit Care Med. 2002;30:2588-92.

51. Teasell R, Dittmer DK. Complications of immobilization and bed rest. Part 2: Other complications. Can Fam Physician. 1993;39:1440-2, 5-6.

52. Rechtine GR, Conrad BP, Bearden BG, et al. Biomechanical analysis of cervical and thoracolumbar spine motion in intact and partially and completely unstable cadaver spine models with kinetic bed therapy or traditional log roll. J Trauma. 2007;62:383-8.

53. Conrad BP, Horodyski M, Wright J, et al. Log-rolling technique producing unacceptable motion during body position changes in patients with traumatic spinal cord injury. J Neurosurg Spine. 2007;6:540-3.

54. Dipaola CP, Conrad BP, Horodyski M, et al. Cervical spine motion generated with manual versus jackson table turning methods in a cadaveric c1-c2 global instability model. Spine (Phila Pa 1976). 2009;34:2912-8.

55. DiPaola CP, DiPaola MJ, Conrad BP, et al. Comparison of thoracolumbar motion produced by manual and Jackson-table-turning methods. Study of a cadaveric instability model. J Bone Joint Surg Am. 2008;90:1698-704.

56. DiPaola MJ, DiPaola CP, Conrad BP, et al. Cervical spine motion in manual versus Jackson table turning methods in a cadaveric global instability model. J Spinal Disord Tech. 2008;21:273-80.

57. Bearden BG, Conrad BP, Horodyski M, et al. Motion in the unstable cervical spine: comparison of manual turning and use of the Jackson table in prone positioning. J Neurosurg Spine. 2007;7:161-4.

58. Cadotte DW, Fehlings LN, Fehlings MG. A series of systematic reviews on the treatment of acute spinal cord injury: a foundation for best medical practice. J Neurotrauma. 2011;28:1329-33.

59. Fehlings MG, Perrin RG. The role and timing of early decompression for cervical spinal cord injury: update with a review of recent clinical evidence. Injury. 2005;36(Suppl 2):B13-26.

60. Fehlings MG, Sekhon LH, Tator C. The role and timing of decompression in acute spinal cord injury: what do we know? What should we do? Spine (Phila Pa 1976). 2001;26:S101-10.

61. Fehlings MG, Vaccaro A, Wilson JR, et al. Early versus delayed decompression for traumatic cervical spinal cord injury: results of the Surgical Timing in Acute Spinal Cord Injury Study (STASCIS). PLoS One. 2012;7:e32037.

CHAPTER

9

Lumbar Disk Disease

☞ INTRODUCTION

Low back pain is one of the most common patient complaints and is the second most common reason for seeing the primary care physician. At some point during life, between 60% and 80% of adults will experience a significant episode of low back pain with a prevalence of 30%.[1] Fortunately, the majority of these cases are self-limiting and can resolve within 6 weeks regardless of treatment.[2] However, it is common for these patients to have repeated episodes. These episodes of low back pain can range from mild lumbar strains that have little impact on the patient's activity to intractable pain that limits the patient's ability to work or perform normal activities of daily living. As a result there are major direct costs related to low back pain including medical and surgical treatment, and indirect costs including missed work and loss of productivity. The total direct and indirect costs of low back pain have been estimated to exceed $100 billion an year.[3]

The evaluation of the patient with low back pain can be very complex and complicated by many factors. While lumbar disk disease has been reported to account for up to 39% of cases of low back pain, it is important to rule out other more serious causes that are detailed in other chapters of this text.[4] Contributing factors to developing low back pain include advanced age, physically demanding occupation, worker's compensation, litigation, sporting activities, cigarette smoking, atherosclerosis, obesity, history of trauma, family history of spinal disorders and previous history of back pain. While some of these factors can be controlled, genetic factors cannot. Previous studies have shown that in the upper lumbar spine 7% of the variability of lumbar disk degeneration was attributable to occupation, 16% by age and 77% to genetic factors.[5] In the lower lumbar spine 2% of variability was attributed to physical loading, 9% to age and 43% to genetics.

The purpose of this chapter is to review the presentation of patients with low back pain and the methods used to diagnose lumbar disk disease as an etiology. Additionally, appropriate surgical and nonoperative treatment options are reviewed.

☞ PATHOPHYSIOLOGY

The intervertebral disk is composed of an inner nucleus pulposus and an outer annulus fibrosus. The nucleus consists of a mesh of type II collagen and an extracellular matrix of proteoglycans that are hydrophilic, maintain a high water content and resist compressive forces. The annulus is comprised of a concentric series of interwoven fibrous lamellae that provide tensile strength to the disk. They attach to the anterior and posterior longitudinal ligaments, and the superior and inferior endplates. The source of neural innervation of the disk lies along the outer annulus where the sinuvertebral nerve innervates the disk, posterior longitudinal ligament and ventral dura.

As individuals age, there is a characteristic degenerative cascade that develops in the intervertebral disks including internal disk disruption, disk herniation and degenerative disk disease. In contrast to the immature spine, the adult disk is largely avascular. This prevents the disk from being able to heal itself once the degenerative process has begun.

Internal disk disruption typically begins in the third decade of life with a change in the proteoglycan content leading to reduced levels of chondroitin sulfate and increased levels of keratin sulfate. These changes diminish the disk's ability to maintain its normal fluid concentration and leads to a decreased ability of the nucleus to resist normal compressive forces. This places additional stress on the outer annular fibers. Pain associated with internal disk disruption is thought to occur due to a combination of mechanical and chemical stimulation of the nerves on the surface of the annulus. In this initial stage of degeneration, there are no imaging findings of disk herniation, instability or loss of disk height. There are also no clinical findings of radicular symptoms or neurologic deficits.

The second stage of the degenerative cascade is lumbar disk herniation. Disk herniations can be categorized as soft or hard. A soft disk herniation is the result of a disruption of the outer annular fibers with protrusion of the inner nucleus material causing compression of the exiting nerve roots. Soft disk herniations are most commonly seen in patients between 30 years and 50 years of age. A hard disk herniation is the result of osteophyte formation or calcification of disk material and typically causes chronic symptoms in patients greater than 55 years of age. Soft disk herniations can be further categorized as a bulge, protrusion, extrusion or sequestration (Figs 1A to D). A disk bulge is caused by the nucleus pushing on the annulus but without any disruption of the annular fibers. A protrusion is a small defect in the outer annular fibers with a portion of the nucleus displaced outside the annulus. The base of the protrusion is wider than the material displaced beyond the borders of the annulus. A disk extrusion consists of further displacement of the nucleus beyond the borders of the annulus where the diameter of the displaced material is greater than at the base. A sequestered disk herniation is a completely free piece of disk that has separated from the remainder of the disk.

The location of the disk herniation determines which nerve root is affected. The majority of lumbar disk herniations occur in a posterolateral location adjacent to the posterior longitudinal ligament. The lumbar nerve roots exit the spinal canal below their same pedicle, so the L4 nerve root exits below the L4 pedicle. The traversing nerve root exits below the caudal next pedicle, so the L5 nerve root traverses the L4-L5 disk space and exits the spinal canal below the L5 pedicle. Posterolateral disk herniations typically affect the traversing nerve root so a posterolateral L4-L5 disk herniation would compress the traversing L5 nerve root (Figs 2A and B). A far lateral lumbar disk herniation would typically affect the exiting nerve root so a far lateral L5-S1 disk herniation would also affect the L5 nerve root (Figs 2A and B).

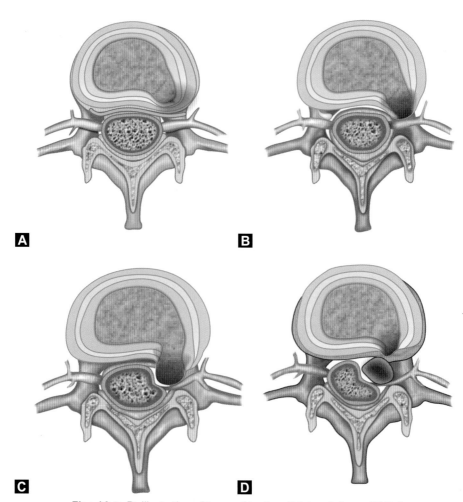

Figs 1A to D: Illustration of types of lumbar disk herniations. (A) Bulge;
(B) Protrusion; (C) Extrusion; and (D) Sequestration

The final stage of the degenerative cascade is degenerative disk disease. This occurs when the disk looses a portion of its normal height. This causes buckling of the ligamentum flavum, facet joint capsules, and annulus into the spinal canal and neuroforamen. This increases the resultant loading of the facet joints and leads to facet joint degeneration. Additional bone spurs can form and cause further narrowing of the spinal canal and foramen. These changes can lead to other spinal disorders including lumbar stenosis and degenerative spondylolisthesis that are discussed further in other chapters.

☞ PATIENT PRESENTATION

The patient with internal disk disruption typically presents with a deep, dull ache in the lower back. It may be aggravated with activity and partially relieved with rest. In this early stage, there may be associated pain in the buttock area, but there is no pain or paresthesias

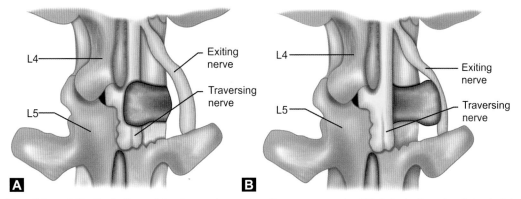

Figs 2A and B: Illustration of the traversing and exiting nerve roots. (A) A typical posterolateral disk herniation as shown at L4-L5 would compress the traversing L5 nerve root; (B) L4-L5 would compress the exiting L4 nerve

into the lower extremities. In some cases, these patients may recall a specific event that occurred prior to the onset of their symptoms, but in many cases patients present with a gradual onset of symptoms without a history of trauma.

In the next stage, lumbar disk herniation, patients more frequently recall an inciting event, but this is not present in all cases. Often patients may have experienced a period of dull lower back pain initially, followed by the more classic symptoms of lumbar disk herniation including radiating pain in a dermatomal distribution in the lower extremity with or without paresthesias. The initial back pain symptoms are often related to the preceding internal disk disruption. Once this advances, and the nucleus herniates through the annulus and compresses the nerve root, the radicular symptoms develop. In some cases, the low back pain subsides after the onset of radicular symptoms, but in some cases both persist. Patients should be questioned on any history of previous similar complaints, history of previous back problems, feelings of weakness in the lower extremities, aggravating and relieving factors, and changes in bowel or bladder control.

Any change in bowel or bladder control should alert the provider to the possibility of cauda equina syndrome. This results from a severe compression in the caudal aspect of the spinal canal. Patients can present with symptoms including unilateral or bilateral leg pain, paresthesias in a saddle distribution, pain in the lower back or lower extremities, bowel incontinence, and initially urinary retention followed by an overflow urinary incontinence. This is considered as surgical emergency, and the patient should have surgery to decompress the area within 24–48 hours to decrease the risk of permanent loss of function.

Physical examination of the suspected lumbar disk herniation should include evaluation of the patient's gait for any signs of weakness, foot drop or Trendelenburg gait pattern. A full neurologic examination can reveal any specific areas of motor or sensory deficits that can be later correlated with imaging findings.

👉 IMAGING

In many cases plain radiographs are the initial imaging modality obtained. These can be evaluated for degenerative changes including loss of disk height, osteophyte formation

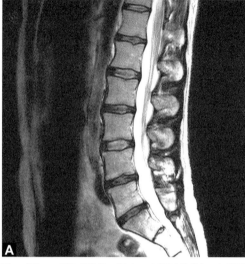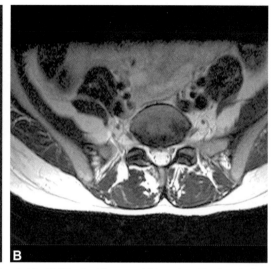

Figs 3A and B: (A) Sagittal and (B) L5-S1 axial T2-weighted MRI of a 39-year-old female with chronic low back pain. Imaging revealed signs of internal disk disruption with loss of fluid signal in the L4-S1 disks and an annular tear at the L5-S1 level

and signs of instability. Computed tomography (CT) provides improved visualization of the osseous structures. It does not provide as good a view of the soft tissues or neural structures as magnetic resonance imaging (MRI), but it is useful for patients where MRI is contraindicated. MRI provides the greatest detail for evaluation of suspected lumbar disk disease. The initial stages of internal disk disruption are visualized on MRI as a loss of fluid content in the disks; annular tears appear as a high-intensity zone (Figs 3A and B). The high-intensity zone refers to a high-intensity signal found on T2-weighted images at the posterior aspect of the annulus and correlates with a radial tear extending from the nucleus to the outer layers of the annulus.

Magnetic resonance imaging is the gold standard imaging modality for evaluation of the patient with a suspected lumbar disk herniation. These images can visualize the exact location of the disk herniation, the degree of central or foraminal compromise and nerve root compression (Figs 4A and B).

Imaging of the final stage of lumbar disk disease, degenerative disk disease, can include plain radiographs and advanced imaging studies. Plain radiographs reveal a loss of normal disk height, osteophyte formation and potential signs of instability. MRI images often reveal Modic changes in the endplates (Figs 5A and B).[6] These changes represent a progressive change in the appearance of the vertebral endplates on MRI as the degree of degeneration advances as shown in the Table 1.

It is important to correlate all imaging findings with the clinical examination of the patient. Many normal, age-related changes can be identified on imaging studies that do not become symptomatic. Boden et al. found that approximately 30% of all individuals had asymptomatic abnormalities found on lumbar spine MRI, and these changes were nearly universal in patients over the age of 60 years.[7] Additionally, these asymptomatic MRI findings have not been found to be predictive of future clinical symptoms.[8]

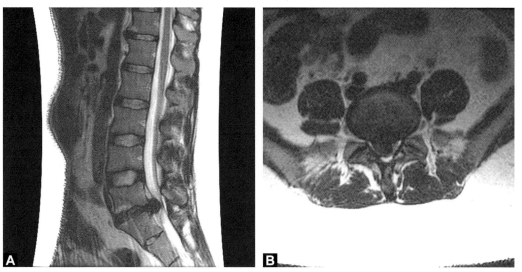

Figs 4A and B: (A) Sagittal and (B) L5-S1 axial T2-weighted MRI of a 27-year-old female with severe right lower extremity pain. Imaging revealed a large L5-S1 disk herniation with severe central and right foraminal stenosis and nerve root compression

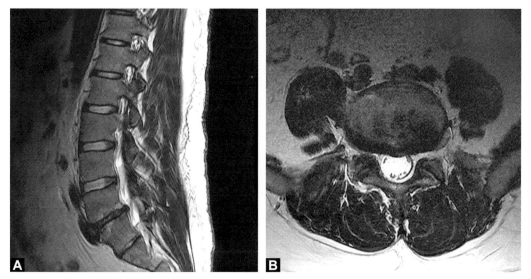

Figs 5A and B: (A) Sagittal and (B) L5-S1 axial T2-weighted MRI images of a 45-year-old male with advanced degenerative disk disease. Images reveal loss of fluid signal in the L5-S1 disk, loss of disk height, endplate edema and a mild, grade 1 spondylolisthesis

Lumbar discography is a technique in which a needle a placed fluoroscopically into the disk space, and contrast fluid is injected into the disk space. The goals are to identify any signs of the contrast flowing through the annulus suggesting a tear and to determine if the increased pressure in the disk recreates the patient's pain. The process is repeated on all disks that appear abnormal on MRI as well as an adjacent level control disk. This technique remains controversial. The main criticisms are the subjective nature of measuring the

Table 1: Description of Modic vertebral endplate changes found on magnetic resonance imaging (MRI)

Modic stage	Anatomic changes	MRI findings
I	Edema	Decreased signal on T1 Bright signal on T2
II	Fatty degeneration in the bone adjacent to the endplates	Bright signal on T1 Intermediate signal on T2
III	Advanced endplate sclerosis	Decreased signal on T1 Decreased signal on T2

patient's pain and the need for injection into a control level. Recent animal studies have used the needle puncture model to create lumbar disk disease. As a result, it has been suggested that the discography technique could create degenerative disk disease in previously normal levels. This has been confirmed by Carragee et al. in a prospective study of 50 discography patients and 52 control subjects.[9] Patients that underwent discography had significantly greater risk of progression of disk degeneration, development of new disk herniation, and loss of disk height and signal intensity.

☞ ELECTRODIAGNOSTIC STUDIES

Electrodiagnostic studies include electromyography (EMG) and nerve conduction studies (NCS). EMG involves the placement of intramuscular needle electrodes to evaluate for muscle function and is used to detect motor dysfunction due to nerve compression. NCS use surface electrodes to measure the amplitude and latency of peripheral nerves. These studies can be useful to help differentiate a nerve root compression associated with cervical disk disease from a peripheral nerve compression. EMG studies have a delay of approximately 4 weeks after nerve injury prior to revealing any abnormality. Additionally, there is a poor correlation between the results of electrodiagnostic studies and MRI findings.[10] As a result, electrodiagnostic studies can aid in refining a differential diagnosis but should not be relied upon without confirmation from other studies.

☞ NONOPERATIVE TREATMENT

Fortunately, the majority of patients with symptoms related to lumbar disk disease will experience a gradual resolution of their symptoms within 6 weeks to 3 months regardless of treatment. During this time, supportive treatment of the symptoms is useful. A short period of relative rest can help decrease the ongoing irritation and inflammation of the involved structures. This should not include bed rest, but instead, avoiding more physically demanding activities that are likely to exacerbate the symptoms. Physical therapy and chiropractic treatment are often utilized for these patients with varied success. Modalities including heat, ultrasound and electrical stimulation can reduce muscle spasms and inflammation, and allow the patient to better perform stretching and strengthening exercises. Strengthening of the core abdominal muscles helps to stabilize the affected areas and is beneficial during exacerbations as well as potential prevention of future episodes.

The efficacy of these programs is highly dependent on patient participation both during and after the structured program. The more effort the patient exerts, and the more the patient continues to implement these exercises into normal routine for the long term, the better the associated results are likely to be.

Medication management typically begins with nonsteroidal anti-inflammatory medication unless the patient has a contraindication to these. Muscle relaxants and narcotics are used for short-term management of pain in some cases but are often avoided due to the risk of dependency and side effects including sedation and constipation. Oral corticosteroids can be effective in relieving symptoms associated with inflammation, but their use should be limited due to potential adverse effects including weight gain and osteonecrosis. Caution should also be used in diabetic patients due to the risk of hyperglycemia. Anticonvulsants including gabapentin and pregabalin have been shown to be effective in reducing symptoms of radiculopathy in patients with disk disease. These medications have numerous potential adverse effects that should be discussed with the patient prior to recommendation for use. Antidepressants should not be considered a primary treatment option for lumbar disk disease, but there is anecdotal support for their use especially in patients with pre-existing symptoms of anxiety or depression that have been exacerbated by their pain complaints.

The use of steroid injections for lumbar disk disease can provide short-term reduction in back pain and radiculopathy in some patients. Patients with tender points in the muscles may benefit from the use of trigger point injections. These injections can be performed in the office setting without the use of fluoroscopy and are felt to be safe, but they provide only short-term benefits. Lumbar epidural steroid injections (LESI) should be performed under fluoroscopic guidance, and they can provide some reduction in radicular symptoms in patients. They are often used during the first 6 weeks to 3 months to reduce patient symptoms while waiting to see if the episode will spontaneously resolve.

OPERATIVE TREATMENT

Indications for surgery for lumbar disk disease include failure of an appropriate course of nonoperative treatment and progressive neurologic deficit. The most serious surgical indication is neurologic deficit. This can present in the form of cauda equina syndrome, which requires surgery within 24–48 hours of the onset of symptoms to reduce the risk of permanent deficit, or the neurologic symptoms can be more gradual. Most cases of neurologic deficit associated with lumbar disk disease will result from a large disk herniation. Neurologic deficits from degenerative disk disease alone are much less common.

Patients with lumbar disk herniation that either have neurologic deficits or failed conservative treatments with intractable pain are considered potential surgical candidates. The most common procedure performed for these patients is a microdiscectomy for removal of the offending portion of disk that is causing nerve root compression. There are newer minimally invasive techniques that have been shown to decrease the amount of soft-tissue dissection and might improve the initial postoperative course. Following surgery, the patient's activities are generally limited for the first 6 weeks to allow for healing and to reduce the risk of a recurrent disk herniation. If the patient develops a single recurrent disk herniation a repeat microdiscectomy is often recommended. In cases of more than one recurrence, a complete discectomy and fusion is often performed.

Surgical treatment of lumbar degenerative disk disease remains more controversial. This is due to the fact that in most cases patients complain predominately of lower back pain, and neurologic findings are less common. Surgical outcomes in general for back pain are less consistent than surgical outcomes for radiculopathy. Part of this is because in some cases it might be difficult to accurately define the specific etiology of a patient's back pain. Symptoms can come from the intervertebral disk, the facet joints, the sacroiliac joint, and the surrounding muscles and other soft tissues.

Historically, a lumbar fusion has been the surgical treatment of choice for these patients. There are many variations that can be chosen from including anterior lumbar interbody fusion (ALIF), posterior lumbar interbody fusion (PLIF), transforaminal lumbar interbody fusion (TLIF), posterior instrumented fusion and posterolateral non-instrumented fusion.

The choice of specific technique for lumbar fusion is based on specific patient characteristics and surgeon experience. The use of instrumentation is believed to increase radiographic fusion success, but not always clinical success. In cases of elderly patients with poor bone quality, instrumentation might be avoided due to the risk of instrumentation failure or pullout. Also in patients with multiple medical comorbidities, instrumentation might be avoided to allow for a shorter operative time. Interbody lumbar fusion techniques allow for a portion or all of the intervertebral disk to be removed, and this provides a large additional fusion surface. It also allows for placement of a structural graft that can help restore the lost disk height and thus increase the foraminal area and reduce nerve root compression. ALIF has the benefit of removing all of the disk material, but it has the limitation of having an increased risk in patients that have had previous abdominal surgery, the need for an approach surgeon, and risk of retrograde ejaculation in male patients. The ALIF can be performed alone or in combination with posterior stabilization. When performed alone, it typically includes anterior instrumentation. In some cases, this involves placement of an anterior lumbar plate in addition to the interbody graft or spacer device. Newer ALIF devices have self-contained stabilization options that allow for placement of screws through the fusion device into the adjacent vertebrae (Figs 6A and B).

Posterior lumbar interbody fusion and TLIF allow for posterior instrumented fusion to be performed with an interbody fusion through a single posterior approach. The difference between the two is the angle at which the approach is taken to the interbody space. In the PLIF the lamina is removed, and the dural sac is retracted centrally to gain access to the disk. In the TLIF a partial to complete facetectomy is performed, and the disk is accessed through Kambin's triangle (Figs 7A and B). The benefit of the TLIF over the PLIF is that eliminates the need for retraction of the neural structures and allows the lamina to remain in place as another potential fusion surface.[11]

The other most recent option for surgery includes motion-sparing technique such as disk arthroplasty devices. The potential benefit of these devices is that they do not eliminate motion at the surgical level, and thus do not place increased mechanical demand on the adjacent levels. It is believed that this could potentially decrease the incidence of adjacent level disk degeneration. However, it remains uncertain how much adjacent level disk degeneration is the result of increased mechanical demands versus natural history.

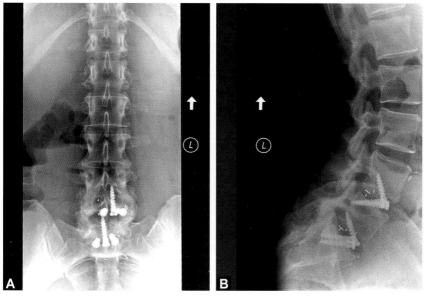

Figs 6A and B: (A) Anteroposterior and (B) lateral postoperative radiographs of the 39-year-old female from Figure 3 that underwent an anterior lumbar interbody fusion (ALIF) at L4-S1

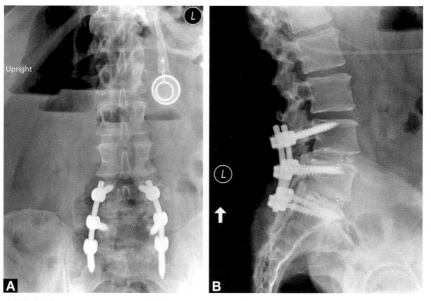

Figs 7A and B: (A) Anteroposterior and (B) lateral postoperative radiographs of the 45-year-old female that underwent transforaminal lumbar interbody fusion (TLIF) at L4-S1 for lumbar degenerative disk disease. The metallic markers embedded in the TLIF cages allow confirmation of their proper placement

REFERENCES

1. Andersson G. Epidemiological features of chronic low-back pain. Lancet. 1999;354:581-5.
2. Waddell G. A new clinical model for the treatment of low-back pain. Spine. 1987;12:632-44.

3. Katz J. Lumbar disc disorders and low back pain: socioeconomic factors and consequences. J Bone Joint Surg Am. 2006;88:21-4.
4. Schwarzer AC, Aprill CN, Derby R, et al. The prevalence and clinical features of internal disc disruption in patients with chronic low back pain. Spine. 1995;20:1878-83.
5. Battie MC, Videman T, Gibbons LE, et al. Determinants of lumbar disc degeneration: a study relating lifetime exposures and magnetic resonance imaging findings in identical twins. Spine. 1995;20:2601-12.
6. Modic M, Steinberg P, Ross J, et al. Degenerative disk disease: assessment of changes in vertebral body marrow with MR imaging. Radiology. 1988;166:193-9.
7. Boden S, McCowin P, Davis D, et al. Abnormal magnetic resonance scans of the lumbar spine in asymptomatic subjects: a prospective investigation. J Bone Joint Surg Am. 1990;72:403-8.
8. Borenstein DG, O'Mara JW Jr, Boden SD, et al. The value of magnetic resonance imaging of the lumbar spine to predict low-back pain in asymptomatic subjects: a seven-year follow-up study. J Bone Joint Surg Am. 2001;83:1306-11.
9. Carragee EJ, Don AS, Herwitz EL, et al. Does discography cause accelerated progression of degenerative changes in the lumbar disc: a ten-year matched cohort study. Spine. 2009;34: 2338-45.
10. Nardin RA, Patel MR, Gudas TF, et al. Electromyography and magnetic resonance imaging in the evaluation of radiculopathy. Muscle Nerve. 1999;22:151-5.
11. Humphreys SC, Hodges SD, Patwardhan AG, et al. Comparison of posterior and transforaminal approaches to lumbar interbody fusion. Spine. 2001;26:567-71.

CHAPTER

10

Lumbar Spinal Stenosis

INTRODUCTION

Spinal stenosis refers to the narrowing of the space available in the spinal canal that can cause compression of the neural elements. It is one of the most common conditions seen in elderly patients. Stenosis can occur in the central spinal canal causing compression of the dural sac or in the lateral recesses or neural foramen causing compression of the exiting nerve roots. Common symptoms include generalized low back pain, buttock pain and lower extremity pain, paresthesias and weakness.

It is important for the treating physician to be able to recognize the symptoms of lumbar spinal stenosis, differentiate it from other potential differential diagnoses, obtain appropriate imaging studies and recommend treatment options. This chapter provides an overview of lumbar spinal stenosis to assist with those goals.

PATHOPHYSIOLOGY

The spinal canal is bordered anteriorly by the vertebral body, intervertebral disk, and posterior longitudinal ligament, laterally by the neural foramen, pedicles and ligamentum flavum, and posteriorly by the lamina, facet joints and ligamentum flavum. Changes in any of these structures can decrease the available space and cause spinal stenosis. Three general shapes of the spinal canal have been identified including round, ovoid and trefoil as shown in Figures 1A to C.[1] The round and ovoid shapes provide the greatest amount of space, while the trefoil shape has the smallest cross-sectional area and greatest incidence of spinal stenosis. It is reported to occur in approximately 15% of patients.

The intervertebral disk is composed of an inner nucleus pulposus and an outer annulus fibrosus. As individuals age changes occur, and there is less of a distinction between these two structures. There is a gradual replacement of Type I collagen with Type II collagen that has less of a water-binding capacity. Decreased fluid content in the disk leads to loss of disk height and ability to withstand mechanical loading. This in turn causes bulging of the disk and the posterior longitudinal ligament into the spinal canal. Degeneration of the disk also affects the surrounding anatomic structures. Loss of disk height causes buckling of the ligamentum flavum into the spinal canal. Subsequent increased loading of the facet

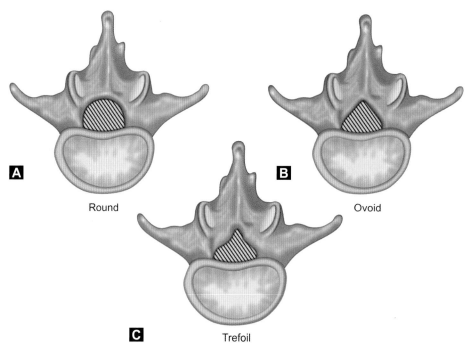

Figs 1A to C: Diagram of the three shapes of spinal canal. (A) Round; (B) Ovoid (C) Trefoil

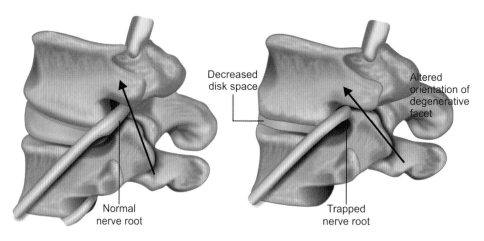

Fig. 2: Diagram of the effect of loss of disk height on facet hypertrophy and overlap causing foraminal stenosis

joints leads to hypertrophy of the facets and further central and lateral recess stenosis. Loss of disk height also causes the facet joints to further overlap, decreasing the foraminal height causing vertical or up-down foraminal stenosis as shown in Figure 2.

The location of the spinal stenosis has important implications for both diagnosis and treatment. Stenosis can occur centrally, in the lateral recess or in the foramen as shown in Figure 3. Central stenosis is typically the result of disk bulging or buckling of the ligamentum flavum and can cause symptoms of neurogenic claudication. In most cases these symptoms

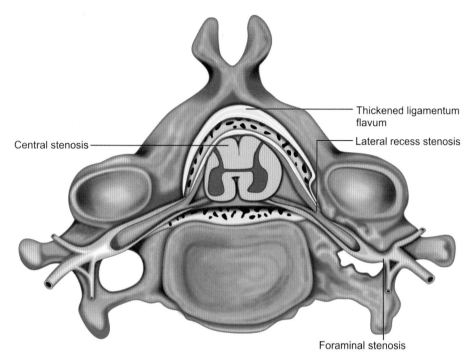

Central stenosis

Thickened ligamentum flavum

Lateral recess stenosis

Foraminal stenosis

Fig. 3: Diagram of potential locations of lumbar spinal stenosis including central, lateral recess or foraminal

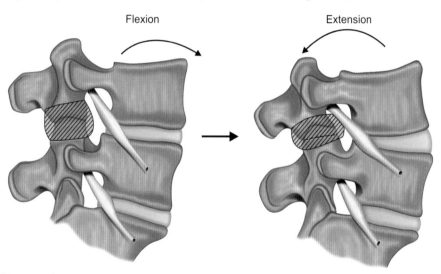

Flexion

Extension

Fig. 4: Diagram of the lumbar spine in flexion and extension showing the increased area available during flexion that explains the improvement of symptoms when the lumbar spine is flexed or the individual is seated

are exacerbated with standing or extension of the spine, and symptoms are relieved with sitting or flexion of the spine. This change in symptoms occurs because during flexion the buckling of the ligamentum flavum is reduced or eliminated, creating additional space in the spinal canal as shown in Figure 4. Stenosis of the lateral recess is caused by disk bulging and facet hypertrophy and leads to symptoms of radiculopathy. Foraminal stenosis can be

Table 1: Causes of lumbar spinal stenosis	
Congenital	Idiopathic
	Achondroplasia
Degenerative	Degenerative disk disease
	Facet arthrosis
Iatrogenic	Postlaminectomy deformity
	Adjacent level degeneration
	Instrumentation malposition
Inflammatory	Acromegaly
	Paget's disease
	Ankylosing spondylitis
Trauma	Burst fracture
	Facet fracture or dislocation
	Lamina fracture
Tumor	Epidural extension of tumor
	Pathologic fracture
Infection	Epidural abscess
	Pathologic fracture

caused by facet hypertrophy, disk herniation, facet cyst, and spondylolisthesis and leads to lumbar radiculopathy symptoms.

While routine age-related degenerative changes are the most common causes of spinal stenosis there are other potential etiologies that should be recognized as detailed in Table 1. Lumbar stenosis can also be dynamic in cases where instability is present.

☞ PATIENT PRESENTATION

Most patients with lumbar spinal stenosis have a degenerative etiology and develop symptoms during their 60s. The most common symptom is buttock and leg pain. Patients with central stenosis may present with signs of neurogenic claudication including pain, heaviness, weakness, burning and cramping in the buttocks that radiates down bilaterally to lower extremities below the knees. The location of the symptoms typically does not follow a dermatomal pattern with central stenosis. Due to extension of the spine, walking downhill produces increased symptoms, while walking uphill places the spine in flexion and produces fewer symptoms. Most patients with central stenosis achieve good relief of symptoms with sitting or when bending forward. The "shopping cart" sign refers to the fact that patients may be very limited in the ability to ambulate, but when bending forward and using a shopping cart they are able to ambulate for further distances with less pain. Patients with central stenosis may also complain of lower back pain that is relieved in flexion and exacerbated with extension.

Patients with lateral recess or foraminal stenosis have compression of individual nerve roots and typically present with symptoms of pain, paresthesias or weakness in a specific dermatomal pattern.

Bowel and bladder dysfunction are less common but can occur. Urinary retention with subsequent overflow incontinence or bowel incontinence could signify cauda equina syndrome and the potential need for emergent imaging and potential surgical decompression. Urinary dysfunction is relatively common in this patient population due to other causes including urinary tract infection, prostate hypertrophy and stress incontinence. These should be ruled out prior to considering a neurologic etiology.

Patients with suspected lumbar spinal stenosis should undergo a complete physical examination. Observation of the patient's stance should assess their sagittal plane posture. Flexion of the lumbar spine or reluctance to fully straighten or extend the spine could be related central stenosis and an attempt to relieve symptoms. The gait should be assessed for ambulatory aids, sagittal plane posture, stability and signs of motor weakness.

Motor function, sensation and reflexes should be tested to identify any areas of deficit as detailed in Chapter 4. The presence of gait changes and hyper-reflexia should raise the concern for myelopathy which is also common in this patient population. Skin discoloration, diminished peripheral pulses and loss of hair on the feet could signify a vascular etiology to the symptoms.

IMAGING

As with most spinal disorders, the imaging of patients with suspected lumbar spinal stenosis typically begins with plain radiographs. These can provide an overall picture of the spine and screen for deformity, trauma, tumor, infection and degenerative changes. Deformity could include degenerative scoliosis or spondylolisthesis which can each occur in conjunction with lumbar stenosis. The radiographs can show loss of disk height, osteophyte formation and foraminal narrowing as shown in Figures 5A and B.

More advanced imaging studies for spinal stenosis include computed tomography (CT) and magnetic resonance imaging (MRI). CT scans provide three-dimensional images of the spine and have the best detail of the osseous structures. The sensitivity of CT in detecting spinal stenosis ranges from 70% to 100%.[2] They can be combined with myelography to provide improved visualization of the neural structures; however, this is an invasive study. CT scans are also useful in patients that cannot have an MRI due to certain metallic implants or the presence of a pacemaker. In patients with more severe spinal deformity CT can provide improved detail over MRI through its ability to image through the disk space despite the deformity.

Magnetic resonance imaging remains the gold standard for imaging of patients with spinal stenosis (Figs 6A and B). It provides excellent detail of the soft tissues and neural structures and can identify central, lateral recess and foraminal stenosis. All imaging results should be interpreted cautiously as the correlation between severity of imaging findings and clinical symptoms is limited.[3,4]

NONOPERATIVE TREATMENT

There is limited information on the natural history of untreated lumbar spinal stenosis. Johnson et al. reported on a series of 32 patients followed for approximately 4 years without

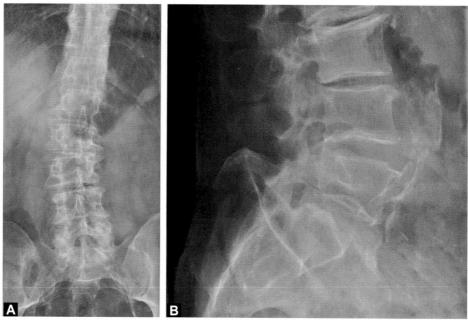

Figs 5A and B: (A) Anteroposterior (AP) and (B) lateral radiographs of 65-year-old with lumbar spinal stenosis. Radiographs show loss of disk height, osteophyte formation and foraminal narrowing with associated degenerative scoliosis

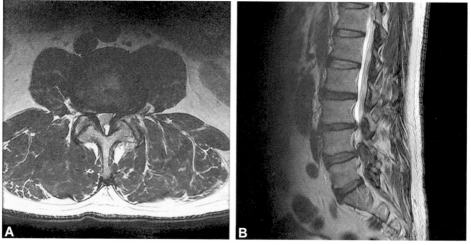

Figs 6A and B: (A) Axial and (B) sagittal MRI of 61-year-old with central and lateral recess stenosis from L2-S1

medical or surgical treatment.[5] In this study the course over time remained relatively steady with 70% of patients remaining unchanged in pain level, 15% reporting improvement and 15% reporting worsened symptoms.

There are numerous options for nonoperative management of patients with lumbar spinal stenosis including medications, physical therapy, chiropractic and injection therapy. The most commonly utilized medications for these patients include nonsteroidal anti-inflammatory medications. These are thought to reduce the inflammation and swelling of the compressed nerve roots; however, there is limited information on their clinical effectiveness. Unfortunately, many older patients with stenosis have various comorbidities that preclude the use of these medications including gastric ulcers, hypertension and cardiovascular disease. Other medication options include acetaminophen, muscle relaxants, narcotics and anticonvulsants. Caution should be used to avoid more than 4 gm daily of acetaminophen to avoid hepatotoxicity. Patients with preexisting liver disorders might need to avoid all acetaminophen. While narcotics and muscle relaxants can in some cases provide reasonable pain relief, caution should be used in this patient population due to the increased risk of sedation, falls and constipation that can be common side effects. Anticonvulsants such as gabapentin have been reported to provide improved pain and functional ability in patients with stenosis, but they are also associated with side effects including sedation, dizziness and increased risk of falls.[6]

The use of physical therapy or chiropractic programs is commonly recommended for patients with spinal stenosis. These programs can include stretching and strengthening exercises, core muscle strengthening, as well as various modalities including heat, ice, massage, ultrasound and electrical stimulation. While these methods are commonly used in conjunction with other treatment options, there is no proven benefit to physical therapy or chiropractic as a standalone treatment option.[7]

Another common nonsurgical treatment for lumbar spinal stenosis is lumbar epidural steroid injection. These injections are typically used to deliver a combination of a long-acting anesthetic with corticosteroids to the area of stenosis. They are felt to be the most beneficial for radicular symptoms as opposed to axial back pain. They can be performed through an interlaminar approach or a transforaminal approach. Each method has been shown to be of benefit for short-term relief of radicular symptoms.[8,9] However, there is conflicting evidence that either approach is superior to the other.[10,11] There is also no strong evidence for their long-term effectiveness. Reported predictors of successful response to epidural steroid injections include relative youth and female sex, while body mass index and MRI severity are not predictive of successful outcomes.[12]

A recent systematic review found low-quality evidence for the use of nonoperative treatment of patients with lumbar spinal stenosis with neurogenic claudication, but failed to identify any moderate- or high-grade evidence.[13]

OPERATIVE TREATMENT

Patients with lumbar spinal stenosis that fail to respond to nonoperative treatment options can be evaluated as potential surgical candidates. Surgery is typically reserved for patients that fail at least 6 weeks of conservative treatment and have intractable symptoms. These patients are often elderly and may have multiple medical comorbidities that increase the relative risks associated with surgery.

The most commonly performed surgery for patients with lumbar spinal stenosis is a lumbar decompression. The goal of this procedure is to alleviate the compression of the nerve roots. There are various methods used to achieve this goal including laminectomy, laminotomy, foraminotomy, placement of interspinous distraction devices and minimally invasive decompression techniques. In the recent Spine Patient Outcomes Research Trial (SPORT), 289 patients with lumbar spinal stenosis were prospectively randomized into either surgical decompression with laminectomy versus nonoperative treatment.[14] Patients receiving surgery maintained significantly greater improvements in pain and functional capacity at 4-year follow-up as compared to the conservative treatment group. The number of involved levels does not appear to affect surgical outcomes with lumbar spinal stenosis alone, but single-level stenosis with degenerative spondylolisthesis fares better than multiple-level stenosis with spondylolisthesis.[15]

In some cases a lumbar spinal fusion with or without instrumentation is combined with the decompression for patient with lumbar spinal stenosis. There are several potential reasons to consider a fusion procedure including deformity, instability and axial back pain. Patients with either degenerative scoliosis or degenerative spondylolisthesis may be considered for a fusion in addition to decompression in an attempt to avoid progression of the deformity. Standing flexion and extension radiographs can be obtained to identify cases of dynamic instability that may also benefit from a fusion. Iatrogenic instability can also occur in cases with more severe facet arthrosis that require a partial or complete facetectomy to decompress the nerve roots. If greater than one half of each facet joint is removed there is a greater risk of postoperative instability, and a fusion is typically recommended. Finally, patients with significant axial back pain from degenerative disk disease might benefit from a fusion to address the axial pain; however, fusion for back pain is considered controversial and less predictable.

The other category of surgery for lumbar spinal stenosis is placement of interbody spacer devices. The goal of these devices is to increase the interspinous distance and provide a mechanical block to extension of the lumbar vertebrae. It is possible that these devices can provide similar clinical results to traditional lumbar decompression procedures through a minimally invasive approach. The results from these devices are limited and conflicting. They can be inserted under local anesthesia without the need for general anesthesia, which is advantageous in the patient with multiple medical comorbidities. However, in a cost-effective analysis comparing nonsurgical care, laminectomy and interspinous process spacers, laminectomy was found to be the most cost-effective treatment for patient with symptomatic lumbar spinal stenosis.[16]

REFERENCES

1. Hillabrand AS, Rand N. Degenerative lumbar stenosis: diagnosis and management. J Am Acad Orthop Surg. 1999;7(4):239-49.
2. Kent DL, Haynor DR, Larson EB. Diagnosis of lumbar spinal stenosis in adults: a meta-analysis of the accuracy of CT, MR, and myelography. AJR Am J Roentgenol. 1992;158(5):1135-44.
3. Haig AJ, Geisser ME, Tong HC, et al. Electromyography and magnetic resonance imaging to predict lumbar stenosis, low back pain, and no back symptoms. J Bone Joint Surg. 2007;89(2): 358-66.
4. Ogikubo O, Forsberg L, Hansson T. The relationship between the cross-sectional area of the cauda equine and the preoperative symptoms in central lumbar spinal stenosis. Spine. 2007;32(13): 1423-8.

5. Johnson EK, Rosen I, Uden A. The natural course of lumbar spinal stenosis. Clin Orthop Rel Res. 1992;279:82-6.

6. Yakso A, Ozgonenel L, Ozgonenel B. The efficacy of gabapentin therapy in patients with lumbar canal stenosis. Spine. 2007;32(9):939-42.

7. Watters WC, Baisden J, Gilbert TJ, et al. Degenerative lumbar spinal stenosis: an evidence-based clinical guideline for the diagnosis and treatment of degenerative spinal stenosis. Spine J. 2008;8(2):305-10.

8. Botwin KP, Gruber RD, Bouchlas CG, et al. Fluoroscopically guided lumbar transforminal epidural steroid injection in degenerative lumbar stenosis. Am J Phys Med Rehabil. 2002;81(12):926-30.

9. Rosenberg SK, Grabinsky A, Kooser C, et al. Effectiveness of transforaminal epidural steroid injections in low back pain: a one-year experience. Pain Physician. 2002;5(3):266-70.

10. Schaufele MK, Hatch L, Jones W. Interlaminar versus transforminal epidural injections for the treatment of symptomatic lumbar intervertebral disc herniations. Pain Physician. 2006;9(4): 199-204.

11. Smith CC, Booker T, Schaufele MK, et al. Interlaminar versus transforaminal epidural steroid injections for the treatment of symptomatic lumbar spinal stenosis. Pain Med. 2010;11(10): 1511-5.

12. Cosgrove JL, Bertolet M, Chase SL, et al. Epidural steroid injections in the treatment of lumbar spinal stenosis. Efficacy and predictability of successful response. Am J Phys Med Rehabil. 2011;90(12):1050-5.

13. Ammendolia C, Stuber K, de Bruin LK, et al. Nonoperative treatment of lumbar spinal stenosis with neurogenic claudication. Spine. 2012;37(10):E609-16.

14. Weinstein JN, Tosteson TD, Lurie JD, et al. Surgical versus nonoperative treatment for lumbar spinal stenosis. Four-year results of the Spine Patient Outcomes Research Trial. Spine. 2010;35(14):1329-38.

15. Park DK, An HS, Lurie JD, et al. Does multilevel lumbar stenosis lead to poorer outcomes? A subanalysis of the Spine Patient Outcomes Research Trial (SPORT) lumbar stenosis study. Spine. 2010;35(4):439-46.

16. Burnett MG, Stein SC, Martels R. Cost-effectiveness of current treatment strategies for lumbar spinal stenosis: nonsurgical care, laminectomy, and X-STOP. J Neurosurg Spine. 2010;13(1): 39-46.

CHAPTER

11

Lumbar Spondylolisthesis

INTRODUCTION

Spondylolisthesis is a relatively common condition of the spine that occurs when one vertebra slips with respect to the neighboring vertebra. It is found in approximately 10% of adults with an overall male-to-female ratio of 2:1, but progression is more commonly seen in females. It can be found in isolation or combined with other spinal disorders such as scoliosis and spina bifida occulta. In the majority of cases the slip is anteriorly and is also known as anterolisthesis, but it can also occur in a posterior direction known as retrolisthesis. It is most commonly found in the lumbar spine, which is the focus of this chapter.

There are various etiologies responsible for spondylolisthesis that will be discussed in detail. Additionally, there are specific patient populations that are at greater risk of developing spondylolisthesis including football linemen, dancers, divers, gymnasts, rowers and wrestlers due to the high levels of hyperextension stress applied to their spines. While this is a relatively common condition, the majority of cases can be effectively treated nonoperatively.

The purpose of this chapter is to review the types and classification of lumbar spondylolisthesis, examination and imaging findings, and operative and nonoperative treatment options.

PATHOPHYSIOLOGY

The lumbar spine is subjected to very high loads that are dependent on an individual's activity level. Approximately 80% of the loads transmitted through the lumbar spine are through the disk space, and 20% are through the facet joints and posterior elements. The anatomy of the lumbar spine helps to prevent the development of spondylolisthesis. Specifically, the facet joints are in a more sagittal orientation in the upper lumbar spine and gradually change to a more coronal orientation in the lower lumbar spine. The iliolumbar ligament provides an additional restraint to forward slip of the L4 and L5 vertebrae (Fig. 1). Any changes in the normal lumbar lordotic curvature, disk or facet joints can alter the ability of the spine to withstand the applied loads and lead to degenerative changes or failure.

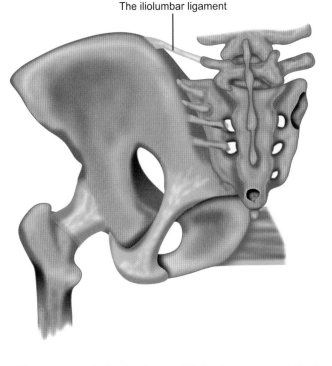

The iliolumbar ligament

Fig. 1: Diagram of the iliolumbar ligament that acts as a restraint to forward slip of the L4 and L5 vertebrae

Type	Etiology	Description
I	Dysplastic/congenital	Congenital anomaly of the sacrum or posterior arch of L5
II	Isthmic	Lesion of the pars interarticularis with three subtypes: *IIA*: Lytic fracture of the pars *IIB*: Elongation of the pars *IIC*: Acute fracture of the pars
III	Degenerative	Degenerative changes of the disk and facet joints
IV	Traumatic	Acute fractures aside from pars fractures
V	Pathologic	Metabolic or neoplastic bone disease
VI	Iatrogenic	Instability from aggressive decompression of the disk and/or facet joints

Table 1: Wiltse classification of spondylolisthesis

The most widely utilized classification system for the etiology of spondylolisthesis is the Wiltse classification as summarized in Table 1.[1] Congenital spondylolisthesis results from a malformation of the neural arches or facets joints of L5 or the sacrum. The neural arch can either remain intact or be disrupted or absent as when found in conjunction with spina bifida occulta. This allows for an early displacement that is typically limited to 50%. There is a 2:1 female-to-male ratio for this form of spondylolisthesis. Neurologic abnormalities are more common with this type when the neural arch remains intact.

Isthmic spondylolisthesis results from a defect in the pars interarticularis in the form of either elongation or fracture known as spondylolysis. The facet joints remain normal in this group. Fewer than 20% of patients with spondylolysis progress to symptomatic spondylolisthesis. There is a 2:1 male-to-female ratio, and it is most commonly found at the L5-S1 level. Both genetic and environmental factors are thought to contribute to the development of isthmic spondylolisthesis. It is most commonly found in Alaskan Inuits and in patients with a positive family history.

Degenerative spondylolisthesis occurs in older adults and is caused by arthritic changes in the facet joints with associated remodeling that allows for abnormal motion to occur. This group of patients frequently has associated disk disease and spinal stenosis.

Many studies have suggested a genetic predisposition for the development of spondylolisthesis. There is a strong familial association with a 25–30% incidence in first- or second-degree relatives.[2,3] In addition to the genetic factors, biomechanical forces are believed to play a role in the development of many cases of spondylolisthesis. Excessive hyperextension forces and persistent lordosis increase the shearing forces applied to the neural arch and can lead to spondylolysis.[4,5] Spondylolysis is likely related to chronic forces across the neural arch leading to a fatigue fracture of the pars interarticularis. An acute traumatic event can complete the pars fracture and cause spondylolisthesis. Athletes with persistent hyperextension are more likely to develop spondylolisthesis including football linemen, dancers, divers, gymnasts, rowers and wrestlers. Persistent lumbar lordosis as seen in patients with coexisting Scheuermann kyphosis have also been reported to have up to a 50% prevalence of spondylolysis.[6]

PATIENT PRESENTATION

Spondylolysis can be discovered either incidentally or as a result of complaints of back pain. In most cases, the pain is isolated to the lower back, with rare cases of pain radiating into the buttocks or lower extremities. There is also frequently a specific traumatic event preceding the development of the lower back pain. Back pain is often exacerbated with standing and hyperextension of the lumbar spine.

Spondylolisthesis often has a similar presentation but is frequently associated with complaints of hamstring tightness. If neurologic signs are present they are most commonly found bilaterally. Pain radiating to the posterior thighs with possible extensor hallucis longus weakness are the most common neurologic findings due to involvement of the L5 nerve root. Patients with degenerative spondylolisthesis are more likely to have associated disk disease and stenosis. As a result radicular findings are more common in this patient group.

Medical history should investigate the duration and location of the patient's pain as well as any exacerbating or relieving factors. Any recent trauma or injury should be discussed. Patient and family history of any spinal disorders should be obtained.

Physical examination should include inspection of the spine for any gross deformity including scoliosis or increased thoracic kyphosis or lumbar lordosis. Additionally, any signs of spina bifida including skin dimpling or hairy patch should be identified. The spine should be palpated for areas of tenderness or step-offs. Flexibility of the spine and

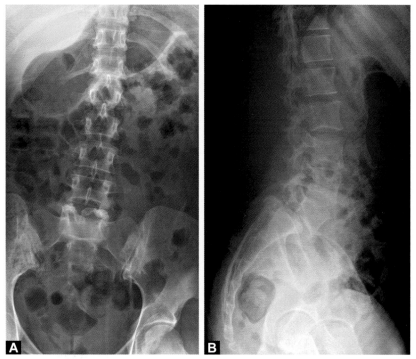

Figs 2A and B: (A) Anteroposterior (AP) and (B) lateral radiographs of a 24-year-old female showing a grade III spondylolisthesis at L5-S1. The AP image also reveals the presence of spina bifida

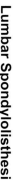

hamstrings should be assessed. A complete neurologic examination should be performed to identify any alteration in muscle strength, sensation or reflexes.

IMAGING

Radiographic evaluation of patients with spondylolisthesis begins with plain radiographs (Figs 2A and B). Standing anteroposterior (AP) and lateral radiographs are able to visualize the majority of cases of spondylolisthesis. Anteroposterior images can also identify the presence of scoliosis or spina bifida. It is important that the radiographs should be obtained during standing as in some cases the slip may partially reduce when in the supine position. As a result computed tomography (CT) or magnetic resonance imaging (MRI) scans might not fully visualize the extent of the spondylolisthesis. Dynamic lateral flexion/extension radiographs are used to identify cases of abnormal motion from instability. Oblique radiographs have been used to identify cases of spondylolysis with a classic presentation of the Scottie dog where the collar around the dog's neck is the location of the defect in the pars interarticularis (Fig. 3). The oblique radiographs have been shown to significantly increase the radiation exposure to the patient as well as the associated cost with minimal benefits.[7] As a result they are no longer ordered on a routine basis.

The degree of spondylolisthesis is most commonly classified according to the Meyerding classification system based on the percentage of forward slip visualized on the lateral radiograph (Table 2). Figure 4 illustrates this grading system.

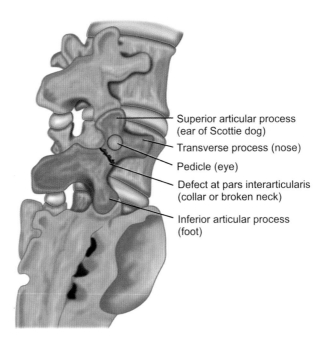

Fig. 3: Diagram of the image seen on an oblique radiograph showing the Scottie dog where the collar is located at the site of a potential fracture of the pars interarticularis

| Table 2: Meyerding classification of spondylolisthesis ||
Grade	Percentage of slip
0	Spondylolysis
I	0–25%
II	25–50%
III	50–75%
IV	75–100%
V	Spondyloptosis

There are several other radiographic measurements that can be obtained from the lateral image that can be used in the assessment of spondylolisthesis including pelvic tilt, pelvic incidence and sacral slope.[8] These measurements are used to assess the sagittal alignment of the pelvis and spine. Pelvic tilt refers to the angle between the line joining the midpoint of the sacral endplate and the axis of the femoral head with a vertical reference line (Fig. 5). Pelvic tilt is closely related to sagittal plane balance. Pelvic incidence refers to the angle between a line joining the midpoint of the sacral endplate to the axis of the femoral head with a line perpendicular to the sacral endplate (Fig. 6). Pelvic incidence is a fixed parameter for each patient that is increased with high-grade spondylolisthesis. It describes the relationship between the sacral endplate and the axis of rotation of the femoral heads. Sacral slope refers to the angle between the sacral endplate and a horizontal reference line (Fig. 7). Sacral slope is used to describe pelvic orientation.

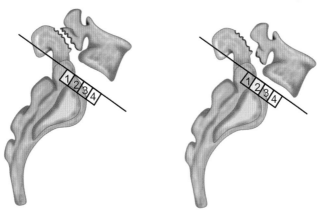

Fig. 4: Diagram of Meyerding classification of spondylolisthesis based on the degree of forward slip

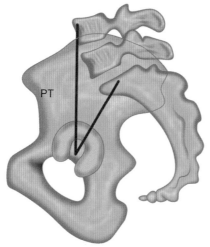

Fig. 5: Diagram showing the measurement of pelvic tilt, which is the angle between the line joining the midpoint of the sacral endplate and the axis of the femoral head with a vertical reference line

Plain radiographs are not always adequate for identifying spondylolysis. Bone scans or single photon emission computed tomography (SPECT) scans can be obtained in these patients with negative radiographs to identify stress fractures in the pars interarticularis.

Computed tomography scans can provide better visualization of the bony anatomy. This can be useful for evaluation of dysplastic facet joints or defects in the pars interarticularis. MRI is very sensitive for evaluation of stress fractures of the pars interarticularis. Increased signal intensity on the T2-weighted or fat saturation images suggest an acute fracture. MRI can also be useful in cases with neurologic findings, especially in those with degenerative spondylolisthesis associated with spinal stenosis.

NONOPERATIVE TREATMENT

Fortunately, the majority of patients with spondylolisthesis can be adequately treated with nonoperative measures. Initial treatment for acute symptoms includes activity modification

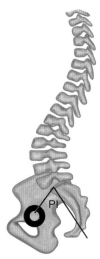

Fig. 6: Diagram showing the measurement of pelvic incidence, which is the angle between a line joining the midpoint of the sacral endplate to the axis of the femoral head with a line perpendicular to the sacral endplate

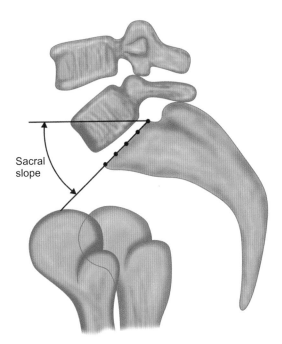

Sacral slope

Fig. 7: Diagram showing the measurement of sacral slope, which is the angle between the sacral endplate and a horizontal reference line

to avoid hyperextension forces, anti-inflammatory medications and a short period of rest. Physical therapy programs provide flexion-based exercise programs with lumbar strengthening exercises and hamstring stretching. In skeletally immature patients with an acute onset of symptoms bracing can be provided for 3–6 months to reduce lumbar lordosis and decrease the forces across the pars interarticularis. If bracing is performed early in acute fractures, the majority of unilateral fractures and 50% of bilateral fractures are reported to heal.[9] Epidural steroid injections are commonly performed in cases with radicular symptoms.

OPERATIVE TREATMENT

Indications for surgery in patients with spondylolisthesis include failed nonoperative treatment with intractable pain and the presence of progressive neurologic deficits. Various options are available for treatments that are dependent of the specific patient characteristics.

Skeletally immature patients with acute fractures that fail conservative treatment can benefit from a direct repair of the pars interarticularis. This is performed by a debridement of the fibrous tissue at the fracture site, application of bone graft material and stabilization. The stabilization can be performed with a variety of methods including a tension band wiring, single lag screw and screw-hook constructs. The benefit of these methods is that a fusion across the disk space is not necessary. Higher rates of pseudoarthrosis occur in skeletally mature patients and in patients with defects greater than 2 mm in length.[10]

Surgical intervention is often recommended for skeletally immature patients with grade III or more spondylolisthesis due to the high risk of further slip. Surgery is also recommended for grade II cases with documented progression. A posterolateral in situ fusion is most commonly performed in these patients. In many cases clinical success is achieved with surgery even in cases with radiographic evidence of pseudoarthrosis.[11] Due to the increased rates of pseudoarthrosis, bending of the fusion mass and continued progression of the slip, skeletally immature patients with a high-grade slip are typically treated with posterior instrumented fusion using pedicle screw fixation. In cases of a high-grade L5-S1 slip, the fusion construct is often extended to the L4 level to increase the fusion rates and better restore a normal lumbar lordosis (Figs 8A and B). Controversy remains over the need for reduction of the slip. Advantages include improved chances of fusion and better restoration of sagittal plane balance. Disadvantages include increased risk of neurologic injury and sacral insufficiency fractures. Free running electromyography performed during surgery can decrease the risk of iatrogenic neurologic injury.

Surgery for adults with spondylolisthesis is reserved for patients that failed conservative treatment and have continued intractable pain and those with progressive neurologic deficits. The ideal surgical treatment for these patients remains unclear. Patients with severe radicular symptoms related to degenerative spondylolisthesis can be treated with a limited decompression procedure without fusion in some cases. Caution is used to avoid further destabilization of the spine and worsening of the slip. This is often a reasonable option for the elderly patient with multiple medical comorbidities. Fusion can be performed though an anterior, posterior or combined approach, with or without instrumentation. There is no consensus on the preferred treatment at this time; however, increased complication rates have been reported in patients with higher-grade slips, degenerative spondylolisthesis and in the elderly. No differences in complication rates were found based on surgical approach or history of previous spine surgery.[12]

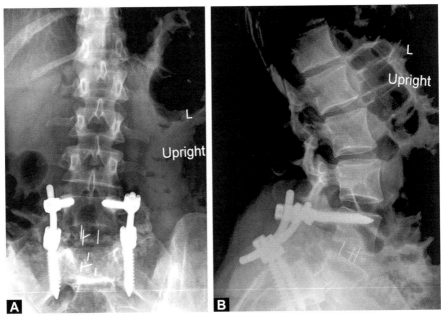

Figs 8A and B: (A) Anteroposterior (AP) and (B) lateral postoperative radiographs of patient from Figure 2 who underwent a posterior lumbar interbody fusion from L4-S1 for a high-grade L5-S1 spondylolisthesis

REFERENCES

1. Wiltse LL. Spondylolisthesis in children. Clin Orthop. 1961;21:156-63.
2. Wiltse L, Rothman S. Spondylolisthesis: Classification, diagnosis, and natural history. Semin Spine Surg. 1989;1:78-94.
3. Wiltse LL, Winter RB. Terminology and measurement of spondylolisthesis. J Bone Joint Surg Am. 1993;65:768-72.
4. Dietrich M, Kurowski P. The importance of mechanical factors in the etiology of spondylolysis. A model analysis of loads and stresses in human lumbar spine. Spine. 1985;10:532-42.
5. Schulitz KP, Niethard FU. Strain on the interarticular stress distribution. Measurements regarding the development of spondylolysis. Arch Orthop Trauma Surg. 1980;96:197-202.
6. Ogilvie JW, Sherman J. Spondylolysis in Scheuermann's disease. Spine. 1987;12:251-3.
7. Scavone JG, Latshaw RF, Weidner WA. Anteroposterior and lateral radiographs: an adequate lumbar spine examination. Am J Roentgenol. 1081;136:715-7.
8. Labelle H, Roussouly P, Bethonnaud E, et al. Spondylolisthesis, pelvic incidence, and spinopelvic balance: a correlation study. Spine. 2004;29:2049-54.
9. Sys J, Michielson J, Bracke P, et al. Nonoperative treatment of active spondylolysis in elite athletes with normal X-ray findings: literature review and results of conservative treatment. Eur Spine J. 2001;10:498-504.
10. Ivanic GM, Pink TP, Achatz W, et al. Direct stabilization of lumbar spondylolysis with a hook screw: mean 11-year follow-up period for 113 patients. Spine. 2003;28:255-9.
11. Lenke LG, Bridwell KH, Bullis D, et al. Results of in situ fusion for isthmic spondylolisthesis. J Spinal Disord. 1992;5:433-42.
12. Sansur CA, Reames DL, Smith JS, et al. Morbidity and mortality in the surgical treatment of 10,242 adults with spondylolisthesis. J Neurosurg Spine. 2010;13:589-93.

CHAPTER

12

Thoracolumbar Spine Trauma

👉 INTRODUCTION

Thoracolumbar (TL) fractures comprise a majority of all fractures in the spine reported yearly.[1,2] The mechanism and energy of injury along with the patient's bone quality play a significant role in what type of injury pattern develops. Treatment can range from observation alone to circumferential decompression and spinal reconstruction. Treatment decision making is broadly based on three main factors: (1) spinal stability, (2) neurology and (3) patient factors. Certain spinal factors such as the presence of osteoporosis and spondyloarthropathies such as ankylosing spondylitis (AS) or diffuse idiopathic skeletal hyperostosis (DISH) must also be recognized. Their presence alters the biomechanical landscape of the spine such that seemingly mild appearing injuries may behave in a more highly unstable fashion.

👉 PATHOPHYSIOLOGY

Injury classification systems serve the purpose of describing and simplifying a complex situation that has multiple variables for the purposes of communication, treatment guidance and prognostication.[3-5] The pathophysiology of TL fractures is best understood from an anatomical and mechanistic standpoint. The combination of these factors along with the resultant stability and neurologic condition form the foundation for historically accepted classification systems.

A review of the historically accepted TL injury classifications is useful. It will help provide understanding of the language that many surgeons continue to use when describing these fractures. It will provide context for understanding how different treatment modalities have evolved, and it will help the reader understand the current best language and most important factors necessary to address in the treatment of TL injury.

Boehler's original classification of TL injuries combined anatomical descriptions of the fracture together with mechanism of injury.[5] He outlined five categories of TL injuries, including (1) compression fractures, (2) flexion-distraction injuries with anterior injury secondary to compression and posterior injury secondary to distraction, (3) extension fractures with injury to the anterior and posterior longitudinal ligaments, (4) shear fractures and (5) rotational injuries.[5]

Watson-Jones described seven fracture types that fit into three general injury patterns. These included (1) simple wedge fracture, (2) comminuted fracture and (3) fracture-dislocation.[6] This system was the first to identify the posterior ligamentous complex (PLC) as a key determinant of stability in TL injuries. It was also meant to be used as a guide for treatment decision making. The Watson-Jones classification system, like so many historical TL classification systems was not validated. It was also mainly a morphologic classification system. This means that it was dedicated to describing the injury and resultant anatomical morphology.

Holdsworth left a lasting mark on TL injury classification systems with the introduction of the "column concept". Holdsworth divided the spine into two major columns: (1) the anterior column, consisting of the vertebral body and intervertebral disk, and (2) the posterior column, consisting of the facet joints and the PLC (interspinous ligament, supraspinous ligament, and ligamentum flavum).[7] Holdsworth highlighted the concept of an intact interspinous ligament and maintained that the posterior column was also important for spinal stability.[7] His classification scheme included both a mechanistic and morphologic description of fractures. He identified anterior compression fractures, fracture dislocations, rotational fracture dislocations, extension injuries, shear injuries and burst fractures. Holdsworth was the first to introduce the concept of a "burst fracture". And stated that both burst and anterior compression fractures were inherently stable given that the posterior column was intact.[7,8]

Kelly and Whitesides preserved the concept of columns but redefined the anterior column as the solid vertebral body and the posterior column as the neural arch and posterior elements. In contrast to others, they proposed that burst fractures were inherently unstable.[9] This concept would be adopted by subsequent developers of classifications such as Denis. Unfortunately the ability to assess and define traumatic spinal stability is not that simple. The authors caution against the development of dogma such as this as it has the potential to mischaracterize an otherwise stable injury based on a nonvalidated, historically popular concept, which is a morphological oversimplification. Denis refined the column concept of TL trauma by describing a middle column consisting of the posterior vertebral body, posterior longitudinal ligament (PLL) and posterior annulus (Fig. 1).[10] Denis did not define rigid parameters of stability and instability. Rather, he stratified the risk of neurologic injury based on two-column involvement and mode of failure of the middle column.[8] Denis' classic article was the first to highlight the importance of neurologic status. He did this through his concept of "degrees of instability". This proposed scale maintained that mechanical and neurologic instability could be present simultaneously or separately. Denis referred to isolated mechanical instability as an injury of the first degree. Second-degree instability involved injuries with a neurologic component but no mechanical instability, whereas third-degree injuries consisted of mechanical instability with neurologic compromise.[5,10] The Denis system was ultimately oversimplified to dictate that if two columns were injured, operative intervention was required. Long-term follow-up studies of burst fractures have demonstrated the successful nonoperative management of these two-column injuries and the classification system has been criticized for its inability to distinguish between stable and unstable burst fractures.[5,10] As an example, two burst fractures may

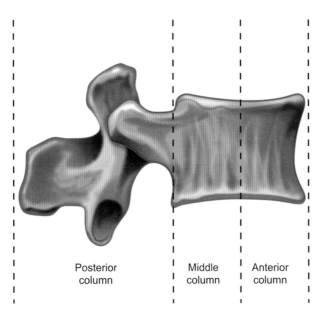

Posterior column | Middle column | Anterior column

Fig. 1: The drawing depicts the anatomic boundaries of the three-column system devised by Denis

have a similar morphology (similar fracture lines, kyphosis and loss of vertebral height), but they may manifest themselves in their characteristics of stability and neurology much differently depending on the energy of injury and bone quality. Low-energy burst fractures rarely result in neurologic deficit, whereas high-energy burst fractures are more likely to have caused bone displacement at the time of injury that can cause neurologic disruption.

Ferguson and Allen disputed the "column" concept developed by Holdsworth and Denis.[11,12] They argued that the term "column" was semantically a poor choice, as the anatomy and biomechanics of the spine did not facilitate such an analogy. They proposed a classification scheme with anterior and posterior spinal "elements", based on injury mechanism and patterns of failure.[11,12] Ferguson and Allen addressed stability using specific criteria that included mechanism of injury, risk of progressive deformity, neurologic function and patient functionality.[11,12]

By understanding both mechanistic classifications, such as those devised by Boehler or Ferguson-Allen, or the morphologic/anatomic classifications, such as those devised by Watson-Jones, Whitesides and Denis, the surgeon is able to couple the knowledge of morphology with mechanism to help define means of reduction and anatomic reconfiguration of the injury. The rationale for understanding mechanism of injury is such that the surgeon is capable of understanding the forces that both created the injury and the necessary forces, and vectors needed for reduction. Also this understanding helps guide the surgeon in choosing reconstruction methods that are needed to resist the deforming forces of injury.

It is clear that several TL fracture classification systems have been described over the years. The most recently presented TL injury classification incorporates three aspects of the patient presentation to guide treatment. The goal of the system is to unify the best understood and accepted elements of the historical classifications, and to incorporate the inherent missing elements that contribute clinical relevance to treatment decision making and prognostication. The key elements of the Thoracolumbar Injury Classification System (TLICS) include: (1) the morphology of the injury based on imaging studies, (2) the integrity of the PLC and (3) the neurologic status of the patient.[13-18] The TLICS assigns point values to each major category based on injury severity. The sum of these points represents the TLICS severity score, which may be used to guide treatment.

Injury morphology is divided into three subtypes, with increasing severity: (1) compression, (2) rotation/translation, and (3) distraction. Although these descriptors share the nomenclature of mechanistic systems, the TLICS is unique in that it defines objective radiographic findings for each injury morphology. Compression injuries are defined by a loss of height of the vertebral body or disruption through the vertebral endplate. This includes traditional compression (i.e. anterior column) and burst (i.e. anterior and middle column) fractures. Sagittal and coronal plane vertebral fractures are difficult to classify using the column descriptors. Rotation/translation injury is identified by horizontal displacement of one TL vertebral body with respect to another. It is typified by unilateral and bilateral dislocations and facet fracture-dislocations, as well as bilateral pedicle or pars fractures with vertebral subluxation.[8] Distraction is identified by anatomic dissociation in the vertical axis, such as a hyperextension injury that causes disruption of the anterior longitudinal ligament (ALL), with subsequent widening of the anterior disk space. Fractures of the posterior elements (i.e. facet, lamina, spinous process) may also be present in distraction injury. Compression injuries receive 1 point, whereas burst fractures receive 2 points. A compression fracture with a coronal plane deformity of greater than 15° is also assigned 2 points. Translational or rotational injuries, inherently more unstable than compression and burst fractures, are assigned 3 points. Distraction injuries, consisting of osseous, ligamentous or a combination of both components, are the most unstable injuries and receive 4 points.[5]

Neurologic status is described in increasing order of urgency: neurologically intact, nerve root injury, complete (motor and sensory) spinal cord or cauda equina injury, and incomplete (motor or sensory) spinal cord or cauda equina injury. In the American Spinal Injury Association (ASIA) classification, injury grades B, C and D are incomplete injuries, whereas grade A represents a complete spinal cord injury.[8] Patients with an intact neurologic examination are assigned 0 points. Patients with a nerve root injury or complete spinal cord injury are allocated 2 points. Patients with an incomplete spinal cord injury or cauda equina syndrome are assigned 3 points secondary to the potential for these patients to benefit from surgical decompression.[5]

In the TLICS, the integrity of the PLC is categorized as intact, indeterminate or disrupted. Assessment can be made based on plain radiographs, computed tomography (CT) scans and magnetic resonance images.[19] Disruption of the PLC is typically indicated by widening of the interspinous space or of the facet joints, empty facet joints, facet perch or subluxation, and dislocation of the spine. When the evidence of disruption is subtle, the integrity of the ligaments is typically defined as either suspected or indeterminate. In some cases, clinical examination may be helpful in determining the status of the PLC; an obvious gap between the spinous processes is indicative of PLC disruption.[8] An intact PLC is assigned 0 points, whereas confirmed ligamentous injury is assigned 3 points. If the condition of the PLC is indeterminate, 2 points are assigned.[5]

The TLICS allows a score to be tallied, and the sum is meant to guide operative versus nonoperative treatment decisions based on the consensus of the expert opinions of the Spine Trauma Study Group.[3-5,8,20] A sum of less than 4 points favors nonoperative treatment, 4 points is intermediate (guided by surgeon judgment) and greater than 4 points indicates consideration for surgical stabilization.

PATIENT PRESENTATION

The evaluation of the patient with suspected TL spine trauma should follow standard advanced trauma life support (ATLS) protocol. The primary survey centers around evaluating and treating issues related to the airway, breathing, circulation, neurologic deficit and exposure (full body assessment). A secondary survey covers a full musculoskeletal examination once the patient has been stabilized. During the secondary survey, a logroll allows inspection and palpation of the posterior spine. The presence of tenderness, swelling or a step deformity can be signs of disruption to the PLC. In the quadriplegic patient, the absence of tenderness will be difficult to interpret because of the loss of sensation. In all patients, with a spine fracture, noncontiguous spinal injuries need to be excluded radiographically.[21] When the main fracture is identified, the authors recommend that at least a full series of plain film X-rays should be performed as a screen for noncontiguous injuries.

The presentation and evaluation of spinal trauma follows similar themes. Much of the patient presentation for TL trauma is similar to the concepts covered in the spinal cord injury chapter. Some key factors specific to TL spine trauma will be reviewed. TL trauma resulting in pure burst fractures typically result from an axial load to the spine. The mechanism may be a fall from height in which the patient lands upon his or her feet. Therefore, a high index of suspicion should be kept to look out for patients with calcaneus fractures with this mechanism. The converse is also true. Patients who present with calcaneus fractures may have associated occult TL injury. A high index of suspicion should be maintained.

Flexion-distraction (chance) type injuries, occur when the center of rotation of the injury is anterior to the spine (i.e. rapid deceleration with lap or shoulder harness providing the fulcrum as shown in Figure 2). These injuries are often associated with small bowel contusions or retroperitoneal injuries.

As the surgeon assesses TL trauma, the account of energy, mechanism and overall health status of the patient cannot be overemphasized. The energy of an injury cannot be exactly measured, but it is often deduced based on circumstances offered by the history. Some high energy type mechanisms may include but are not limited to: industrial accidents such as logging or machining injuries, crushing injuries from heavy equipment, ejection from vehicle, vehicle rollover, major auto deformity (damage into passenger area) auto-pedestrian or auto-bicycle impact, high-speed vehicle crash (> 40 mph adult and > 20 mph child), motorcycle or all-terrain vehicle (ATV) crash, fatality in same vehicle, prolonged extrication (> 20 minutes), and fall more than 20 feet for adult and more than 10 feet for a child. These factors should be interpreted on a case by case basis with appropriate context applied. Low-energy mechanisms tend to result in injuries that are more stable in healthy individuals but can still cause very severe consequences because of the frailty of the patient (i.e. osteoporosis or a AS generates inherent weakness in the spine).

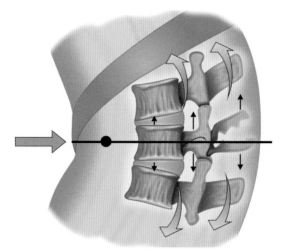

Fig. 2: The illustration depicts a mechanistic interpretation of a flexion-distraction thoracolumbar spinal injury

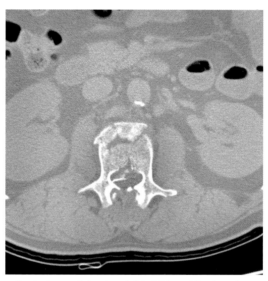

Fig. 3: Axial CT scan of a patient who sustained a stable L1 burst fracture from a motorcycle accident. The patient was able to carry his motorcycle over 50 feet from the scene of the accident. He was able to be treated without a brace with activity modification and pain medications as needed

One of the most important factors in the assessment of TL trauma is to ask the patient what they did immediately after the injury. Did they walk away? If so, how far? A patient's ability to ambulate after injury, and their demonstration of spinal load bearing is one of the best determinants of spinal injury stability. For example, the author evaluated a 42-year-old healthy man involved in a motorcycle collision. He presented with an L1 burst fracture with moderate comminution and normal neurology (Fig. 3). He reported that he carried his broken motorcycle over 50 feet after the accident. This was perhaps the best indicator of injury stability that we could have to guide treatment course. The patient was discharged from the emergency department after upright X-rays, and no brace was prescribed.

Patient factors such as age, medical comorbidities and general assessment of frailty are also key considerations in treatment planning. Assessment of preinjury function such as ambulatory status will shape a patient's and clinician's expectations for the goals of treatment.

IMAGING

When a TL fracture is suspected, X-rays are typically the first and quickest radiographic evaluation. The incidence of noncontiguous spinal fractures has been reported to range from 1.6% to 19%.[22-24] Therefore, when a spine fracture is diagnosed in one region of the spine, the authors recommend full radiographic spinal survey. This can be done with plain X-rays. The use of CT scan for trauma patients has increased dramatically over the last decade. Patients who present to trauma centers are receiving CT scans to rule out cervical spine, chest, abdomen and pelvis injuries.[25] Often, reconstruction views of the entire spine are available to assess for spinal fractures. The role for CT as a screening tool is evolving, but it is well accepted as the best method currently to assess the three-dimensional anatomy of bony spinal column injuries. When spinal fractures are identified and require surgery, the authors find CT scan useful in preoperative planning for instrumentation placement, assessing areas of canal compromise due to bone fragment retropulsion and areas of joint disruption such as facet fracture or dislocation.

Standing or weight-bearing X-rays are typically utilized in two scenarios. The first is to assess the stability of a nonoperatively treated fracture. After the fracture has been determined "stable" and acceptable for nonoperative treatment (brace or no brace), the patient should receive standing or upright X-rays. This is done to assess the alignment of the fracture and global spinal alignment prior to discharge from the hospital or clinic. Upright X-rays are also typically utilized after the patient has begun mobilizing post surgery. These X-rays are used to determine spinal alignment and instrumentation position after the patient has had a chance to "load" the spine.

The role of magnetic resonance imaging (MRI) in assessing TL trauma is evolving. It is best accepted as a method for assessing the neural elements including nerve roots and spinal cord. MRI can identify spinal cord compression, edema, contusion or hemorrhage.[19] It can also identify areas of bone edema and inflammation that may not be evident on CT scan. It is also useful in identifying epidural masses, abnormal marrow signal and pathologic fracture or bone lesions from tumor. MRI is much more sensitive than CT and plain films at identifying ligamentous and soft tissue injury. However, the reliance of MRI alone as a means of diagnosing posterior ligamentous complex injury is not as accurate as surgeons had hoped.[26-30] MRI tends to "overcall" PLC injuries in the spine, and thus this modality should be used in concert with other morphologic assessments such as CT and physical examination.[5-9]

NONOPERATIVE TREATMENT

The majority of thoracic and lumbar spine fractures can be treated nonoperatively. The reason for this is that the majority of fractures in this region are low energy, stable fractures, the most common of which include compression fractures. The vast majority of these fractures heal without any intervention. Since injury morphology is only one component of the evaluation, particular attention should be applied to assessment of neurology and patient factors. Some compression fractures are pathologic and can lead to progressive deformity and neurologic deficit. Suspicion should be maintained for tumor or bone marrow pathology despite the majority of vertebral compression fractures being a result of osteoporosis. A comprehensive review of the management of vertebral compression fractures is beyond the scope of this chapter. It should be noted that most but not all vertebral compression fractures can be treated conservatively. Of those that demonstrate persistent pain, percutaneous vertebroplasty or kyphoplasty can offer significant relief.[31] Other minor injuries to the TL spine include transverse process fractures, isolated spinous process and isolated facet fractures without subluxation or malalignment. A healthy dose of caution and skepticism should always be exercised when the surgeon encounters these injuries so as not to miss a potentially unstable injury. Upright and delayed flexion extension X-rays can be helpful if questions about stability persist. However, most of these injuries only require symptomatic treatment.

Wood et al. performed a well-designed randomized controlled trial to compare operative and nonoperative treatment of TL burst fractures without neurologic deficit.[2] Their rationale for the study was that there was an ongoing lack of consensus amongst surgeons as to the optimum management of these injuries. Their original hypothesis was that operative treatment would lead to superior long-term clinical outcomes. Patients were randomized to one of two treatment groups: operative (posterior or anterior arthrodesis and instrumentation) or nonoperative treatment (application of a body cast or orthosis). Radiographs and CT scans were analyzed for sagittal alignment and canal compromise. All patients completed a questionnaire to assess any disability they may have had before the injury, and they indicated the degree of pain at the time of presentation with use of a visual analog scale. At the conclusion of the study no significant differences could be identified between operative and nonoperative groups for radiographic parameters such as canal compromise and kyphosis or for clinical parameters such as patient's reported pain, function and work status.[2] They concluded that operative treatment of patients with a stable TL burst fracture and normal findings on the neurological examination provided no major long-term advantage compared with nonoperative treatment.[2]

Bailey et al. sought to answer the question of whether orthosis treatment makes a difference in the clinical outcomes of neurologically intact patients with stable burst fractures.[32] The study was designed as a multicenter prospective randomized clinical equivalence trial. The primary outcome measure was the score based on the Roland-Morris Disability Questionnaire assessed at 3 months post injury. Sixty-nine patients were followed to the primary outcome time point, and 47 were followed for up to 1 year. No significant difference was found between treatment groups for any outcome measure at any stage in the follow-up period. Bailey et al. demonstrated equivalence between treatment with a thoracolumbosacral orthosis (TLSO) and no orthosis for thoracolumbar AO type A3 burst fractures. The authors contend that a TL burst fracture, in exclusion of an associated PLC injury, is inherently a very stable injury and may not require a brace.[32]

A subset of flexion-distraction ("chance" type) injuries can also be treated nonoperatively. The flexion-distraction mechanism generates a failure in tension from posterior to anterior. Any combination of bone, PLC and disk can be affected and various amounts of displacement or fracture comminution may result. The patient should be neurologically intact in order to consider nonoperative treatment. An attempt can be made to treat nonoperatively for injuries that involve primarily bone and have not caused severe kyphosis, or are reduced by postural mechanisms (bracing or hyperextension maneuvers). Any number of braces can be chosen. Typically an extension force is recreated with the brace to counteract the mechanism of injury. "Clam shell" type custom molded TLSO, casting and Jewett braces have all been used. Operative treatment is more apt to be considered in cases with neurologic injury, dislocation of facet joints and in injuries that affect mostly discoligamentous structures. Also operative treatment is recommended when there is excessive widening of the posterior elements for which a reduction cannot be achieved and in cases where anterior support has been disrupted by shearing or compression to the point that mechanical instability is present.

In the case of primary discoligamentous injuries (without much or any bone injury to heal) flexion-distraction injuries are less likely to heal in a stable configuration and thus operative treatment is favored.

☞ OPERATIVE TREATMENT

The factors outlined in the TLICS classification (injury morphology, patient neurology and integrity of the PLC) are key factors in helping the surgeon determine the role for surgical treatment. They are not the only parameters. Special consideration should be given to any patient who exhibits signs of inflammatory spondyloarthropathy that generate increased rigidity of the spine, such as DISH or AS. These spinal diagnoses should be considered "wild cards" in the assessment of operative necessity. Typically benign appearing injuries tend to be mechanically unstable due to the enormous biomechanical lever arms presented. Patients with AS are also known to have bone that is quite frail and may have a propensity to developing epidural hematoma. Therefore these factors should be anticipated.[33]

"Patient factors" hold the ultimate "veto power" in the assessment of surgical necessity. No matter what classification system is utilized to assess spinal stability, the patient's survival prognosis, medical comorbidities, preoperative clinical function and potential to generate adverse events operatively must all be taken into account as the ultimate determinants.

The surgical management of TL injuries has evolved substantially over the past three decades, aided by an increased understanding of spinal biomechanics, improved methods of imaging and classification, and an expansive growth of spinal instrumentation technology. The key components to treating TL injuries include achieving or maintaining stability of the injured region and decompressing compromised neural elements when applicable. The TLICS (along with appropriate consideration of patient and intrinsic spinal factors) aids the surgeon in determining when to operate.[3,4,8] Typically patients that score 5 or greater should be given a strong consideration for surgery due to a combination of problems associated with spinal malalignment, neurologic injury and disruption to the PLC. Various techniques are available to employ to decompress and reconstruct the spine.

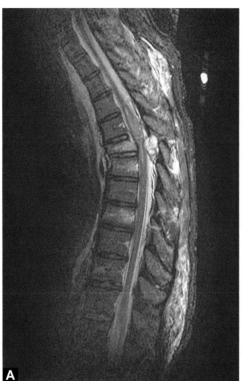 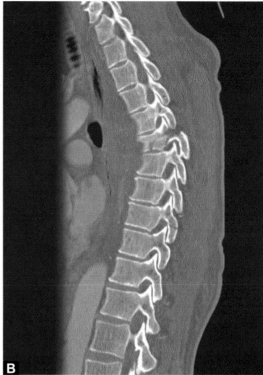

Figs 4A and B: The images are from a 25-year-old male involved in a high speed motorcycle accident. He sustained a T6-T7 fracture dislocation and T9 bony flexion-distraction type injury with T6 American Spinal Injury Association (ASIA) impairment scale A neurologic injury. (A) Sagittal MRI demonstrating spinal cord compression with posterior hematoma and posterior ligamentous complex injury; (B) Sagittal CT demonstrating T6-T7 level facet fracture-dislocation with nondisplaced T9 inferior articular process fracture

Posterior Instrumentation

The utilization of posterior pedicle screw instrumentation remains the mainstay of modern day TL fracture fixation. By virtue of their translational, rotational or kyphotic malalignment, TL fractures (especially those with dislocations as illustrated in Figures 4A and B) are, generally speaking, best treated with posterior pedicle screw instrumentation.[18] The forces necessary to generate anatomic realignment of kyphosis, translation and dislocations are best generated by current posterior instrumentation systems. The ability to correct severe translation or rotational malalignment is difficult (if not impossible in some cases) from the anterior approach alone. Biomechanically, the posterior pedicle screw instrumentation is better able to resist shear and rotational forces at play in these injuries, and it allows reconstruction of the posterior tension band.[18] For some injuries without anterior comminution, such as flexion-distraction (chance type), posterior instrumentation is ideally suited for restoring the posterior tension band.

Posterior instrumentation has also demonstrated the ability through indirect methods of distraction to generate ventral decompression of the thecal sac as long as the PLL is intact.[18,34,35] This technique can reduce canal compromise by as much as 50% but is typically capable of about 20% canal compromise clearance.[36-38] The danger in doing this relates to the kyphosis that can be induced with distraction and the potential for failing to decompress the neural elements with an incomplete reduction.

Patients with complete thoracic spinal cord injury with little chance of recovery may also benefit from posterior instrumentation and fusion for immediate stabilization, maintenance of alignment and to aid in nursing care.[18] An all posterior approach in the polytrauma patient also is beneficial in that it avoids violation of the intrathoracic or intra-abdominal space which may be injured in the polytrauma patient.[18]

There are few specific contraindications to posterior instrumentation in TL fractures. For pure burst fractures, where the PLC is intact, one could argue that in these cases, there is little reason to approach the spine posteriorly and potentially disrupt it. However, there may be reasons in such cases to avoid an anterior approach. In general, stabilization achieved with posterior fixation allows for immediate patient mobilization, the benefits of which are obvious in a polytrauma setting. Physiologic instability and the inability to ventilate while in the prone position may make it difficult to technically perform the surgery, however. Indirect reduction and posterior stabilization of burst fractures may be more difficult after 72 hours post injury.[36,39] This appears to happen because the mobility of the structures (i.e. bony fragments disks and ligamentous structures) become less mobile over time in the early phases of fracture healing. Indirect reduction techniques also tend to be less successful in patients with greater than 67% canal compromise.[40]

The obvious advantage of the posterior approach is its familiarity to all spine surgeons, the relative ease at placing pedicle screw instrumentation, and the biomechanical strength of posterior pedicle screw constructs. It avoids potential injury to intra-abdominal or retroperitoneal structures that are at risk during anterior exposures, and the potential morbidity of performing a thoracotomy and/or taking down the diaphragm to access injuries at the TL junction.

The main disadvantage to the posterior approach in TL burst fracture management is in the potential for failing to adequately decompress the neural elements when depending on ligamentotaxis and indirect reduction of the burst fragment. Direct visualization of the burst fragment and its removal is not possible with this technique unless a posterolateral or transpedicular approach is employed. If a surgeon is employing a posterolateral or transpedicular approach he/she may consider adding anterior column support due to the possible need to perform facetectomy and further destabilize the spine. Whether the addition of levels in a posterior construct is worse than the morbidity of a thoracoabdominal approach and take-down of the diaphragm to perform a shorter segment anterior construct is unknown.

The ultimate goal of instrumenting the spine is to create immediate stability to facilitate fracture healing and bony fusion. It has been traditionally taught that it is also necessary to perform a fusion in addition to instrumentation for proper healing. If proper stability is achieved, bone grafting and fusion may not be necessary in properly selected cases. Dai et al. compared fusion versus nonfusion in patients with a Denis type-B burst fracture involving the TL spine and a load-sharing score of less than or equal to 6[41,42] that were managed with posterior pedicle screw instrumentation. They found that radiographic and clinical parameters were not different between groups.[41] However, if there is concern that healing may be compromised, and there is advanced comminution then fusion should also be added. Injuries that are purely or mostly discoligamentous in nature should be fused because of the inability for these structures to heal with their original integrity.

There are multiple options to enhance bony fusion. Local bone from laminectomy or facet osteotomy can also be used in the fusion bed. Iliac crest autograft, harvested from the posterior ileum is the gold standard for posterior spinal fusion in the setting of trauma. However, the morbidity of harvesting iliac crest autograft has been well established,[43,44] and thus alternative synthetic biologic products are currently on the market such as recombinant human bone morphogenetic protein (BMP) variants that may also be useful alternatives or adjuncts to autograft. It should be noted that the efficacy and safety of these products have yet to fully be determined in TL trauma.

Special Considerations

When lamina fractures occur in conjunction with burst fractures or fracture dislocations, the possibility of dural tears or entrapped nerve roots must be addressed.[45-47] A lamina fracture in a comminuted burst fracture can be a sentinel sign for dural laceration. In the case of neurologic injury (especially in the cauda equina region), nerve root entrapment is a possible source of ongoing neurologic compression. The posterior approach allows access to decompression and dural repair in this case. Most cases benefit from direct dural repair with a water tight closure. But this is not always possible with complex tears or those that are ventral. In this case, biologic patches and fibrin glue may help achieve a good seal. A distal lumbar drain is always an option for persistent cerebrospinal fluid leak. Figures 5A to E present a case of a 45-year-old male who was involved in a high-speed motor vehicle crash while intoxicated. He suffered a T6-T7 fracture dislocation, T6 ASIA impairment scale A neurologic injury. He was surgically fixed with posterior pedicle screw instrumentation. Intraoperatively he was found to have a transected spinal cord. Facetectomies and a spinal shortening osteotomy were done to achieve bony apposition. The spinal cord and dura were beyond repair. A water tight fascial and skin closure was performed, and the patient healed uneventfully. Four months postoperatively he was found to have a fluctuance in the subcutaneous space deep to his incision. He was otherwise asymptomatic. He was diagnosed with pseudomeningocele, and it was resolved with no intervention after 3 months. This finding was initially worked up at an outside hospital for infection by imaging, laboratories and aspiration which were all found to be negative. His MRI reveals classic noncontrast enhancing high T2 signal subcutaneous fluid collection contiguous with the epidural space.

It has been discussed earlier that the incidence of noncontiguous spinal fractures is upward of 20%.[48,49] Severe, devastating injuries can often be distracting to the surgeon upon initial evaluation. They may be a point of distraction away from more subtle noncontiguous injuries. Figures 6A to D demonstrate an example of a 36-year-old male involved in a logging accident. He suffered a complete neurologic injury as a result of fractures at T7, T8 and T9. A much more subtle appearing T4 vertebral body fracture was also identified. Intraoperatively, it was found that he had severe ligamentous disruption up to the T4 level. Surgical fixation was extended above this level.

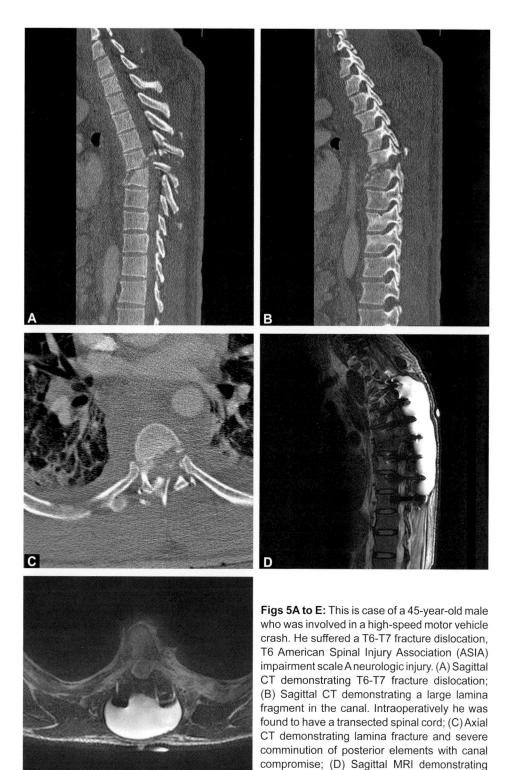

Figs 5A to E: This is case of a 45-year-old male who was involved in a high-speed motor vehicle crash. He suffered a T6-T7 fracture dislocation, T6 American Spinal Injury Association (ASIA) impairment scale A neurologic injury. (A) Sagittal CT demonstrating T6-T7 fracture dislocation; (B) Sagittal CT demonstrating a large lamina fragment in the canal. Intraoperatively he was found to have a transected spinal cord; (C) Axial CT demonstrating lamina fracture and severe comminution of posterior elements with canal compromise; (D) Sagittal MRI demonstrating classic findings of large pseudomeningocele; (E) Axial MRI of pseudomeningocele

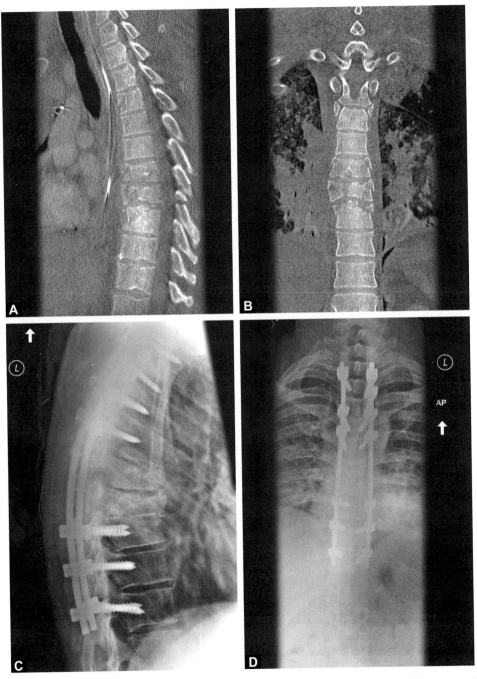

Figs 6A to D: A 36-year-old male involved in a logging accident; T7 American Spinal Injury Association (ASIA) impairment scale A. (A) Sagittal CT illustrating fractures at T7, T8 and T9 as well as a much more subtle appearing T4 vertebral body fracture; (B) Coronal CT; (C) Postoperative imaging of fracture fixation T3-T11 pedicle screw construct. Bony union of fractures is identified; (D) Anteroposterior postoperative X-ray

Pedicle screw complications can occur by malposition or mechanical failure. The incidence of iatrogenic neurologic deficit with the use of pedicle screw instrumentation is reported to be about 1%. This may occur as a result of misplaced screws or because of manipulation of the spinal cord or roots.[50] Visceral or vascular structures are at risk during pedicle screw insertion if screws are inserted too laterally or anteriorly.[18] Screw pullout of pedicle fracture may occur intraoperatively (early failure) or postoperatively (late failure), especially when the patient has osteopenia or osteoporosis. It has been shown in multiple studies that resistance to loosening and pull-out of pedicle screws is directly related to bone mineral density.[51]

Anterior Spinal Reconstruction

It can no longer be said that if there is bony compromise of the canal from retropulsed vertebral fragments, with neurologic injury, that the TL spine must be approached from anterior. The anterior spine (a zone consisting of the elements from the ALL to PLL) can be accessed from a variety of approaches (anterior, posterior AKA "posterolateral" or "extracavitary", direct lateral or a combination). There are benefits and risks of each approach. Patients with incomplete fracture reduction after a posterior approach may be candidates for anterior decompression if neurologic recovery is incomplete, and residual compression persists. However, no single approach has been found to be superior with respect to generating neurologic recovery. Each approach has its own technical nuances, but all of them can accomplish the job of direct neurologic decompression and stabilization of the anterior spine.[52]

The typical anterior approaches to the spine involve either transthoracic or retroperitoneal exposures. Each of these approaches allows access to the anterior and middle columns of the spine to the ventral spinal canal. They afford access to decompress the ventral spinal cord and dura, and allow the surgeon to reconstruct a comminuted vertebral body. Various reconstructive materials are available to gain immediate stability including structural autograft, allograft, fixed and expandable titanium cages and polyetheretherketone (PEEK) cages. Implant types commonly used anteriorly for fracture indications include rigid and nonrigid plate and screw, and rod constructs. Most studies report the use of either rigid screw and rod constructs or rigid plate constructs. Semi-rigid or dynamized constructs using screws and rods have been reported with satisfactory outcomes. Implants should be placed laterally to avoid contact with the aorta because such contact has been reported to cause late vascular disruption and death. In addition, to avoid problems with the iliac vessels, anterior plate-and-screw or rod-and-screw constructs should not be used below L4.[52]

Relative contraindications to the anterior (retroperitoneal or transthoracic/transpleural) approach include chest or abdominal injuries or pre-existing pulmonary pathology. The anterior approach is more difficult for low lumbar fractures (i.e. L4 and L5) because of anatomic constraints, especially for restoring alignment and attaining satisfactory fixation. However, these injuries rarely require surgery and generally should be managed posteriorly in patients in whom stabilization is required. Because of the large ratio of canal to neural element area, low lumbar fractures behave differently from upper lumbar fractures, and generally do well with nonsurgical management, except in cases of instability.

Anterior decompression is rarely used alone for injuries other than burst fractures. Most other fracture types are either well treated nonsurgically (i.e. compression fractures) or managed with a posterior approach to restore the integrity of the posterior elements and prevent kyphosis (i.e. flexion-distraction injuries). In certain limited circumstances, these injuries may require an adjunctive anterior decompression because of herniated disk, marked comminution of the middle column, or concern about additional displacement of fragments into the canal.[52]

The authors have found the posterolateral or extracavitary approaches to be highly useful for the purposes of both neurologic decompression and anterior reconstruction. Most thoracic fractures do not require anterior reconstruction. Typically enough stability can be obtained with posterior instrumentation, and the comminuted vertebral bone has excellent healing potential. In the cases where neurologic decompression is necessary costotransversectomy or transpedicular approaches can be taken to remove or ventrally redirect dorsally displaced bone fragments. This approach allows direct visualization and nearly 360° control of the neural elements throughout the operation. By staying "extrapleural" this approach avoids the morbidity of a chest tube. Likewise in the lumbar region avoiding a separate anterior exposure decreases the risk of ileus and other associated morbidity. In the thoracic spine, nerve roots can be sacrificed if necessary to insert anterior inter-body reconstruction devices. In the lumbar region, sacrifice of nerve roots is undesirable. The authors prefer the use of expandable cages in this case (Figs 7A to D) or utilization of the direct lateral or anterior (retroperitoneal) approaches in such cases.[53]

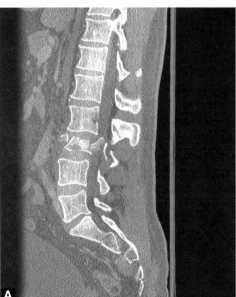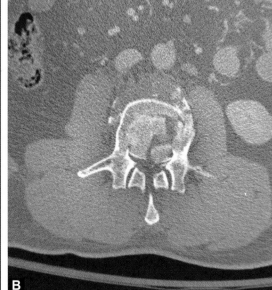

Figs 7A and B

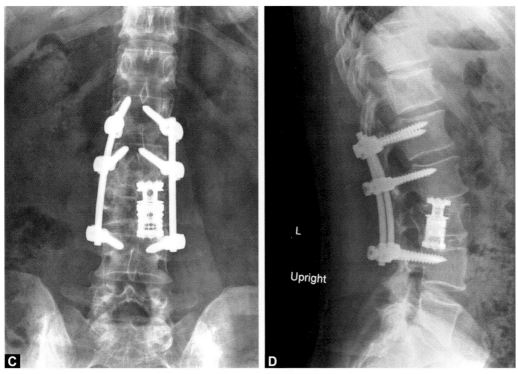

Figs 7A to D: A 36-year-old male was involved in a snowmobile accident and suffered an L3 burst fracture. He sustained a unilateral neurologic injury with incomplete motor and sensory deficit to his left leg. He had bilateral leg pain (left > right). (A) Sagittal CT; (B) Axial CT; (C) A 4-month postoperative anteroposterior and (D) lateral X-ray demonstrating healing of the fracture and fusion

☞ REFERENCES

1. Gertzbein SD. Scoliosis Research Society. Multicenter spine fracture study. Spine (Phila Pa 1976). 1992;17:528-40.
2. Wood K, Buttermann G, Mehbod A, Garvey T, et al. Operative compared with nonoperative treatment of a thoracolumbar burst fracture without neurological deficit. A prospective, randomized study. J Bone Joint Surg Am. 2003;85-A:773-81.
3. Patel AA, Dailey A, Brodke DS, et al. Thoracolumbar spine trauma classification: the Thoracolumbar Injury Classification and Severity Score system and case examples. J Neurosurg Spine. 2009;10:201-6.
4. Patel AA, Hurlbert RJ, Bono CM, et al. Classification and surgical decision making in acute subaxial cervical spine trauma. Spine (Phila Pa 1976). 2010;35:S228-34.
5. Sethi MK, Schoenfeld AJ, Bono CM, et al. The evolution of thoracolumbar injury classification systems. Spine J. 2009;9:780-8.
6. Watson-Jones. The results of postural reduction of fractures of the spine. J Bone Joint Surg Am. 1938;20:567-86.
7. Holdsworth F. Fractures, dislocations, and fracture-dislocations of the spine. J Bone Joint Surg Am. 1970;52:1534-51.
8. Patel AA, Vaccaro AR. Thoracolumbar spine trauma classification. J Am Acad Orthop Surg. 2010;18:63-71.

9. Kelly RP, Whitesides TE Jr. Treatment of lumbodorsal fracture-dislocations. Ann Surg. 1968;167:705-17.

10. Denis F. The three column spine and its significance in the classification of acute thoracolumbar spinal injuries. Spine (Phila Pa 1976). 1983;8:817-31.

11. Allen BL Jr, Ferguson RL, Lehmann TR, et al. A mechanistic classification of closed, indirect fractures and dislocations of the lower cervical spine. Spine (Phila Pa 1976). 1982;7:1-27.

12. Ferguson RL, Allen BL Jr. A mechanistic classification of thoracolumbar spine fractures. Clin Orthop Relat Res. 1984;77-88.

13. Vaccaro AR, Baron EM, Sanfilippo J, et al. Reliability of a novel classification system for thoracolumbar injuries: the Thoracolumbar Injury Severity Score. Spine. 2006;31:S62-9.

14. Vaccaro AR, Kim DH, Brodke DS, et al. Diagnosis and management of thoracolumbar spine fractures. Instr Course Lect. 2004;53:359-73.

15. Vaccaro AR, Lee JY, Schweitzer KM Jr, et al. Assessment of injury to the posterior ligamentous complex in thoracolumbar spine trauma. Spine J. 2006;6:524-8.

16. Vaccaro AR, Lehman RA Jr, Hurlbert RJ, et al. A new classification of thoracolumbar injuries: the importance of injury morphology, the integrity of the posterior ligamentous complex, and neurologic status. Spine. 2005;30:2325-33.

17. Shah RV, Albert TJ, Bruegel-Sanchez V, et al. Industry support and correlation to study outcome for papers published in Spine. Spine. 2005;30:1099-104.

18. Whang PG, Vaccaro AR. Thoracolumbar fracture: posterior instrumentation using distraction and ligamentotaxis reduction. J Am Acad Orthop Surg. 2007;15:695-701.

19. Bozzo A, Goulet B, Marcoux J, et al. The role of magnetic resonance imaging in the management of acute spinal cord injury. J Neurotrauma. 2011;28:1401-11.

20. Vaccaro AR, Lim MR, Hurlbert RJ, et al. Surgical decision making for unstable thoracolumbar spine injuries: results of a consensus panel review by the Spine Trauma Study Group. J Spinal Disord Tech. 2006;19:1-10.

21. Schouten R, Albert T, Kwon BK. The spine-injured patient: initial assessment and emergency treatment. J Am Acad Orthop Surg. 2012;20:336-46.

22. Henderson RL, Reid DC, Saboe LA. Multiple noncontiguous spine fractures. Spine (Phila Pa 1976). 1991;16:128-31.

23. Miller CP, Brubacher JW, Biswas D, et al. The incidence of noncontiguous spinal fractures and other traumatic injuries associated with cervical spine fractures: a 10-year experience at an academic medical center. Spine (Phila Pa 1976). 2011;36:1532-40.

24. Wittenberg RH, Hargus S, Steffen R, et al. Noncontiguous unstable spine fractures. Spine (Phila Pa 1976). 2002;27:254-7.

25. Fisher CG, Noonan VK, Dvorak MF. Changing face of spine trauma care in North America. Spine (Phila Pa 1976). 2006;31:S2-8.

26. Dekutoski MB, Hayes ML, Utter AP, et al. Pathologic correlation of posterior ligamentous injury with MRI. Orthopedics. 2010;33:53.

27. Rihn JA, Anderson DT, Sasso RC, et al. Emergency evaluation, imaging, and classification of thoracolumbar injuries. Instr Course Lect. 2009;58:619-28.

28. Rihn JA, Fisher C, Harrop J, et al. Assessment of the posterior ligamentous complex following acute cervical spine trauma. J Bone Joint Surg Am. 2010;92:583-9.

29. Rihn JA, Yang N, Fisher C, et al. Using magnetic resonance imaging to accurately assess injury to the posterior ligamentous complex of the spine: a prospective comparison of the surgeon and radiologist. J Neurosurg Spine. 2010;12:391-6.

30. Vaccaro AR, Rihn JA, Saravanja D, et al. Injury of the posterior ligamentous complex of the thoracolumbar spine: a prospective evaluation of the diagnostic accuracy of magnetic resonance imaging. Spine (Phila Pa 1976). 2009;34:E841-7.

31. Klazen CA, Lohle PN, de Vries J, et al. Vertebroplasty versus conservative treatment in acute osteoporotic vertebral compression fractures (Vertos II): an open-label randomised trial. Lancet. 2010;376:1085-92.

32. Bailey CS, Dvorak MF, Thomas KC, et al. Comparison of thoracolumbosacral orthosis and no orthosis for the treatment of thoracolumbar burst fractures: interim analysis of a multicenter randomized clinical equivalence trial. J Neurosurg Spine. 2009;11:295-303.

33. Caron T, Bransford R, Nguyen Q, et al. Spine fractures in patients with ankylosing spinal disorders. Spine (Phila Pa 1976). 2010;35:E458-64.

34. Aebi M. Thalgott JS, Webb JK. AO ASIF Principles in Spine Surgery. New York: Springer; 1998.

35. Chang KW. A reduction-fixation system for unstable thoracolumbar burst fractures. Spine. 1992;17:879-86.

36. Crutcher JP Jr, Anderson PA, King HA, et al. Indirect spinal canal decompression in patients with thoracolumbar burst fractures treated by posterior distraction rods. J Spinal Disord. 1991;4:39-48.

37. Harrington RM, Budorick T, Hoyt J, et al. Biomechanics of indirect reduction of bone retropulsed into the spinal canal in vertebral fracture. Spine. 1993;18:692-9.

38. Sjostrom L, Karlstrom G, Pech P, et al. Indirect spinal canal decompression in burst fractures treated with pedicle screw instrumentation. Spine. 1996;21:113-23.

39. Willen J, Lindahl S, Irstam L, et al. Unstable thoracolumbar fractures. A study by CT and conventional roentgenology of the reduction effect of Harrington instrumentation. Spine. 1984;9:214-9.

40. Gertzbein SD, Crowe PJ, Fazl M, et al. Canal clearance in burst fractures using the AO internal fixator. Spine. 1992;17:558-60.

41. Dai LY, Jiang LS, Jiang SD. Posterior short-segment fixation with or without fusion for thoracolumbar burst fractures. a five to seven-year prospective randomized study. J Bone Joint Surg Am. 2009;91:1033-41.

42. Parker JW, Lane JR, Karaikovic EE, et al. Successful short-segment instrumentation and fusion for thoracolumbar spine fractures: a consecutive 41/2-year series. Spine (Phila Pa 1976). 2000;25:1157-70.

43. Arrington ED, Smith WJ, Chambers HG, et al. Complications of iliac crest bone graft harvesting. Clin Orthop Relat Res. 1996:300-9.

44. Goulet JA, Senunas LE, DeSilva GL, et al. Autogenous iliac crest bone graft. Complications and functional assessment. Clin Orthop Relat Res. 1997:76-81.

45. Aydinli U, Karaeminogullari O, Tiskaya K, et al. Dural tears in lumbar burst fractures with greenstick lamina fractures. Spine. 2001;26:E410-5.

46. Denis F, Burkus JK. Diagnosis and treatment of cauda equina entrapment in the vertical lamina fracture of lumbar burst fractures. Spine. 1991;16:S433-9.

47. Wing P, Aebi M, Denis F, et al. Management of an unstable lumbar fracture with a laminar split. Spinal Cord. 1999;37:392-401.

48. Korres DS, Boscainos PJ, Papagelopoulos PJ, et al. Multiple level noncontiguous fractures of the spine. Clin Orthop Relat Res. 2003;31:95-102.

49. Shear P, Hugenholtz H, Richard MT, et al. Multiple noncontiguous fractures of the cervical spine. J Trauma. 1988;28:655-9.

50. Katonis P, Christoforakis J, Kontakis G, et al. Complications and problems related to pedicle screw fixation of the spine. Clin Orthop Relat Res. 2003:86-94.

51. Halvorson TL, Kelley LA, Thomas KA, et al. Effects of bone mineral density on pedicle screw fixation. Spine (Phila Pa 1976). 1994;19:2415-20.

52. Kirkpatrick JS. Thoracolumbar fracture management: anterior approach. J Am Acad Orthop Surg. 2003;11:355-63.

53. Eck JC. Minimally invasive corpectomy and posterior stabilization for lumbar burst fracture. Spine J. 2011;11:904-8.

CHAPTER

13

Adolescent
Idiopathic Scoliosis

🔹 INTRODUCTION

Adolescent idiopathic scoliosis (AIS) is the most common form of spinal deformity accounting for 80% of all scoliosis cases. Idiopathic scoliosis can be divided into categories based on the age of onset. The infantile group occurs from birth to less than 3 years, juvenile scoliosis occurs from 3 years to less than 10 years, and AIS first develops in patients from 10 years of age up to less than 18 years of age. AIS is by far the most common of these groups and is the topic of this chapter.

In order to make the diagnosis of scoliosis, a coronal plane Cobb angle of at least 10° is necessary. The prevalence of scoliosis among adolescents is reported to be less than 3%, and approximately 5% of those progress to greater than 30° in magnitude.[1] The prevalence of scoliosis is similar among boys and girls, but girls frequently have more progressive curves that require treatment.[2]

The purpose of this chapter is to provide the reader with a better understanding of the pathophysiology of AIS as well as the clinical evaluation and operative and nonoperative treatment options.

🔹 PATHOPHYSIOLOGY

Unfortunately, despite many recent advances in the diagnosis and treatment of AIS, the underlying etiology remains uncertain. It is generally agreed upon that AIS is a multifactorial disorder that is influenced by various factors including genetics, the nervous system, hormonal factors and metabolic dysfunction, skeletal growth, biomechanical factors and environmental factors.

Much of the initial research on genetic factors related to AIS came from twin studies. Kesling and Reinker performed a meta-analysis of the literature comparing the concordance of AIS in monozygotic versus dizygotic twins.[3] They reported that the concordance among monozygotic twins was 73% versus 36% among dizygotic twins (p < 0.003).

Despite good evidence for a familial cause of scoliosis, there is still debate over the specific genetic mechanism involved with AIS. Previous investigators have suggested various inheritance patterns including autosomal dominance, X-linked, or multifactorial.[4]

Table 1: Summary of hormonal and metabolic abnormalities more commonly seen with adolescent idiopathic scoliosis (AIS)
Elevated levels of growth hormone between 7 years and 12 years of age
Low levels of estrogen
Low levels of melatonin in progressive AIS
Impaired melatonin-signaling transduction in osteoblasts, myoblasts and lymphocytes
Elevated levels of osteopontin
Increased levels of calmodulin in platelets with progressive AIS
Osteopenia
Low levels of leptin

Axenovich et al. performed a segregation analysis to help clarify the genetic model while studying families with AIS and suggested that it was the result of a single autosomal dominant locus (p < 0.001).[5]

Advances in genetic testing methods have allowed for the development of prognostic genetic testing. The AIS prognostic test (AIS-PT), also known as ScoliScore (DePuy Spine, Raynham, MA) has been previously validated and certified for use in white patients with AIS over 10 years of age.[6] This is a saliva-based genetic test that provides a score for the risk of progression between 0 and 200. Patients with scores below 50 have less than 1% risk of progression of their curve to a severe range if left untreated. Patients with scores above 180 have a high risk of progression and are often recommended for surgical intervention. Patients in the intermediate range between 51 and 179 have a risk of progression and are recommended for close monitoring with possible treatment.

Many researchers have reported on potential abnormalities of the central nervous system that could contribute to AIS. These have included hindbrain problems with syrinx, low-lying cerebellar tonsils, postural and dynamic balance problems, asymmetry of the paraspinous musculature, and disharmony expressed in the spine between the autonomic and somatic nervous system. This research remains relatively limited and inconclusive at this time.

Various hormonal and metabolic abnormalities have been reported in patients with AIS as summarized in Table 1. Many of these abnormalities are still being actively investigated in an attempt to correlate their effects on patients with AIS.

Additionally, various skeletal growth abnormalities have been reported to be more common in patients with AIS. These include an association between skeletal growth velocity and curve progression.[7] Others have suggested that AIS progression is not the result of growth velocity but instead related to a rapid enlargement of the skeletal size exceeding the capacity of postural mechanisms to control an initiating deformity.[8] While many studies have reported patients with AIS to be taller than age-matched controls, Cheung et al. reported girls with AIS to be shorter prior to menarche but to become taller with longer arm span during their growth spurt than controls.[9]

Biomechanical factors have been suggested to play a role in AIS through the principles of the Hueter-Volkmann Law. This states that skeletal growth is accelerated under tensile forces and retarded under compressive forces. AIS can produce asymmetric loading of the spine that can cause further asymmetric growth.

Table 2: Summary of the Risser grading scale for skeletal maturity	
Risser grade	*Radiographic finding*
0	No iliac apophysis visible
1	Initial appearance of the iliac apophysis
2	Migration half way across the iliac wing
3	Three quarters of the apophysis is formed
4	Ossification has occurred across the iliac wing but it is not fused to the ileum
5	Complete ossification of the iliac apophysis with fusion to the ileum

The final component thought to be involved with the development of AIS is environmental factors. These can include diet, calcium and vitamin D levels and level of exercise. However, additional research is necessary to confirm the specific roles of each of these factors in AIS.

PATIENT PRESENTATION

As with all other spinal disorders, the patient with AIS first undergoes a thorough medical and family history, and physical examination. The history should obtain information on when an abnormal spinal curvature was first identified and how, whether or not there has been any progression of the curve, pain in the back or extremities, paresthesias or weakness in the extremities, aggravating or relieving factors, history of recent growth spurt, age of onset of menarche for girls, and family history of scoliosis or other spinal disorders.

The physical examination should include measurement of height and weight. The skin should be examined for the presence of dimples or hair patches over the lower spine associated with spina bifida. Café au lait spots could suggest neurofibromatosis. The patient's coronal and sagittal plane balance should be assessed. Asymmetry of the shoulders and pelvis, and leg-length discrepancy should be noted. Curve rotation should be evaluated with the Adams forward bending test. The rigidity of the curve should also be evaluated along with the ability to passively correct the curvature. A complete neurologic examination should also be performed.

IMAGING STUDIES

Posteroanterior (PA) and lateral 36 × 14 inch radiographs should be obtained to measure the degree of curvature and assess coronal and sagittal plane balance. The Cobb angle is measured as the angle between lines drawn across the superior endplate of the cranial most vertebra of the curve and the inferior endplate of the caudal most vertebra of the curve on the PA radiograph (Fig. 1). A Cobb angle greater than 10° is necessary to be classified as scoliosis. The radiographs should also include the iliac apophyses to allow for evaluation of the Risser sign which is a radiographic indicator of skeletal maturity (Fig. 2). Table 2 summarizes the Risser grading scale. The PA radiograph should be used to determine the end vertebra, neutral vertebra and the stable vertebra for use in measurement and potential future surgical planning (Fig. 3). The degree of axial rotation should also be assessed and can be classified based on the Nash-Moe rotation scale (Fig. 4). The coronal plane balance

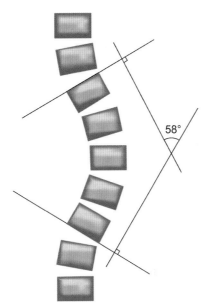

Fig. 1: Diagram of Cobb angle measurement

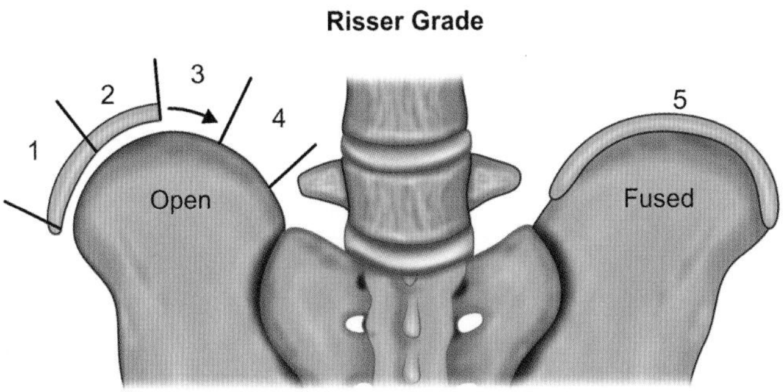

Risser Grade

Fig. 2: Diagram of the Risser scale for skeletal maturity

can be measured on the PA radiograph as the horizontal distance between the central sacral vertical line (CSVL) and a horizontal line drawn down through the center of the C7 vertebra (Fig. 5). The sagittal plane balance can be measured from the lateral radiograph as the horizontal distance from the posterior superior aspect of the S1 vertebra to a vertical line drawn down from the center of the C7 vertebra (Fig. 6). A positive sagittal balance signifies that the C7 vertebra lays ventral to the sacrum causing a relative forward flexed posture, while a negative sagittal balance signifies that the C7 vertebra lays dorsal to the sacrum causing a relative extended posture.

There are several classification systems used for AIS. Historically the King and Moe system was the most widely utilized and is summarized in Table 3. More recently, the Lenke classification has become the standard system used and is summarized in Table 4.

Magnetic resonance imaging (MRI) is recommended for atypical curve types with the apex to the left as well as cases with excessive axial back pain or neurologic abnormality. The MRI can be used to evaluate for possible infection, malignancy, intraspinal lesion, syrinx

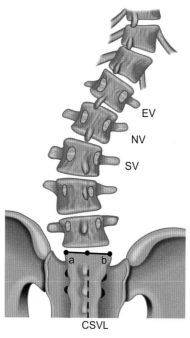

EV

NV

SV

a   b

CSVL

Fig. 3: Diagram of the posteroanterior radiograph showing the end, neutral and stable vertebrae. The end vertebra is the most tilted vertebra at the cephalad and caudal ends of the curve. The neutral vertebra is the most cephalad vertebra below the apes of the curve in which the pedicles are symmetric. The stable vertebra is the most cephalad vertebra that is most closely bisected by the central sacral vertical line (CSVL), which is a vertical reference line drawn through the middle of the S1 vertebra

EV: end vertebra; NV: Neutral vertebra; SV: Stable vertebra

Left (concave)

Right (convex)

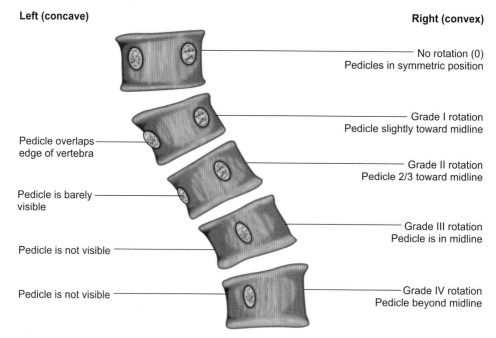

No rotation (0)
Pedicles in symmetric position

Grade I rotation
Pedicle slightly toward midline

Pedicle overlaps edge of vertebra

Grade II rotation
Pedicle 2/3 toward midline

Pedicle is barely visible

Grade III rotation
Pedicle is in midline

Pedicle is not visible

Pedicle is not visible

Grade IV rotation
Pedicle beyond midline

Fig. 4: Diagram of the Nash-Moe vertebral axial rotation classification

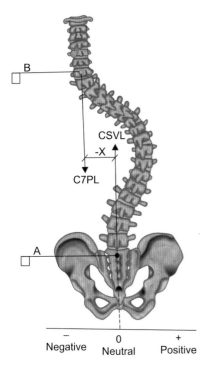

Fig. 5: Diagram of the measurement of coronal plane balance (X) as the distance between the central sacral vertical line (CSVL) and a vertical line drawn down through the center of the C7 vertebra

or tethered spinal cord. Computed tomography (CT) scans can be used to evaluate for a possible osteoid osteoma or osteoblastoma that can cause localized back pain and scoliosis.

NONOPERATIVE TREATMENT

Decisions for treatment of patients with AIS are based on the degree of curve, amount of curve progression over time, and the age and skeletal maturity of the patient. Previous studies have reported the risk of needing surgery for AIS is 16% for curves less than 20° at the onset of puberty, 75% for curves 20–30° at the onset of puberty and 100% for curves greater than 30° at the onset of puberty.[10] In general terms, there are three options for treatment including observation, bracing and surgery.

Observation of the curve is typically recommended for patients with small magnitude curves. Patients with minimal spinal asymmetry less than 10° should be followed by the primary care physician, and radiographs should not be obtained unless there is clinical progression of the curve based on physical examination. Skeletally immature patients with curves measuring between 10° and 20° should have repeat physical examination and radiographs every 6–12 months until skeletal maturity is achieved or curve progression occurs. Skeletally immature patients with curves measuring between 20° and 30° should be monitored more closely every 4–6 months for radiographic evidence of curve progression. The majority of patients with AIS can be effectively managed with this observation alone.

For curves between 30° and 45° or greater than 25° with documented progression of greater than 5° bracing is a potential option in skeletally immature patients. Since bracing

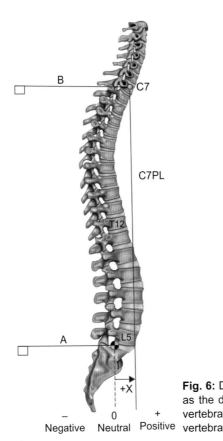

B

C7

C7PL

T12

A

L5

+X

− 0 +
Negative Neutral Positive

Fig. 6: Diagram of the measurement of sagittal plane balance (X) as the distance between the posterior superior aspect of the S1 vertebra, and a vertical line drawn down from the center of the C7 vertebra

Table 3: King and Moe classification system		
Curve location	Type	Description
Thoracic	I	Primary lumbar, compensatory thoracic curve
	II	Primary thoracic, compensatory lumbar curve
	III	Thoracic curve only with apex at or above T10
	IV	Long thoracic curve extends to L4
	V	Double thoracic curve
Double major		Equally structural curves in the thoracic and lumbar spine
Lumbar		Apex in the lumbar spine
Thoracolumbar		Apex at the thoracolumbar junction

is not effective for the correction of scoliosis it is not recommended for patients who have reached skeletal maturity. The goal of bracing treatment is to slow down progression of the curve during remaining skeletal growth. Several types of braces are available including a standard thoracolumbosacral orthosis (TLSO). This brace is typically recommended for curves with an apex caudal to T7 and used 23 hours daily. Other braces including the Charleston bending brace is molded for additional corrective force across the spine

Type	Proximal thoracic	Main thoracic	Thoracolumbar/lumbar	Curve type
Table 4: Lenke classification system				
1	Nonstructural	Structural	Nonstructural	Main thoracic
2	Structural	Structural	Nonstructural	Double thoracic
3	Nonstructural	Structural	Structural	Double major
4	Structural	Structural	Structural	Triple major
5	Nonstructural	Nonstructural	Structural	Thoracolumbar/lumbar
6	Nonstructural	Structural	Structural	Thoracolumbar/lumbar, main thoracic
		Modifiers		
Lumbar modifier	*Location of central sacral vertical line (CSVL) at lumbar apex*		*Thoracic sagittal modifier*	*Sagittal profile T5–T12*
A	Between pedicles		–	Hypokyphotic < 10°
B	Touches apical body		N	Normal 20–40°
C	Lateral to body		+	Hyperkyphotic > 40°

and is for nighttime use only. Bracing is recommended for use until skeletal maturity has been achieved with radiographs being obtained every 4–6 months to monitor for curve progression.

The use of bracing for AIS remains somewhat controversial. The main reason for the continued controversy over the effectiveness of bracing for AIS is the difficulty of monitoring patient compliance with the brace. Miller et al. performed a study on the effectiveness of electronic monitoring of brace compliance.[11] They determined that if patients were informed that their brace was monitored for compliance in wearing the compliance improved from 56.5% to 85.7% with a mean increase of 5.24 hours of brace wear daily (p = 0.029).

While the psychological effect of bracing is difficult to accurately measure, many patients with AIS are either noncompliant or refuse to wear a brace due to issues associated with self-esteem and appearance. Danielsson et al. evaluated adults with a history of AIS for their perceptions on body appearance and quality of life, and compared groups of patients that had been treated with bracing or observation alone without bracing.[12] Patients treated with a brace reported less quality of life, worse feelings of body asymmetry and less satisfaction compared to those with just observation despite similar curve size and trunk rotation. The authors concluded that wearing the brace might have caused a "scar in the mind" leading to these perceptions.

☞ OPERATIVE TREATMENT

Surgical treatment for patients with AIS should be reserved for patients with a curve greater than 40° in skeletally immature patients or those with documented progression despite bracing treatment.

The most common surgical technique for patients with AIS is a posterior fusion with segmental pedicle screw instrumentation (Figs 7A to D). Historically, hook and rod

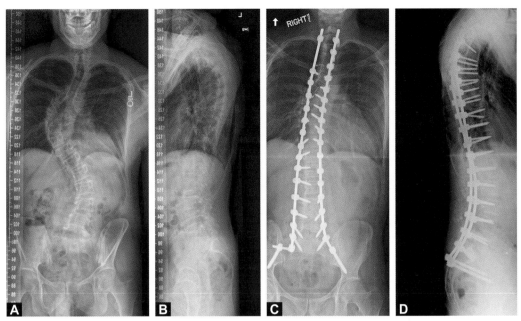

Figs 7A to D: (A) Preoperative posteroanterior and (B) lateral radiographs of female with adolescent idiopathic scoliosis; (C) Postoperative posteroanterior and (D) lateral radiographs reveal good correction of deformity following T2-ileum posterior segmentation instrumented fusion

constructs were used posteriorly, but they did not provide a rigid support or sufficient ability to de-rotate and correct the abnormal spinal curvature. The specific levels of instrumentation are based on specific curve characteristics and the degree of flexibility. In some cases the fusion levels span sufficiently to include the neutral and stable vertebrae. However, with stronger pedicle screw instrumentation techniques and the flexibility typically associated with younger patients with AIS, additional motion segments can often be maintained. In most cases, it is not necessary to instrument caudal to the L4 level in patients with AIS, as opposed to patients with degenerative scoliosis where extension down to the pelvis is much more common.

Anterior spinal decompression and fusion has been previously performed for AIS, but it is much less commonly performed since the more routine use of pedicle screws in the thoracic spine. These anterior procedures could be performed either through a traditional thoracotomy or through less invasive techniques including video-assisted thoracoscopy. A major benefit of the anterior fusion over historical posterior hook and rod constructs was the ability to prevent the crankshaft phenomenon. This refers to a continued growth of the anterior spinal column after solid posterior column fusion that led to continued axial rotational deformity. The use of thoracic pedicle screws has been shown to effectively eliminate the need for anterior instrumentation for concerns over the crankshaft phenomenon.

The newest development for AIS surgery involves minimally invasive techniques in which pedicle screws are placed fluoroscopically under image-guidance, and fusion is performed either through interbody devices or facet joint fusions.[13] The proposed benefits of these techniques include less blood loss, less postoperative pain, quicker mobilization and return to function.

Regardless of the specific techniques utilized, there are potential risks associated with surgery for AIS. These include infection, spinal cord injury, injury to the nerves and blood vessels, failure of spinal fusion or instrumentation, malpositioned instrumentation, inadequate correction, adjacent level degeneration or deformity, incidental durotomy, and incidental thoracotomy. Spinal cord injury and the potential for postoperative paralysis is one of the most devastating potential complications. In most cases surgeons use neurophysiologic monitoring intraoperatively including somatosensory evoked potentials and motor evoked potentials to decrease these risks.

REFERENCES

1. Bunnell WP. The natural history of idiopathic scoliosis before skeletal maturity. Spine. 1986;11: 773-6.
2. Kane WJ, Moe JH. A scoliosis-prevalence survey in Minnesota. Clin Orthop Rel Res. 1970;69: 216-8.
3. Kesling KL, Reinker KA. Scoliosis in twins. A meta-analysis of the literature and report of six cases. Spine. 1997;22:2009-15.
4. Miller NH. Idiopathic scoliosis: cracking the genetic code and what does it mean? J Pediatr Orthop. 2011;31:S49-S52.
5. Axenovich TI, Zaidman AM, Zorkoltseva IV, et al. Segregation analysis of idiopathic scoliosis: demonstration of a major gene effect. Am J Med Genet. 1999;86:389-94.
6. Ogilvie JW. Update on prognostic genetic testing in adolescent idiopathic scoliosis (AIS). J Pediatr Orthop. 2011;31:S46-8.
7. Cheung J, Veldhuizen AG, Halberts JP, et al. Geometric and electromyographic assessments in the evaluation of curve progression in idiopathic scoliosis. Spine. 2006;31:322-9.
8. Burwell RG, Aujila RK, Grevitt MP, et al. Pathogenesis of adolescent idiopathic scoliosis in girls – a double neuro-osseous theory involving disharmony between the two nervous systems, somatic and autonomic expressed in the spine and trunk: possible dependency on sympathetic nervous system and hormones with implications for medical therapy. Scoliosis. 2009;4:24.
9. Cheung SK, Lee TK, Kit TY, et al. Abnormal peri-pubertal anthropometric measurements and growth pattern in adolescent idiopathic scoliosis: a study of 598 patients. Spine. 2003;28:2152-7.
10. Dimeglio A, Canavese F, Charles YP. Growth and adolescent idiopathic scoliosis: when and how much? J Pediatr Orthop. 2011;31:S28-S36.
11. Miller DJ, Franzone JM, Matsumoto H, et al. Electronic monitoring improves brace-wearing compliance in patients with adolescent idiopathic scoliosis. A randomized clinical trial. Spine. 2012;37:717-21.
12. Danielsson AJ, Hasserius R, Ohlin A, et al. Body appearance and quality of life in adult patients with adolescent idiopathic scoliosis treated with a brace or under observation alone during adolescence. Spine. 2012;37:755-62.
13. Sarwahi V, Wollowick AL, Sugarman EP, et al. Minimally invasive scoliosis surgery: an innovative technique in patients with adolescent idiopathic scoliosis. Scoliosis. 2001;6:16.

CHAPTER

14

Adult Scoliosis

👉 INTRODUCTION

Adult patients with scoliosis are distinctly different from pediatric scoliosis patients in terms of presenting symptoms, history, comorbidities and treatment options. These patients can not be effectively treated as just an adult version of the patient with adolescent idiopathic scoliosis (AIS). In general, the curves are more rigid and it is difficult to achieve correction without more aggressive techniques including osteotomies. The patient's older age brings additional medical comorbidities that can increase the risk of surgery. The patient's symptoms differ from the adolescent and can include more degenerative complaints including radiculopathy, myelopathy and chronic back pain.

There are two main categories of patients with adult scoliosis. These are based on whether or not the patient had scoliosis as an adolescent. For those patients who had AIS as a child that continued to progress and became more symptomatic as an adult, it is referred to as adult idiopathic scoliosis. This group can present with or without degenerative changes. The other group of patients is those who did not have a history of AIS as a child but instead developed scoliosis after skeletal maturity. This condition is referred to as adult *de novo* scoliosis.

This chapter reviews each of these categories of adult scoliosis including the pathophysiology, patient presentation, imaging studies and treatment options.

👉 PATHOPHYSIOLOGY

Scoliosis refers to an abnormal curvature of the spine with a Cobb angle greater than 10° (Fig. 1). In the normal spine the plumb line should pass through the center of the sacrum on the anteroposterior (AP) view. On the lateral view the plumb line should pass from the C7 vertebral body through the posterior portion of the L5-S1 disk space (Fig. 2). Adult scoliosis is a relatively common condition with a prevalence of 15% or greater.[1,2] It is increasingly common as the general population continues to age.

There are two general categories of adult scoliosis: (1) Type I refers to the patient with a history of AIS that continued to progress to symptomatic scoliosis as an adult. (2) Type II refers to the patient who had no history of scoliosis until after reaching skeletal maturity.

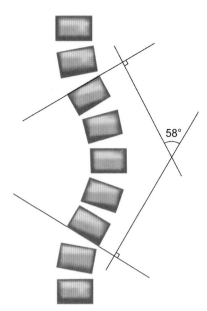

Fig. 1: Diagram of Cobb angle measurement

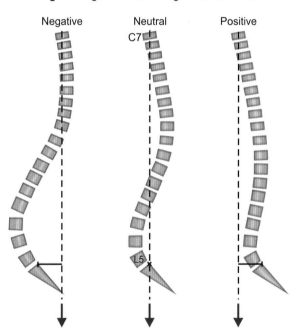

Fig. 2: On the lateral view the plumb line should pass from the C7 vertebral body through the posterior portion of the L5–S1 disk space. If the line passes anterior to this point it is called positive sagittal balance. If the line passes posterior to this point it is called negative sagittal balance

The pathophysiology and natural history of these two groups are very different. As with AIS, Type I adult scoliosis can affect the thoracic or lumbar spine. It can present as merely a progression of the AIS curve, or it can be combined with degenerative changes as well. Sagittal plane deformity is much less common in Type I adult scoliosis as compared to

Type II. Previous investigators have reported that nearly 70% of patients with AIS for greater than 40 years had some progression of their curve.[3] In that study large thoracic curves greater than 50° progressed on average 1° per year, while thoracolumbar curves progressed 0.5° per year, and lumbar curves progressed 0.24° per year. These numbers can be used to council young patients on their risk of curve progression and the potential benefits of surgery earlier in life.

In contrast, Type II adult scoliosis most commonly affects the lumbar or thoracolumbar spine. The apex of the curve is most commonly found at L3–L4. The most common etiology for this curve is widespread asymmetric degenerative changes in the spine that affect the disk, facet joints and ligamentum flavum. Other less common causes of Type II adult scoliosis include neuromuscular disorders, metabolic bone disease with pathologic fractures, leg-length discrepancy and pelvic obliquity. While sagittal imbalance is relatively uncommon in Type I adult scoliosis, it is much more common in Type II and is often a major cause for chronic back pain in these patients. The magnitude of the curve also varies between these two types, and curves greater than 60° are rare in Type II adult scoliosis. The rate of curve progression, however, is often greater in Type II with a mean rate of progression of 3° per year. The rate of progression in Type II curves is based on the severity of degenerative changes. Previous studies have identified risk factors for curve progression to include lumbar curves greater than 30°, greater than 30% apical vertebral rotation, 6 mm or more lateral listhesis, and degenerative disk disease located at the thoracolumbar junction.[4]

🖝 PATIENT PRESENTATION

The medical history should identify any previous history of scoliosis in the patient and at what age it was first identified. Patients should be questioned regarding any prior spinal disorders, trauma, or previous complaints of back or leg pain including duration of those symptoms and any changes that have over time. Aggravating and relieving factors and any previous treatments should be discussed. The past medical history should be reviewed for diabetes, vascular disorders, osteoporosis and other metabolic disorders, thyroid disorders, nutritional deficiencies and chronic pain syndromes. Any family history of scoliosis or other spinal disorders should be identified.

Patients with adult scoliosis typically present with complaints of chronic low back pain that is activity related. Standing and walking exacerbate the pain, while there is little to no pain with sitting or lying down. Patients with a positive sagittal balance have greater complaints of lower back pain because these patients are using their back muscles to try to hold themselves upright and develop fatigue pain. Unilateral or bilateral radicular complaints including pain and paresthesias are common and result from degenerative changes of the disk, facet joints, osteophytes and hypertrophy of the ligamentum flavum causing central or foraminal stenosis and nerve root compression. Vascular studies might be necessary to rule out vascular claudication in some cases.

The physical examination begins with inspection of the patient. The overall balance from the front and side should be assessed to determine if the head is well seated over the pelvis in both planes. The patient's back should be examined for any gross curvature, rib

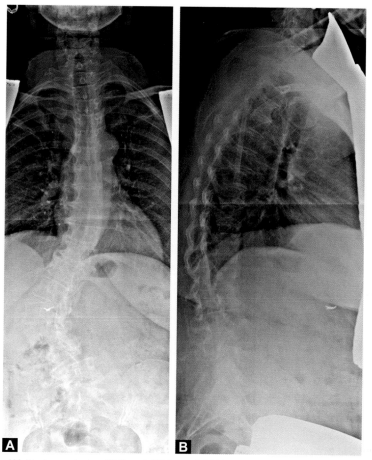

Figs 3A and B: (A) Posteroanterior (PA) and (B) lateral full length scoliosis radiographs of a 57-year-old female with Type II adult scoliosis; Images reveal widespread degenerative changes in the lumbar spine with a 55° curve from T12-L4 and an apex at the L2-L3 disk space. There is a lateral listhesis of L3 on L4 of 17 mm. There is a loss of the normal lordotic curvature with resulting positive sagittal balance

prominence, step-offs, skin changes and previous surgical scars. Observations of the patient ambulating and getting out of the chair can help assess for proximal leg strength, balance and any gait abnormalities. Patients with progressive gait changes should be evaluated for cervical spondylotic myelopathy. Skin discoloration or loss of hair on the legs and feet could signify vascular disorders. The spine should be palpated for any areas of point tenderness or changes in muscle tone. Having the patient bent can assess for the flexibility of the curvature. A full neurologic examination should be performed to identify any motor or sensory deficits or reflex abnormalities.

IMAGING

Imaging of the patient with adult scoliosis begins with 36-inch full length posteroanterior (PA) and lateral scoliosis plain radiographs (Figs 3A and B). These can be used to assess for the magnitude of spinal curvature, sagittal and coronal plane balance, instability, lateral

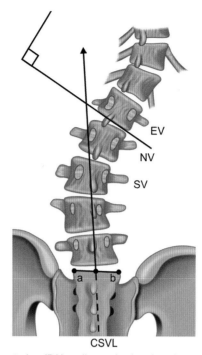

Fig. 4: Diagram of the posteroanterior (PA) radiograph showing the end, neutral and stable vertebrae. The end vertebra (EV) is the most tilted vertebra at the cephalad and caudal ends of the curve. The neutral vertebra (NV) is the most cephalad vertebra below the apes of the curve in which the pedicles are symmetric. The stable vertebra (SV) is the most cephalad vertebra that is most closely bisected by the central sacral vertical line (CSVL), which is a vertical reference line drawn through the middle of the S1 vertebra

listhesis, spondylolisthesis, spondylotic changes and pelvic obliquity. The PA radiograph should be used to determine the end vertebra, neutral vertebra and the stable vertebra for use in measurements and potential future surgical planning (Fig. 4). Flexion-extension lateral radiographs can be used to assess for dynamic spondylolisthesis. Side-bending radiographs can be used to assess the flexibility of the curve. The degree of vertebral body rotation at the apex of the coronal plane curvature provides information of the rigidity of the curve. The greater degree of vertebral rotation at the apex correlates to greater rigidity of the curve (Fig. 5).

Advanced imaging studies are frequently performed in patients with adult scoliosis including computed tomography (CT), CT with myelogram and magnetic resonance imaging (MRI). Both CT and MRI can be used to evaluate for compression of the neural structures in patients with an abnormal neurologic examination and to obtain measurements of pedicle sizes for surgical planning. Computed tomography has the advantage of superior bony detail and the ability to change the gantry and allow for axial imaging through the disk space regardless of the degree of curvature of the spine. Magnetic resonance imaging provides improved visualization of the soft tissues and neurologic structures but is often limited in severe deformities by being unable to image in a plane through the disk space.

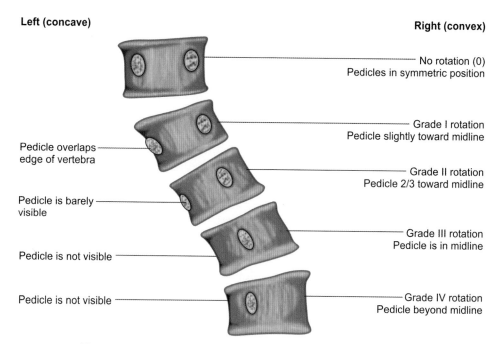

Left (concave)   **Right (convex)**

No rotation (0)
Pedicles in symmetric position

Grade I rotation
Pedicle slightly toward midline

Pedicle overlaps edge of vertebra

Grade II rotation
Pedicle 2/3 toward midline

Pedicle is barely visible

Grade III rotation
Pedicle is in midline

Pedicle is not visible

Grade IV rotation
Pedicle beyond midline

Pedicle is not visible

Fig. 5: Diagram of the Nash-Moe vertebral axial rotation classification

NONOPERATIVE TREATMENT

Nonoperative treatment options for patients with adult scoliosis include medications, physical therapy, massage therapy, chiropractic treatment and steroid injections. None of these treatment options is a cure for the disorder or even a treatment for the spinal curvature. Instead, each can provide some degree of symptomatic relief for the patient. The most commonly utilized medications for these patients include nonsteroidal anti-inflammatory medications. These are thought to reduce the inflammation and swelling; however, there is limited information on their clinical effectiveness. Unfortunately, many older patients with scoliosis have various comorbidities that preclude the use of these medications including gastric ulcers, hypertension and cardiovascular disease. Other medication options include acetaminophen, muscle relaxants, narcotics and anticonvulsants. Caution should be used to avoid more than 4 g daily of acetaminophen to avoid hepatotoxicity. Patients with pre-existing liver disorders might need to avoid all acetaminophen. While narcotics and muscle relaxants can in some cases provide reasonable pain relief, caution should be used in this patient population due to the increased risk of sedation, falls and constipation that can be common side effects. Anticonvulsants such as gabapentin can provide improved pain and functional ability in patients with stenosis, but they are also associated with side effects including sedation, dizziness and increased risk of falls.

The use of physical therapy or chiropractic programs is commonly recommended for patients with scoliosis. These programs can include stretching and strengthening exercises, core muscle strengthening, as well as various modalities including heat, ice, massage, ultrasound and electrical stimulation. While these methods are commonly used in conjunction with other treatment options, there is no proven benefit to physical therapy or chiropractic as a stand alone treatment option. By increasing the strength of the muscles patients are better able to compensate for their abnormal curvature with less muscle fatigue pain.

Another common nonsurgical treatment for patients with adult scoliosis associated with radicular symptoms is lumbar epidural steroid injection. These injections are typically used to deliver a combination of a long-acting anesthetic with corticosteroids to the area of stenosis. They are felt to be the most beneficial for radicular symptoms as opposed to axial back pain. They can be performed through an interlaminar approach or a transforaminal approach. Local trigger point injections into inflamed muscles can provide some short-term relief of muscle pain but is not expected to provide long-term relief.

As opposed to young patients with AIS, there is no benefit for the use of bracing for adults with scoliosis. Bracing in adults is not capable of correcting the curve or halting any further progression of the curve. Instead, bracing shields the muscles and can lead to muscle atrophy and increased levels of muscle fatigue pain.

Unfortunately, there is no strong evidence for the use of any of these nonoperative treatment options over the others for patients with adult scoliosis.[5] Each of these treatments remains an option for reducing symptoms related to adult scoliosis.

☛ OPERATIVE TREATMENT

The decision to perform surgery on patients with adult scoliosis is difficult due to the presence of medical comorbidities, magnitude of the surgery, potential risks of surgery, and wide variation of patient's symptoms and imaging findings. In this patient population all patients can not be treated alike.

Potential indications for surgery include progressive curvature, presence of neurologic deficits, intractable pain, poor cosmesis and failure of conservative treatment. It is crucial to correlate the patient's symptoms, physical examination findings and imaging results prior to any decision to offer surgery. Surgery for patients with AIS is typically aimed at achieving the maximum curve correction that is safely possible. This is not always the case for adult scoliosis. In some cases, the major complaint is related to the coexisting stenosis causing radicular symptoms. For these patients that have failed conservative options, a limited decompression of the stenotic areas might be sufficient to treat the patient. Care must be taken with this approach to avoid destabilizing the spine and causing an iatrogenic spondylolisthesis or worsening degree of scoliosis. In most cases of adult scoliosis decompression without fusion should be avoided over multiple levels at the apex of the curve or at a level with lateral listhesis. If those levels correspond to the location of symptomatic stenosis, a limited decompression and fusion with or without instrumentation might be effective. The benefit of this approach is that it can help alleviate the neurologic symptoms while avoiding iatrogenic destabilization of the spine. Care should be taken to avoid ending a fusion at the apex of a curve or adjacent to a level with listhesis. In these cases it might not be necessary to address the entire curve or to achieve any curve correction.

In cases of intractable back pain, instability, multilevel stenosis and sagittal imbalance, the limited surgical options discussed above are generally not sufficient. Instead, a wide decompression of the affected levels with fusion across the curve is necessary. The decision to use an anterior, posterior or combined approach depends on many factors including magnitude of sagittal plane deformity, bone quality and flexibility of the curve. With the use of osteotomies and vertebral column resection the majority of adult scoliosis cases can be treated from a single posterior approach. This avoids the added morbidity of the anterior approach and potential need for thoracotomy and chest tubes. These techniques, however, do increase the associated risks of surgery and are technically demanding. Anterior column support can be achieved from a posterior approach through either a posterior or transforaminal interbody fusion technique. Anterior lumbar interbody fusion does offer improved anterior release for deformity correction and improved fusion surface area compared to the posterior approaches to the interbody space. This can be especially important in long fusion constructs that extend to the sacrum.

The decision on specific levels to include in the fusion construct is beyond the scope of this chapter, but there are several rules that are typically followed. Fusions are generally not ended at a junctional zone such as C7-T1 or T12-L1 or at the apex of a kyphotic curve. This is to reduce the risk of adjacent level kyphosis occurring postoperatively. Fusion should also not be ended adjacent to a level with spondylolisthesis, rotatory subluxation or severe stenosis. If a long fusion extends across the L5-S1 level either extension to the ileum or anterior interbody fusion is typically performed to reduce the risk of pseudoarthrosis at L5–S1 or instrumentation failure with pullout of the S1 screws.

The most recent advancement in the surgical treatment of adult scoliosis is the use of minimally invasive techniques. This is a technically demanding approach with a large learning curve. A full understanding of the complex anatomy and skill with open procedures should be obtained along with the use of minimally invasive techniques in more basic cases prior to using them on complex deformity cases. While there are limited outcomes data in this patient population the early results appear promising to provide decreased blood loss, decreased pain and shorter hospital stays.[6]

There are many potential risks associated with surgery for patients with adult scoliosis. In a large systematic review of the literature 38% of patients were reported to have surgical complications after fusion for adult scoliosis with less than 1% mortality.[7] The most common complications included dural tear, wound infection, and pulmonary, renal and neurologic complications. The risk for pseudoarthrosis has been reported to be approximately 13% in these patients.[8] Others have reported overall complication rates ranging from 40% to 86%.[9,10]

REFERENCES

1. Schwab F, Dubey A, Gamez L, et al. Adult scoliosis: prevalence, SF-36, and nutritional parameters in an elderly volunteer population. Spine (Phila Pa 1976). 2005;30:1082-5.
2. Schwab F, Dubey A, Pagala M, et al. Adult scoliosis: a health assessment analysis by SF-36. Spine. 2003;28:602-6.

3. Weinstein SL, Dolan LA, Spratt KF, et al. Health and function of patients with untreated idiopathic scoliosis: a 50-year natural history study. JAMA. 2003;289:559-67.
4. Korovessis P, Piperos G, Sidiropoulos P, et al. Adult idiopathic lumbar scoliosis. A formula for prediction of progression and review of the literature. Spine. 1994;19:1926-32.
5. Everett CR, Patel RK. A systematic literature review of nonsurgical treatment in adult scoliosis. Spine (Phila Pa 1976). 2007;32:S130-4.
6. Mundis GM, Akbarnia BA, Philips FM. Adult deformity correction through minimally invasive lateral approach techniques. Spine (Phila Pa 1976). 2010;35:S312-21.
7. Drazin D, Shirzadi A, Rosner J, et al. Complications and outcomes after spinal deformity surgery in the elderly: review of the existing literature and future directions. Neurosurg Focus. 2011;31(4):E3.
8. Yadla S, Maltenfort MG, Ratliff JK, et al. Adult scoliosis surgery outcomes: a systematic review. Neurosurg Focus. 2010;28(3):E3.
9. Ganocy TK, Ohtomo M, Boachie-Adjei O. Complication rates for combined anterior-posterior adult deformity surgery. SRS Meeting, Quebec City, Quebec, Canada, 2003.
10. Lapp MA, Bridwell KH, Lenke LG, et al. Long-term complications in adult spinal deformity patients having combined surgery: a comparison of primary to revision patients. Spine. 2001;26:973-83.

CHAPTER

15

Inflammatory Disorders of the Spine

🖝 INTRODUCTION

The majority of arthritic conditions affecting the spine are the result of degenerative arthritis. There are, however, other types of arthritis of the spine that can occur less frequently. The most common of these is the category of inflammatory arthritis. This group of disorders includes rheumatoid arthritis (RA) and the seronegative spondyloarthropathies. The seronegative spondyloarthropathies include ankylosing spondylitis (AS), diffuse idiopathic skeletal hyperostosis (DISH), reactive arthritis, psoriatic arthritis and enteropathic arthritis.

Rheumatoid arthritis is a chronic inflammatory disease that affects the synovial lining of joints leading to widespread joint destruction. The most common locations of involvement include the hands, the feet and the cervical spine. Fortunately, due to improvements in pharmacologic management of RA, the involvement of spine has become less severe and less common.

Patients with inflammatory arthritis present unique challenges from both a diagnostic and management perspective. They should be properly distinguished from the patient with traditional degenerative arthritis. Failure to do so can lead to poor results and severe complications. This chapter presents a review of patients with inflammatory arthritis including discussions on pathophysiology, patient presentation, clinical workup, and conservative and surgical treatment options.

🖝 RHEUMATOID ARTHRITIS

Pathophysiology

Rheumatoid arthritis is a chronic, systemic, inflammatory disease that causes destruction of the synovial joints throughout the body. It results from an immune response of T-lymphocytes to unknown antigens. This activates macrophages and leads to an increased production of monokines such as interlukin-1 and tumor necrosis factor-α (TNF-α), and the subsequent attraction of lymphocytes, neutrophils and angiogenesis. The synovial destruction results from the release of activated metalloproteinases such as procollagenase and progelatinase.[1]

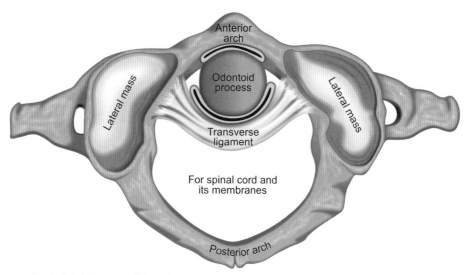

Fig. 1: Axial diagram of the atlantoaxial joint showing the transverse ligament that can be disrupted with rheumatoid arthritis (RA) leading to instability

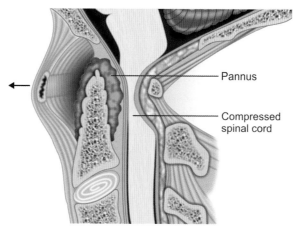

Fig. 2: Lateral diagram of the atlantoaxial joint in a patient with rheumatoid arthritis (RA) that developed a pannus surrounding the odontoid causing spinal cord compression

Involvement of the spine is most often found in the upper cervical spine. Rheumatoid arthritis affects the synovial joints in the region including the atlanto-occipital, atlantoaxial, zygapophyseal and uncovertebral joints. It can also affect the disks and the bursal and ligamentous structures. The most common site of involvement is the atlantoaxial joint leading to instability and subluxation.[2] Involvement of the transverse ligament (Fig. 1) can lead to ligamentous laxity, atlantoaxial instability and anterior subluxation. Anterior subluxation of 0–3 mm is normal in adults, but 3–6 mm of subluxation suggests instability due to disruption of the transverse ligament, and 9 mm or more suggests disruption of the periodontoid ligamentous and capsular structures with gross instability.[3,4] Instability can lead to formation of a pannus posterior to the odontoid that can cause spinal cord compression (Fig. 2). Posterior subluxation can result from erosion or fracture of the odontoid process.

Involvement of the lateral atlantoaxial joints around the foramen magnum can lead to superior subluxation. Erosion of the lateral masses and odontoid process can lead to lateral subluxation.

The next most frequent location of RA involvement of the spine is the subaxial cervical spine. Destruction of the zygapophyseal joints and bursal structures leads to anterior subluxation and kyphosis of the subaxial cervical motion segments. Subluxation of more than 3.5 mm is generally considered to be unstable.

The subluxation and kyphosis caused by RA in the cervical spine can cause severe pain as well as neurovascular complications. Patients can develop spinal cord compression and myelopathy as well as compression of the vertebral arteries and anterior spinal artery that can cause paralysis, coma, stroke or sudden death.

Patient Presentation

The most common location for spinal involvement is the cervical spine, and involvement of the thoracic or lumbar spine is much less frequent. Clinical symptoms of RA of the cervical spine are often delayed well beyond the presence of radiographic evidence of the disease.

Patients most commonly complain of neck pain and stiffness that is worst in the morning and improves with activity. Involvement of the upper cervical region with compression of the posterior rami of the greater and lesser occipital nerves (C1 and C2, respectively) can trigger occipital headaches. Subluxation of the joints can cause a feeling of the head falling forward and difficulty maintaining an upright position of the head and neck. More severe involvement can present with loss of consciousness, syncope and vertigo. Neurologic symptoms can include paresthesias in the upper extremities due to nerve root traction or compression. Signs of cervical myelopathy and urinary incontinence can be present due to spinal cord compression from subluxation or odontoid pannus formation. Vertebral artery compression can present with cranial nerve palsies, visual disturbances, dizziness, cerebellar ataxia, Horner's syndrome and dysarthria.

Physical examination begins with the overall appearance of the patient. In most cases of significant RA involvement of the spine the patient has already been diagnosed with RA based on peripheral skeletal involvement as described in Table 1.[5] To be properly diagnosed with RA the patient should have at least four of the seven criteria with criteria 1–4 being present for at least 6 weeks. Characteristic findings in the patient's hands include ulnar deviation of the digits, nodules over the extensor surfaces, joint tenderness, bogginess, swelling and limited range of motion.

Examination of the cervical spine may reveal the head in a forward flexed position or tilted to one side. It may be difficult for the patient to actively extend the neck to neutral or beyond. Local tenderness over the spinous processes is commonly present. The Ranawat criteria provide a scale for pain and neurologic function in patients with RA of the cervical spine as detailed in Table 2.[6]

Imaging Studies

Imaging of the patient with RA of the spine begins with plain radiographs of the cervical spine including anteroposterior (AP), lateral with flexion and extension, and open-mouth

Table 1: American Rheumatism Association 1987 revised criteria for the classification of rheumatoid arthritis[5]

Clinical finding	Description
Morning stiffness	Morning stiffness in and around the joints, lasting 1 hour before maximal improvement
Arthritis of three or more joint areas	At least three joint areas simultaneously have soft tissue swelling or fluid
Arthritis of the hand joints	At least one area swollen in the wrist, metacarpophalangeal (MCP) or proximal interphalangeal (PIP) joint
Symmetrical arthritis	Simultaneous involvement of PIP, MCP or metatarsophalangeal joints is acceptable without absolute symmetry
Rheumatoid nodules	Subcutaneous nodules over bony prominences, extensor surfaces or juxta-articular regions
Serum rheumatoid factor	Demonstration of abnormal amounts of serum rheumatoid factor by any method for which the result has been positive in less than 5% of normal control subjects
Radiographic changes	Radiographic change typical of rheumatoid arthritis on posteroanterior hand and wrist radiographs, which must include erosions or unequivocal bony decalcification localized in or most marked adjacent to the involved joints (osteoarthritis changes alone do not qualify)

Table 2: Ranawat criteria for pain and neural assessment[6]

Pain assessment	
Grade	Description
0	None
1	Mild; intermittent, requiring only aspirin analgesia
2	Moderate; a cervical collar was needed
3	Severe; pain could not be relieved by either aspirin or collar
Neural assessment	
Class	Description
I	No neural deficit
II	Subjective weakness with hyperreflexia and dysesthesias
IIIA	Objective findings of paresis and long tract signs but walking possible
IIIB	Quadriparesis with resultant inability to walk or feed oneself

odontoid views. Specific radiographic features have been identified that suggest the diagnosis of RA of the cervical spine as detailed in Table 3.[7] The flexion-extension views are used to measure the anterior atlantodental interval (AADI) and posterior atlantodental interval (PADI) as shown in Figure 3. The AADI is the distance from the anterior aspect of the odontoid to the posterior aspect of the anterior ring of the atlas. The PADI is the distance from the posterior aspect of the odontoid to the anterior aspect of the posterior ring of the atlas. As discussed above, the AADI can be used to determine the severity of anterior atlantoaxial subluxation. Less than 3 mm is considered normal, 3–6 mm is considered

Table 3: Radiographic criteria for the diagnosis of rheumatoid arthritis of the cervical spine[7]

Atlantoaxial subluxation of 2.5 mm or more

Multiple subluxations of C2-C3, C3-C4, C4-C5 and C5-C6

Narrow disk spaces with little or no osteophytosis

Erosion of the vertebrae, especially the vertebral endplates

Small, pointed odontoid with erosion of the cortex

Basilar impression

Apophyseal joint erosion with blurred facets

Cervical spine osteoporosis

Wide (> 5 mm) space between the posterior arch of the atlas and the spinous process of the axis

Secondary osteosclerosis of the atlantoaxial occipital complex

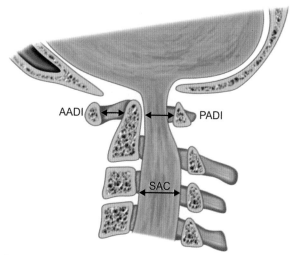

Fig. 3: Lateral diagram of the atlantoaxial joint showing the measurements for the anterior atlantodental interval (AADI) and posterior atlantodental interval (PADI)

unstable, and greater than 9 mm has been recommended for surgery. This measurement is often limited due to erosion of the normal anatomic structures that prevents an accurate measurement. It is also limited in that is does not account for the possible presence of a pannus posterior to the odontoid that can cause spinal cord compression. As a result of these limitations of the AADI, the PADI has become a more reliable predictor of neurologic outcome in these patients. Patients with a PADI of 14 mm or more have been reported to have an increased likelihood of neurologic recovery following stabilization, while those with a PADI less than 10 mm had no neurologic recovery.[8]

Cranial settling can have severe neurologic complications including sudden death. There are several measurements that can be used to identify the presence of cranial settling as shown in Figure 4. Chamberlain's line is drawn from the posterosuperior tip of the hard palate to the posterior lip of the foramen magnum (opisthion). Cranial settling is present

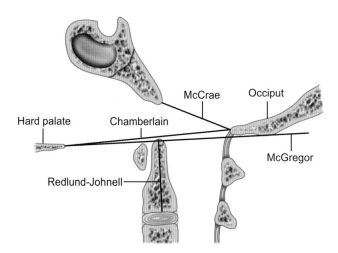

Fig. 4: Drawing showing the lines for measurement of cranial settling including McCrae's line, Chamberlain's line, McGregor's line and the Redlund-Johnell line

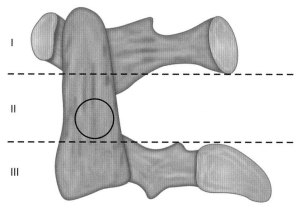

Fig. 5: Drawing the sagittal view of the atlas and axis showing the station of the atlas. If the ring of the atlas is in station I there is no cranial settling, in station II there is mild settling, and in station III there is severe settling

if the tip of the odontoid is more than 6 mm above this line. McCrae's line connects the basion to the opisthion. Cranial settling is present if the tip of the odontoid is above this line. McGregor's line is drawn from the posterosuperior tip of the hard palate to the caudal base of the occiput. Cranial settling is present if the tip of the odontoid is greater than 4.5 mm above this line. The Redlund-Johnell method draws a vertical line from the midpoint of the caudal margin of C2 to bisect McGregor's line. Cranial settling is present if the distance is greater than 34 mm in males and 29 mm in females. The station of the atlas is determined by dividing the odontoid into thirds in the sagittal plane as shown in Figure 5. The ring of the atlas should lie in the cephalad third (station I). Mild cranial settling is present if the ring is in station II, and severe cranial settling is present if the ring lies in station III.

Advanced imaging studies including CT scan and magnetic resonance imaging (MRI) are often obtained as well. The CT scan provides superior bony detail compared to plain radiographs. It is useful for surgical planning and for measurements for spinal instrumentation. MRI is obtained in cases with neurologic abnormalities to assess for brainstem, spinal cord and nerve root compression. The extent of pannus formation can also be assessed on MRI.

Nonoperative Treatment

Nonoperative management of patients with RA of the cervical spine is recommended unless there is a neurologic deficit or signs of instability. Symptomatic treatment can consist of intermittent use of a soft collar, trials of physical therapy and pharmacologic treatment. Rigid collars are not typically tolerated well in this patient population. Close clinical follow-up is crucial to identify any new signs or symptoms that suggest neurologic compromise or instability.

There are numerous pharmacologic treatment options for RA. While most of these are managed by the primary physician or rheumatologist, it is important for the spine specialist to have an understanding of the available options. Nonsteroidal anti-inflammatory drugs (NSAID's) can reduce the pain and inflammation associated with RA, but should be used with caution due to the risk of gastrointestinal bleeding and potential cardiovascular risks. Corticosteroids can be used intermittently for deceasing inflammation, but are not typically used long-term due to side effects. Disease modifying antirheumatic agents (DMARD's) are recommended for patients with documented joint damage that have failed NSAID's. This class of medications has a delayed onset of action but has been shown to effectively decrease inflammation and slow the progression of RA. There are multiple options of medications in this class with different mechanisms of action including pyrimidine inhibitors, anti-TNF-α inhibitors and immunosuppressive agents. Many of these have a higher potential for serious side effects and require close monitoring.

Operative Treatment

Patients with RA of the cervical spine may be candidates for surgery if they develop instability, myelopathy or neurologic deficits. Unfortunately, these patients present unique surgical challenges due to their frequent medical comorbidities, immunosuppression, poor bone quality, and poor soft tissue and skin coverage. These factors put the patient at increased risk of complications including infection, wound dehiscence, ulcer formation, instrumentation pullout or failure, adjacent level degeneration or insufficiency fracture, dysphasia, esophageal perforation or stricture, upper airway obstruction, and other medical and anesthesia-related complications.

There are numerous surgical options available depending on the specific needs of the patients. In most cases the goals are to decompress the spinal cord and exiting nerve roots, and stabilize the unstable spine. This often requires extension of the fusion to the occiput and possibly to the upper thoracic spine. In most cases this involves placement of a combination of lateral mass and pedicle screws for fixation. Due to the frequent problems with poor bone quality additional levels of fixation are often added. In some cases further fixation can be added with posterior wiring techniques.

The most common location for instability in these patients is the atlantoaxial joint. Options for fixation include posterior wiring constructs, postoperative halo bracing, posterior transarticular screws, posterior C1 lateral mass and C2 pedicle screw constructs. Additional options for fixation include C2 pars interarticularis screws and laminar screws. If a large pannus has formed posterior to the odontoid a transoral resection of the odontoid can be performed, but it is often not necessary. In most cases once stability is achieved, the pannus begins to reabsorb.

An example case is shown in Figures 6A to E of a 61-year-old female with a history of RA since age 18. She had undergone a previous posterior cervical decompression and instrumented fusion from C2-C7 10 years ago. She had sustained multiple falls since then and complained of severe neck pain, headaches and difficulty holding her head upright. Her initial images revealed the previous surgical decompression and fusion with severe cranial settling and kyphotic deformity. She underwent a removal of her previous spinal instrumentation, C1-C4 decompression, osteotomies from C2-C5 and posterior instrumented fusion from the occiput to T2. This case details the need for multiple points of fixation due to poor bone quality and complexity of these cases requiring multiple cervical osteotomies.

☛ SERONEGATIVE SPONDYLOARTHROPATHIES

Pathophysiology

The group of disorders known collectively as seronegative spondyloarthropathies include AS, DISH, reactive arthritis, psoriatic arthritis and enteropathic arthritis. These disorders share a common genetic predilection and similar characteristics. They are typically associated with sacroiliitis with or without spondylitis, peripheral inflammatory arthritis, tendency for familial aggregation and a negative rheumatoid factor. The genetic predilection is associated with the presence of the HLA-B27 antigen. This is present in more than 90% of white patients with AS, but it is found in only 7–8% of the white population without AS.[9] The exact correlation between HLA-B27 and seronegative spondyloarthopathies remains uncertain, but a bacterial association has been suggested.

These are inflammatory disorders in which the affected joints become arthritic, erode, and eventually can progress to autofusion. The sacroiliac joints are often the first joints to be affected, followed by the vertebral apophyses and the costovertebral joints. The major differentiation between the seronegative spondyloarthropathies and RA is that they affect the bony insertions of ligaments and tendons, while RA affects the synovial joints. Also, the seronegative spondyloarthropathies often affect the entire axial skeleton, while RA is typically confined to the cervical spine. While all of the seronegative spondyloarthropathies cause sacroiliitis, there are unique features of each in terms of the involvement of the peripheral skeleton.

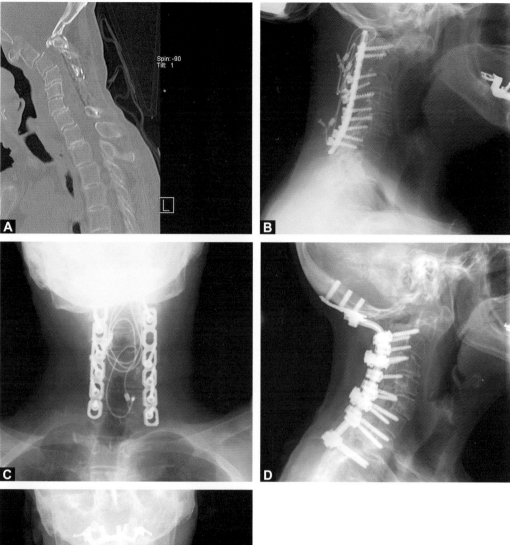

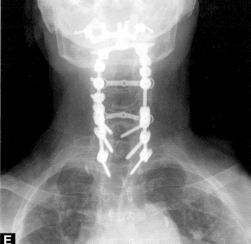

Figs 6A to E: Case example of patient with severe kyphotic deformity and cranial settling with rheumatoid arthritis (RA) that had progressed following a previous surgery 10 years ago. Preoperative images include (A) Sagittal CT scan; (B) Lateral radiograph and (C) Anteroposterior (AP) radiograph; (D) Postoperative lateral and (E) AP radiographs reveal the occiput-T2 fusion performed after C2-C5 osteotomies, C1-C4 decompression and removal of previously placed instrumentation

Table 4: Diagnostic criteria for ankylosing spondylitis (AS)		
	Rome criteria	*New York criteria*
Clinical criteria	• Low back pain and stiffness for > 3 months not relieved by rest	• Limitation of motion of the lumbar spine in flexion, extension and lateral bending
	• Pain and stiffness in the thoracic region	• History of presence of pain at the thoracolumbar junction or lumbar spine
	• Limited motion in the lumbar spine	• Limitation of chest expansion to 1 inch or less
	• Limited chest expansion	• Sacroiliitis
	• History of iritis or its sequelae	
Radiographic criteria	Radiograph showing bilateral sacroiliac changes characteristic of AS	

Patient Presentation

Patients with seronegative spondyloarthropathies typically develop symptoms between the ages of 15 and 40, but patients with psoriatic arthritis are typically at least 30 years old. There is a 3:1 male predominance for AS, but others are found equally among both genders. A dull low back pain with stiffness is often the initial complaint. The back pain often improves with exercise. With AS and DISH there can be a gradual flattening of the lumbar lordotic curvature. As the thoracic spine becomes more involved, there is loss of motion in the spine and in the chest cavity that can lead to a decrease in pulmonary function. With AS involvement of the cervical spine there is further loss of motion and a gradual protrusion of the head forward into a flexed position with eventual inability to extend the head. Table 4 summarizes the Rome criteria and New York criteria for the diagnosis of AS.

In contrast, the other seronegative spondyloarthropathies are more commonly associated with pain and loss of motion that can be intermittent. Reactive arthritis can be self-limiting in many cases. The severity of enteropathic arthritis is directly related to the severity of the bowel disease; however, there is no direct correlation between skin symptoms and joint symptoms in patients with psoriatic arthritis.

Spinal cord and nerve root impingement can lead to neurologic findings in some patients. Atlantoaxial subluxation can occur with AS. Vertebral fracture is a serious complication for patients with AS. The spine can become rigid in advanced cases, and the bone becomes very brittle and prone to fracture. Patients with a fracture may have mild symptoms after the trauma, and a high level of suspicion is necessary to make the proper diagnosis. Any new position of the spine or increased range of motion should be considered to be related to a fracture until proven otherwise as there is no other method for the ankylosed spine to change position. Unfortunately, AS patients with spinal fractures have much higher morbidity than other spine fracture patients. There is a greater risk of neurologic and pulmonary complications as well as death.

Imaging Studies

The most universal plain radiographic finding in patients with seronegative spondylo-arthropathies is the presence of sacroiliitis on the pelvic imaging. In more advanced

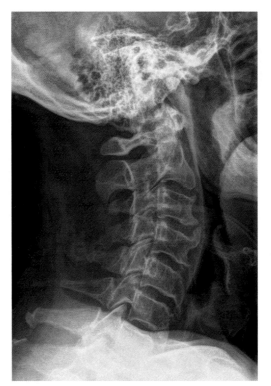

Fig. 7: Lateral radiograph of patient with diffuse idiopathic skeletal hyperostosis (DISH) showing the characteristic large anterior flowing syndesmophytes

cases the sacroiliac joints become ankylosed. The formation of anterior syndesmophytes is commonly seen in this group of disorders on plain spine radiographs. The most characteristic radiographic findings occur with DISH and AS. In DISH the patient develops large anterior, nonmarginal syndesmophytes that limit range of motion as demonstrated in Figure 7. When found in the cervical spine these syndesmophytes can lead to dysphasia or stridor. Four contiguous vertebral bodies need to be affected for a proper diagnosis of DISH.

Plain radiographs of the spine in patients with AS show thin, marginal syndesmophytes that lead to a characteristic bamboo spine appearance as demonstrated in Figures 8A and B. Over time the spine becomes gradually forward flexed and completely ankylosed in more advanced cases. Full length scoliosis radiographs are useful to better assess for sagittal balance in these cases.

In most cases advanced imaging is reserved for evaluation of neurologic deficits or after trauma. Neurologic findings can be caused by the formation of large syndesmophytes or ossification of the posterior longitudinal ligament that can lead to signs of myelopathy. This can be best evaluated by MRI.

In patients with DISH or AS even minor trauma needs to be carefully evaluated with advanced imaging studies. These rigid spines can become very fragile and at risk for fracture. In some cases the fractures can be very obvious as in Figures 9A to C.

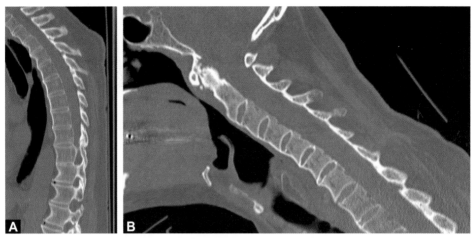

Figs 8A and B: (A) Lateral radiograph of the thoracic and (B) cervical spine of a patient with ankylosing spondylitis (AS) showing the characteristic thin, marginal syndesmophytes and bamboo spine appearance. Additionally, the cervical image shows the forward flexed posture that becomes fixed with more advanced cases

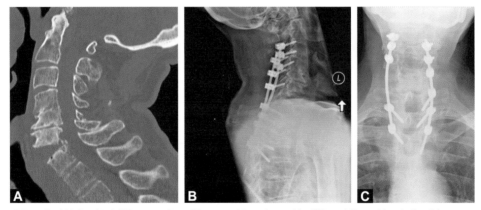

Figs 9A to C: (A) Sagittal CT scan of an 88-year-old patient with diffuse idiopathic skeletal hyperostosis (DISH) after a fall down the stairs that revealed a hyperextension injury at the C6-C7 level. The patient underwent a reduction and posterior instrumented fusion from C3-T2 as shown in the (B) postoperative lateral and (C) anteroposterior (AP) radiographs

Nonoperative Treatment

The primary goals of treatment of patients with seronegative spondyloarthropathies are to control pain, maximize range of motion, reduce deformity and maintain function. This involves a comprehensive program including patient education, medications and physical therapy. Patients should be educated about their disorder including the benefits of exercise and stretching. Patients with AS should be cautioned to avoid the use of multiple pillows while sleeping, which can push the head and neck into further flexion. They should also be warned that any new position or increased range of motion after even minor trauma could represent a fracture in more advanced cases of complete ankylosis. The goals of

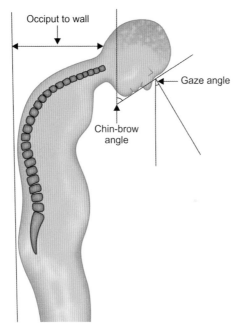

Fig. 10: Diagram of chin-brow angle

physical therapy are to maximize the range of motion in both the spine and peripheral joints. Patients often report less pain and improved function with greater levels of activity. Multiple medication options are available for these patients. NSAIDs and corticosteroids can help reduce the levels of inflammation and help control pain. DMARD's such as anti-TNF-α inhibitors can help slow the course of the disease.

Operative Treatment

Operative management of patients with seronegative spondyloarthropathies is typically reserved for cases of progressive deformity, neurologic deficits and trauma. Patients with AS can develop a progressive forward flexed deformity that can lead to a fixed chin on chest deformity. This can interfere with hygiene, eating, and ability to ambulate and function independently. This can be measured using the chin-brow to vertical angle as shown in Figure 10. Surgical intervention involves performing osteotomies and fusions to realign the spine in a more functional position. In cases of cervical flexion deformities a pedicle subtraction osteotomy can be performed at either C7 or T1 depending on the location of the vertebral arteries. In cases of global positive sagittal imbalance lumbar pedicle subtraction osteotomy can be performed to restore sagittal balance as shown in Figures 11A to D.

As discussed previously, patients can sustain fractures even with minor trauma due to the relative fragility of the spine. A high level of suspicion is necessary to identify these injuries. In patients with AS the fractures are treated more like a long bone fracture in that they require multiple points of fixation on both sides of the fracture site. This is because of the long lever arms that are created by the spinal segments being ankylosed.

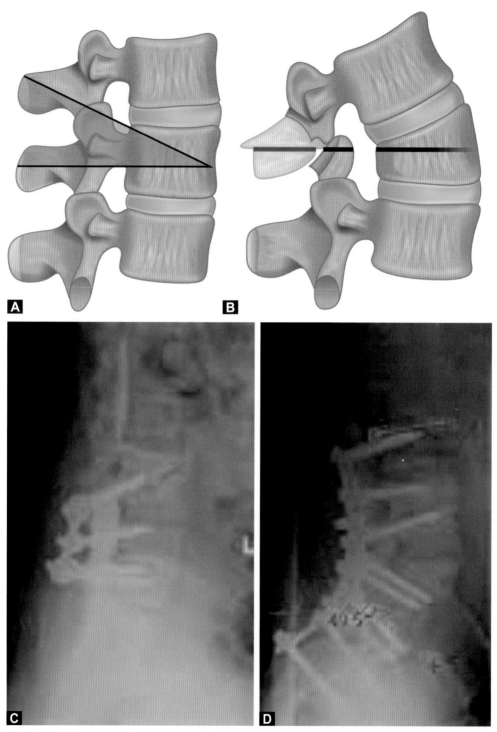

Figs 11A to D: Illustration of the pedicle subtraction osteotomy where the pedicles of a vertebra along with a wedge of vertebral body can be removed and closed down to restore between 20° and 40° of lordosis per level

REFERENCES

1. Panayi GS. The immunopathogenesis of rheumatoid arthritis. Br J Rheumatol. 1993;32 (Suppl 1):4-14.
2. Reiter MF, Boden SD. Inflammatory disorders of the cervical spine. Spine. 1998;23(24):2755-66.
3. Rana NA, Hancock DO, Taylor AR, et al. Atlanto-axial subluxation in rheumatoid arthritis. J Bone Joint Surg Br. 1973;55(3):458-70.
4. Weissman BN, Aliabadi P, Weinfeld MS, et al. Prognostic features of atlantoaxial subluxation in rheumatoid arthritis patients. Radiology. 1982;144(4):745-51.
5. Arnett FC, Edworthy SM, Block DA, et al. The American Rheumatism Association 1987 revised criteria for the classification of rheumatoid arthritis. Arthritis Rheum. 1988;31(3):315-24.
6. Ranawat CS, O'Leary P, Pellicci P, et al. Cervical spine fusion in rheumatoid arthritis. J Bone Joint Surg Am. 1979;61(7):1003-10.
7. Bland JH, Van Buskirk FW, Tampas JP, et al. A study of roentgenographic criteria for rheumatoid arthritis of the cervical spine. AJR Am J Roentgenol. 1965;95(4):949-54.
8. Boden SD, Dodge LD, Bohlman HH, et al. Rheumatoid arthritis of the cervical spine: A long term analysis with predictors of paralysis and recovery. J Bone Joint Surg Am. 1993;75(9):1282-97.
9. Schlosstein L, Terasaki PI, Bluestone R, et al. High association of an HL antigen, W27, with ankylosing spondylitis. N Engl J Med. 1973;288(14):704-6.

CHAPTER

16

Osteoporosis of the Spine

☞ INTRODUCTION

Osteoporosis is the most common metabolic bone disorder affecting the spine. Its effects vary greatly depending on the severity of the disease but can include generalized or localized back pain, vertebral compression fractures, progressive kyphosis or scoliosis, pulmonary dysfunction and cardiac compromise. The prevalence of osteoporosis continues to rise as the population ages. In 1989, there were an estimated 700,000 osteoporotic vertebral compressions annually in the United States.[1,2] Approximately, 26% of women over the age of 50 years and 40% of women over the age of 80 years were reported to have sustained a vertebral compression fracture.[1,3] In 2011, 10 million individuals over the age of 50 years were reported to have osteoporosis, with an additional 34 million with osteopenia.[4] By 2020, the numbers are expected to rise to 14 million with osteoporosis and 47 million with osteopenia. The direct medical costs of osteoporosis in the United States ranged from $17.3 to $20.3 billion in 2005, and are expected to rise to $25.3 billion by 2025.[5]

Due to its widespread occurrence and associated cost to society, it is crucial for the spine specialist to have an understanding of the underlying bone biology that leads to the disorder as well as the appropriate medical and surgical treatment options. This chapter provides an overview of normal bone biology as well as the pathophysiology associated with osteoporosis. Patient presentation and the appropriate medical workup and imaging evaluation will be reviewed, followed by medical and surgical treatment options.

☞ BONE BIOLOGY

The normal functions of bone can be divided into structural and physiologic categories. The structural functions of bone include providing a structural scaffold for the body, giving the body shape, providing an attachment site for muscles, tendons and ligaments and protecting the underlying internal organs. The physiologic functions of bone include hematopoiesis, storage site for calcium, phosphate and other minerals, and regulation of extracellular calcium concentration.

Bone is a dynamic structure that is constantly being formed, resorbed and remodeled in response to mechanical stress and physiologic and biochemical demands. This progress is made possible through the interaction of three types of bone cells: (1) osteoclasts,

(2) osteoblasts and (3) osteocytes. Osteoclasts are multinucleated giant cells that are primarily responsible for the resorption of bone. They release protons that lower the local pH, activate acid proteases and degrade the extracellular matrix of bone. They have surface receptors for and act in response to calcitonin, colchicine, interlukin-1, interlukin-6, prostaglandin E_2 and γ-interferon. Osteoclasts do not have receptors for parathyroid hormone (PTH) or 1,25-dihydroxyvitamin D_3. Instead, the osteoclasts act in a paracrine response to these cells through inhibition of resorption by osteoblastic cells.

Osteoblasts are the cells responsible for forming bone. They are active in protein synthesis and secrete unmineralized bone matrix known as osteoid. They also help to control the transport of calcium and phosphate in and out of bone cells. They have high concentrations of alkaline phosphatase and can produce Type I collagen and osteocalcin. They have surface receptors for PTH and 1,25-dihydroxyvitamin D_3. Osteoblasts respond to these cells and in turn regulate both phases of bone remodeling by inhibiting osteoclastic bone resorption and by controlling bone formation.

An osteocyte is the mature bone cell that forms after the osteoid secreted by the osteoblast becomes mineralized. They have numerous cell processes that act to communicate with other osteocytes and osteoblasts.

The extracellular matrix of bone is composed of water, collagen and hydroxyapatite crystals formed from calcium and phosphate. The hydroxyapatite provides the rigidity and compressive strength to bone.

Parathyroid hormone plays an active role in bone metabolism and acts in response to serum calcium levels. If the serum calcium levels are low, PTH acts on the osteoblasts, as well as the kidneys to increase the flow of calcium back into the serum partially through increased bone resorption. Vitamin D is converted to 25-hydroxyvitamin D_3 in the liver and subsequently to 1,25-dihydroxyvitamin D_3 in the kidneys. This is the active form of vitamin D, and it plays a role in the synthesis of calcium-binding proteins that increase the ability to absorb calcium during digestion. The conversion to its active form in the kidneys is regulated by PTH. Calcitonin is a hormone secreted by the thyroid gland in response to elevated serum calcium levels and acts to inhibit osteoclasts to prevent further release of calcium. The roles of PTH, vitamin D and calcitonin in the medical treatment of osteoporosis has been discussed later in the chapter.

The spine is often one of the first areas of the skeleton to be affected by osteoporosis. This is largely due to the relative composition of cortical and trabecular bone in the spine. Cortical bone is the strong, dense outer layer of bone, while trabecular bone is the less dense inner portion of bone. Trabecular bone is metabolized at a rate eight times faster than cortical bone.[6] In the appendicular skeleton the ratio of cortical to trabecular bone is approximately 4:1, while in the spine the ratio is 1:2.[6,7] As a result the loss of trabecular bone mass associated with osteoporosis has a greater effect on the vertebrae than the appendicular skeleton due the greater percentage of trabecular bone. Osteoporosis can lead to a marked loss of trabecular bone mass and subsequent loss of strength in the vertebrae as shown in Figures 1A and B.

Previous investigators have attempted to determine how the normal architecture of the vertebrae is altered with osteoporosis. Thomsen et al. identified that there is a greater loss of horizontal versus vertical trabecular bone is patients with osteoporosis.[8] However, in a study

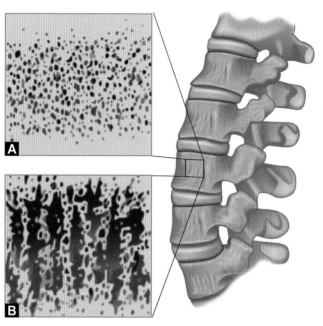

Figs 1A and B: (A) Diagram of normal and (B) osteoporotic vertebral body showing the loss of trabecular bone associated with osteoporosis

of isolated trabecular bone, the fracture of vertical trabeculae was found to contribute more to the overall mechanical strength of the bone than the bone volume fraction of the bone.[9] In a study on the failure characteristics of trabecular bone the vertical trabeculae were found to fail most commonly due to the fact that they sustained a greater portion of the applied loads.[10] Fields et al. investigated the influence of vertical trabeculae on the compressive strength of human vertebrae using high-resolution microcomputed tomography and microfinite element analysis and determined that the bone volume fraction of the vertical trabeculae accounted for substantially more of the compressive strength than the bone volume fracture of all trabeculae ($r^2 = 0.83$ vs 0.59, $p < 0.005$).[11] Finite element analysis showed that removal of the cortical shell did not appreciably alter these results, and that the major load pathways occurred through parallel columns of vertically oriented bone. As a result, it was determined that the variation in compressive strength of vertebrae is primarily due to variation in the bone volume fraction of vertical trabeculae ($r^2 = 0.93$). This is a stronger predictor than previous studies that have reported on measurements of bone mineral content through bone mineral density using dual-energy X-ray absorptiometry (DEXA) scans ($r^2 = 0.86$).[6]

☞ PATHOPHYSIOLOGY

Osteoporosis results from an imbalance in the normal mechanism of bone remodeling that leads to a decrease in bone strength and subsequent increased risk for fracture. An individual typically achieves a peak level of bone mass between the ages of 18 and 25 years. There are numerous factors that affect the value of an individual's peak bone mass including

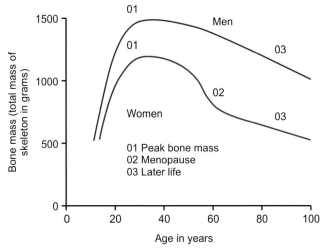

Fig. 2: Graph of bone mass as a function of age for men and women. Note that women have a lower peak bone mass than men, and that after menopause women have a more rapid decline in bone mass due to estrogen deficiency. This explains the higher rates of osteoporosis in women than men

genetics, nutrition, endocrine abnormalities, physical activity, smoking and generalized health.[12] More than 20 specific genes have been identified that play a role in the development of osteoporosis and have been shown to contribute to up to 80% of the variation in peak bone mass in twin studies.[13]

Osteoporosis can occur either through an individual's failure to achieve a normal peak bone mass or through excessive bone resorption. It is well known that postmenopausal women are at the greatest risk of developing osteoporosis due to estrogen deficiency. The deficiency in estrogen results in a more marked decrease in bone mass as shown in Figure 2.

PATIENT PRESENTATION

In most cases the patient with osteoporosis is initially asymptomatic prior to diagnosis. The onset of pain associated with a fracture is often the first indication that a patient has osteoporosis. Unfortunately, even after a patient sustains a fracture they often remain undiagnosed due to failure of the treating physicians to perform a proper evaluation. It is the responsibility of the physician to identify risk factors, recognize a potential osteoporotic fracture and perform the appropriate screening evaluation to identify osteoporosis.

Osteopenia, or low bone density, is a precursor to osteoporosis and has been shown to be a risk factor for the development of osteoporosis and osteoporotic fractures.[14] There are numerous biologic and lifestyle factors that increase the risk for osteoporosis and osteoporosis-related fractures as summarized in Table 1. Osteoporosis can be either primary or secondary. Primary osteoporosis does not have an identifiable cause, while secondary osteoporosis results from another coexisting disorder. Table 1 lists many other diseases that can lead to the development of secondary osteoporosis.

Table 1: Summary of risk factors for developing osteoporosis or osteoporosis-related fractures
Biologic risk factors
Low bone mass (osteopenia)
Older age
Female gender
Rheumatic and autoimmune disorders (ankylosing spondylitis, lupus, rheumatoid arthritis)
History of fracture as an adult
Parental history of fracture
Family history of bone disease
Ethnicity
Small, thin stature
Hypogonadal disorders (androgen insensitivity, hyperprolactinemia, premature ovarian failure, athletic amenorrhea)
Hematologic disorders (hemophilia, sickle cell disease, thalassemia, leukemia, lymphoma)
Genetic disorders (cystic fibrosis, hemochromatosis, glycogen storage diseases, porphyria, homocystinuria, hypophosphatemia)
Endocrine disorders (adrenal insufficiency, diabetes mellitus, Cushing's syndrome, hyperparathyroidism, hypothyroidism, thyrotoxicosis)
Gastrointestinal disorders (celiac disease, gastric bypass, malabsorption, pancreatic disease, primary biliary cirrhosis, inflammatory bowel disease)
Weight loss of more than 1% per year in the elderly
Late onset of sexual development
Height loss or progressive spinal curvature
Medications (anticoagulants, anticonvulsants, barbiturates, chemotherapy, glucocorticoids, gonadotropin-releasing hormone agents, immunosuppressants, lithium, long-acting progestin, proton-pump inhibitors)
Lifestyle risk factors
Smoking
Low calcium intake
Vitamin D deficiency
Alcohol (> 3 drinks daily)
Inadequate physical activity
Low body mass index
High caffeine intake

When a patient presents with a suspected osteoporotic fracture the medical history can provide some important information for diagnosis. A complete list of past medical problems, family medical history, ethnicity, smoking status, diet, exercise or activity level and medications can identify many potential risk factors for osteoporosis. In most cases osteoporosis-related fractures occur following a minor trauma or no trauma at all. The patient may not be able to recall any specific inciting event prior to his or her onset of pain. As a result fracture without trauma is a potential warning sign for osteoporosis. Any change in the patient's height, posture, or balance should be investigated. Vertebral compression fractures cause a loss of height as well as increased thoracic kyphosis. This hyperkyphosis can result in a positive sagittal balance and place the patient at a higher risk for subsequent falls and further injury. Any history of previous fractures and their causes should be identified. A history of multiple fractures with minimal trauma suggests a potential problem with the strength of the bone.

The physical examination should assess for any abnormal spinal curvature or areas of tenderness to palpation. A complete neurologic evaluation should be performed to assess for any motor or sensory deficits. Typical osteoporotic vertebral compression fractures do not result in neural compromise, so neurologic findings are not commonly found. The results of the history and physical examination can help direct the physician to order the most appropriate laboratory and imaging studies.

🖝 LABORATORY STUDIES

Due to the fact that there are numerous primary and secondary causes of osteoporosis there are many potential laboratory studies that can help identify or confirm a diagnosis as summarized in Table 2. These can assess for hematologic disorders, electrolyte imbalances, and renal or hepatic dysfunction. While the ordering and interpretation of these laboratory studies may fall outside the realm of the spine specialist it is important to have an understanding of their role and be able to refer the patient to the appropriate care provider for this evaluation if necessary.

Table 2: Laboratory studies to identify potential causes of osteoporosis
Complete blood count (CBC)
Electrolytes
Creatinine
Blood urea nitrogen (BUN)
Calcium
Phosphorus
Total protein
Albumin and prealbumin
Alkaline phosphatase
Liver enzymes (LFT)
24-hour urinary calcium
Serum and urine protein electrophoresis (SPEP/UPEP)
Thyroid function tests
Prolactin
Parathyroid hormone (PTH)
25-Hydroxyvitamin D_3
1,25-Dihydroxyvitamin D_3
Osteocalcin

☞ IMAGING STUDIES

Plain Radiographs

The radiographic evaluation of the patient with a suspected osteoporotic fracture typically begins with a plain radiograph of the symptomatic site to assess for a fracture. An anteroposterior (AP) and lateral view of the spine is often sufficient to identify a fracture. In a healed compression fracture the fracture fragments are often more rounded or there may be an autofusion with the adjacent vertebra. However, it is not always possible to determine the acuity of the fracture on plain radiographs alone. The age of the fracture is better determined by either a bone scan or magnetic resonance imaging (MRI) which would reveal increased uptake and edema, respectively, in an acute fracture. It is often difficult to determine the precise level of the fracture in the thoracic spine with plain radiographs alone. Also it may not be possible to determine the presence of osteoporosis on plain radiographs as up to 25–50% loss of bone mass is necessary to identify this.

If a fracture is identified it is important to differentiate the type of fracture. In patients with osteoporosis the most common spine fracture is a vertebral compression fracture as shown in Figures 3A and B. This involves a compression of the anterior and possibly middle column of the spine without disruption of the posterior cortex of the vertebral body or

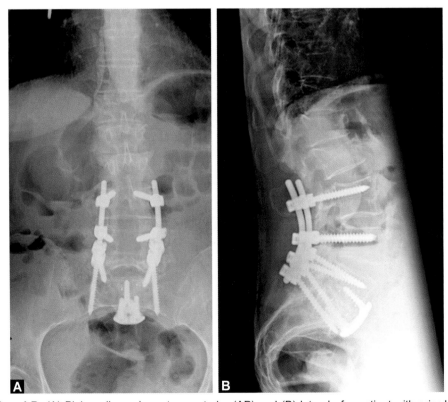

Figs 3A and B: (A) Plain radiographs anteroposterior (AP) and (B) lateral of a patient with prior L3-S1 instrumented fusion who sustained vertebral compression fractures from osteoporosis at T12, L1 and L2

Essentials of Spinal Disorders

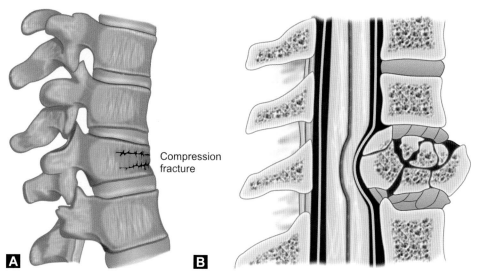

Figs 4A and B: Diagram of (A) vertebral compression fracture and (B) burst fracture. Note that the burst fracture involves a disruption of the posterior cortex of the vertebral body while the compression fracture does not

involvement of the posterior elements. As a result these are stable fractures and should be differentiated from a burst fracture that involves disruption of the posterior cortex of the vertebral body and possible involvement of the posterior elements as shown in Figures 4A and B. On the AP radiograph the horizontal distance between the pedicles should gradually increase with each more caudal level. In the case of a burst fracture the distance between the pedicles is typically widened more than the distance at the neighboring levels. In some cases this differentiation may not be possible without axial imaging studies.

In addition to the fracture, many other findings may be present on the plain radiographs including increased kyphosis, degenerative scoliosis, degenerative disk disease and spondylolisthesis. These other findings could contribute to the patient's symptoms and need to be considered prior to treatment.

Magnetic Resonance Imaging

An MRI is a useful modality for evaluation of a patient with a suspected osteoporotic fracture. With an acute fracture of less than 3-month duration there will be increased edema at the site of the fracture in response to the increased blood flow that occurs as part of the healing process as shown in Figures 5A to C. Disruption of the posterior cortex of the vertebral body is also more definitive with MRI as compared to plain radiographs. Other potential pain generators including stenosis, degenerative disk disease and spondylolisthesis can also be identified.

Even in a patient with a vertebral compression fracture and a known history of osteoporosis, it is crucial to verify there is not another potential cause of the fracture. Vertebral compression fractures from metastatic disease, lymphoma or multiple myeloma can have a very similar appearance on imaging studies. In many cases of metastasis to the spine, there will be more extensive bone destruction and neighboring soft tissue involvement. Often a vertebral biopsy is necessary to make a definitive diagnosis.

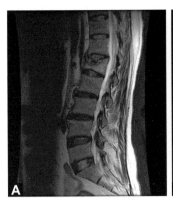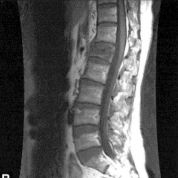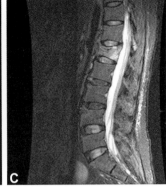

Figs 5A to C: MRI of a patient with an L1 osteoporotic compression fracture. There is a typically wedge deformity of the vertebral body without disruption of the posterior cortex of the vertebral body. (A) The T2-weighted image shows an increased signal intensity and (B) the T1-weighted image shows decreased signal intensity; (C) STIR image is often more sensitive to the presence of a fracture and shows a more pronounced change in signal intensity

Computed Tomography

Computed tomography (CT) can also provide axial imaging of the spine and is useful to distinguish between a vertebral compression fracture and a burst fracture. It provides more detail than the plain radiograph but may not be able to definitively distinguish between an acute versus chronic fracture. As with MRI, it can assess for other spinal disorders including stenosis, degenerative disk disease and spondylolisthesis. CT is a good alternative for patients who are unable to obtain an MRI.

Bone Densitometry

One of the most commonly performed imaging studies for the identification of osteoporosis is bone densitometry. This includes both dual-energy X-ray absorptiometry (DEXA) and dual-energy quantitative CT (QCT). With QCT a lateral CT is obtained of 2–4 lumbar vertebrae, and a quantitative measurement of the trabecular bone is obtained. This value is compared with known values to determine the relative amount of loss of bone mass compared to normal. Only approximately one-tenth of the radiation of a typical CT scan is required for the QCT, and it takes about 20 minutes to perform.[15] The DEXA scan has become the gold standard for the diagnosis of osteoporosis. With DEXA, an X-ray beam is emitted that can assess for the mineral content of the scanned bone divided by its surface area. This value is compared to normal scores for a young, healthy adult of the same gender to provide the T-score. The DEXA value is also compared to the age- and gender-matched population to provide the Z-score. These two scores provide a measurement of the number of standard deviations from the control population. These scans are often obtained of the lumbar spine, hip, distal radius and calcaneus. Caution should be used for values obtained from a spine with deformity as the overlap of the vertebrae can lead to a falsely elevated reading. The World Health Organization (WHO) provides guidelines for the diagnosis of osteopenia and osteoporosis as shown in Table 3.

Table 3: World Health Organization guidelines for the diagnosis of osteoporosis

Diagnosis	DEXA score	Description
Normal bone mass	T-score ≥ -1	Bone density not more than 1 standard deviation below the mean for a young adult of the same gender
Osteopenia	T-score between -1.0 and -2.5	Bone density between 1 and 2.5 standard deviations below the mean for a young adult of the same gender
Osteoporosis	T-score < -2.5	Bone density more than 2.5 standard deviations below the mean for a young adult of the same gender
Established or severe osteoporosis	T-score < -2.5	Osteoporosis plus the presence of one or more fragility fractures

Table 4: Recommendations for screening individuals for osteoporosis based on gender, age and potential risk factors

National Osteoporosis Foundation	U.S. Preventative Services Task Force	American Association of Clinical Endocrinologists
Women > 65 years Men > 70 years Regardless of risk factors	Women > 65 years with previous fracture or risk factors	Women > 65 years
Postmenopausal women and men 50–59 years with risk factors	Women < 65 years with risk factors	Postmenopausal women with history of fracture, radiographic evidence of osteopenia or on steroid treatment
Perimenopausal women with risk factors	No screening recommended for men	Perimenopausal or postmenopausal women with risk factors
Patients > 50 years with a previous fracture		Secondary osteoporosis
Patients with medical disorder or taking medications associated with low bone mass		No screening recommended for men
Patients being considered for pharmacologic treatment of osteoporosis		
Postmenopausal women discontinuing estrogen		

Screening Recommendations

There are numerous different organizations that have provided recommendations for screening individuals for osteoporosis based on age, gender and potential risk factors. There is some discrepancy among these recommendations as shown in Table 4. In addition, the WHO task force has developed a country-specific tool to identify individuals at high risk for osteoporosis-related fractures called the fracture risk assessment tool (FRAX).[16] This

Table 5: Recommended daily allowance of calcium

Age	Calcium intake (mg/day)
Infants	
Birth to 6 months	210
6 months to 1 year	270
Children	
1–3 years	500
4–8 years	800
9–13 years	1,300
Young adults	
14–50 years	1,000
Adults	
51 and older	1,200
Pregnancy	
< 18 years	1,300
19–50 years	1,000
Lactation	
< 18 years	1,300
19–50 years	1,000

tool combines data from clinical risk factors and bone density measurements to determine a 10-year relative risk of a patient sustaining a hip fracture or major osteoporotic fracture of the hip, spine, humerus or wrist.

In addition to these clinical guidelines for screening, patients being considered for instrumented spinal fusion with risk factors for osteoporosis should potentially undergo screening. Patients with low bone density have a higher risk of instrumentation failure or pullout of screws and adjacent level fragility fractures. This needs to be carefully considered prior to proceeding with surgery in these patients.

NONOPERATIVE MANAGEMENT

The first management option for osteoporosis to be considered is prevention. Low bone mass associated with osteoporosis is a function of both an inability to achieve a high enough peak bone mass as a young adult and an excessive amount of loss of bone mass later in adult life. Maximizing the peak bone mass in young adults can reduce their later risk of developing osteoporosis. This includes focusing on adequate nutrition, smoking cessation, avoiding excessive alcohol intake and physical exercise. The optimal daily recommended allowance of calcium for various age groups is summarized in Table 5. This should be combined with at least 800–1,000 IU of vitamin D daily.

There are numerous pharmacologic options available for the treatment of patients with osteoporosis. While the administration of these medications does not typically fall to the spine specialist, it is important to have an understanding of these medications, their mechanisms, and know when to recommend potential treatment. Table 6 provides an overview of the various classes of medications for osteoporosis.[17,18]

Table 6: Pharmacologic treatment options for osteoporosis		
Category	Mechanism	Reported efficacy
Bisphosphonates	Reduces resorptive activity of osteoclasts	Reduced vertebral fractures 50–70%; maximum effect in 3–36 months
Selective estrogen receptor modulator (SERM)	Inhibits bone resorption	Reduced vertebral fractures by 35%
Recombinant human parathyroid hormone (PTH)	Reduces osteoblastic apoptosis and increases number of osteoblasts	Reduced vertebral fractures by 65%
PTH analogs	Reduces osteoblastic apoptosis and increases number of osteoblasts	Reduced vertebral fractures by 47%
Strontium	Inhibits bone resorption Increases bone formation	Reduced vertebral fractures by 40%
Humanized monoclonal antibody (Denosumab)	Inhibits osteoclast formation	Reduced vertebral fractures 68%

For patients that develop osteoporotic vertebral compression fracture, many can be treated successfully with nonoperative measures. These can include pain medications, activity modification and in some cases short-term bracing. Narcotic medications should be used very cautiously or avoided in these patients due to the increased risk of falling and constipation in this patient population. Bracing is not typically necessary from a structural perspective, but can assist with immobilization of the fracture and pain control. The pain associated with vertebral compression fractures gradually dissipates as the fracture heals over a period of approximately 3 months. Bracing should only be used during the initial 3 months from the time of the fracture to avoid further muscle deconditioning beyond that point.

OPERATIVE MANAGEMENT

Fortunately, operative management of osteoporotic vertebral compression fractures is often not required. These patients typically are older and have various medical comorbidities, and surgery should be avoided if possible. In some cases patients are unable to tolerate the pain with conservative treatment alone. Historically, open fracture stabilization was the only available surgical option for these patients. This had significant associated risks due to patient comorbidities and the risk of instrumentation failure and pullout due to the poor bone quality.

More recently, percutaneous techniques for injection of viscous polymethylmethacrylate (PMMA) cement into the vertebral body were developed.[19] There are two main categories of percutaneous treatment for these fractures including vertebroplasty and kyphoplasty. In vertebroplasty, less viscous cement is injected and fills the gaps in the trabecular bone. In kyphoplasty, a cavity is created by inflation of a percutaneously-placed balloon, and the cement is then injected in a more viscous state into the cavity as shown in Figures 6A to E. Potential risk factors for these techniques include cement leakage, adjacent level compression fracture, infection, pulmonary embolus, hypoxia and pneumonia.

Table 7: Reported benefits and drawbacks of vertebroplasty and kyphoplasty		
	Vertebroplasty	*Kyphoplasty*
Cost	Less expensive	More expensive
Fracture height reduction	Less fracture reduction	Improved fracture reduction
Cement leakage	Increased risk (19.7%)	Reduced risk (7.0%)
Adjacent level fracture	Increased risk (17.9%)	Reduced risk (14.1%)

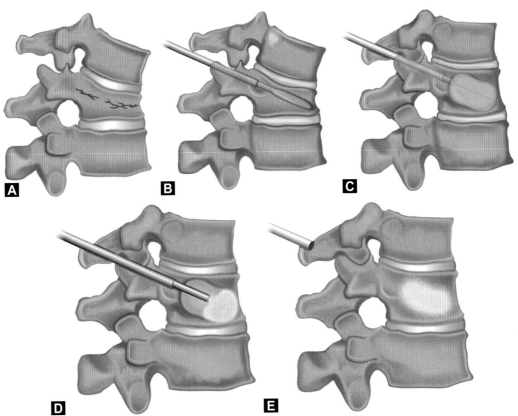

Figs 6A to E: Illustration of the kyphoplasty technique. (A) Patient develops a vertebral compression fracture; (B) Needle is passed through the pedicle, and a balloon is inserted; (C) Balloon is inflated in vertebral body, partially restoring the normal shape; (D) Balloon is deflated which creates a cavity in the vertebral body, and the cement is injected; (E) The needle is then removed

A previous meta-analysis compared the efficacy and limitations of vertebroplasty versus kyphoplasty for the treatment of vertebral compression fractures, and the relative benefits and drawbacks of each technique are summarized in Table 7.[20]

While the majority of vertebral augmentation techniques use PMMA, there are more recent reports of using alternative substances including bioactive substances.[21] Vertebroplasty using both substances was found to provide effective pain relief, but the bioactive substance was reported to have better pain relief at 3 months and improved function at 24 months. Additional studies are needed to further investigate the utility of these substances.

As mentioned previously in this chapter the other instance in which osteoporosis becomes a major issue for the spine surgeon is when an instrumented fusion is being planned. Due to the poor bone quality there is an increased risk for adjacent level fragility fractures and screw pullout in patients with osteoporosis. Numerous attempts have been made to reduce these risks including vertebral augmentation at the ends of the instrumentation construct and adjacent levels, expandable pedicle screws, hydroxyapatite-coated pedicle screws, and fenestrated pedicle screws to allow for injection of cement through the screws.[22-25] While most of these techniques have been shown to provide increased biomechanical stability, this remains a very challenging patient population, and additional work is needed to improve outcomes with reduced risks.

REFERENCES

1. Melton LJ, Kan SH, Frye MA, et al. Epidemiology of vertebral fractures in women. Am J Epidemiol. 1989;129(5):1000-11.
2. Wasnich RD. Vertebral fracture epidemiology. Bone. 1996;18(3 Suppl):179S-83S.
3. Silverman SL. The clinical consequences of vertebral compression fracture. Bone. 1992;13(Suppl 2): S27-31.
4. Dempster DW. Osteoporosis and the burden of osteoporotic-related fractures. Am J Manag Care. 2011;17:S164-9.
5. Roche JJ, Wenn RT, Sahota O, et al. Effect of comorbidities and postoperative complications on mortality after hip fracture in elderly people: prospective observational cohort study. BMJ. 2005;331(7529):1374.
6. Einhorn TA. Osteoporosis and metabolic bone disease. Adv Orthop Surg. 1984;8:175-84.
7. Hansson T, Roos B, Nachemson A. The bone mineral content and ultimate compressive strength of lumbar vertebrae. Spine. 1980;5:46-55.
8. Thomsen JS, Ebbsen EN, Mosekilde L. Age-related differences between thinning if horizontal and vertical trabeculae in human lumbar bone as assessed by a new computerized method. Bone. 2002;31(1):136-42.
9. Liu XS, Sajda P, Saha PK, et al. Complete volumetric decomposition of individual trabecular plates and rods and its morphological correlations with anisotropic elastic moduli in human trabecular bone. J Bone Miner Res. 2008;23:223-35.
10. Liu XS, Bevill G, Keaveny TM, et al. Micromechanical analysis of vertebral trabecular bone nased on individual trabecular segmentation of plates and rods. J Biomech. 2009;42:249-56.
11. Fields AJ, Lee GL, Liu XS, et al. Influence of vertical trabeculae on the compressive strength of the human vertebra. J Bone Miner Res. 2011;26(2):263-9.
12. Becker DJ, Kilgore ML, Morrisey MA. The societal burden of osteoporosis. Curr Rheumatol Rep. 2010;12(3):186-91.
13. Ralston SH, Uitterlinden AG. Genetics of osteoporosis. Endocr Rev. 2010;31:629-62.
14. Khosla S, Melton LJ. Osteopenia. N Engl J Med. 2007;356(22):2293-300.
15. Johnston CC, Slemenda CW, Melton LJ. Clinical use of bone densitometry. N Engl J Med. 1991;342:1105-9.
16. Kanis JA, Johnell O, Oden A, et al. FRAX and the assessment of fracture possibility in men and women from the UK. Osteoporos Int. 2008;19:385-97.
17. Langdahl BL, Rajzbaum G, Jakob, et al. Reduction in fracture rate and back pain and increased quality of life in postmenopausal women treated with teriparatide: 18-month data from the European Forteo Observational Study (FEOS). Calcif Tissue Int. 2009;85(6):484-93.

18. Sandhu SK, Hampson G. The pathogenesis, diagnosis, investigation and management of osteoporosis. J Clin Pathol. 2011;64:1042-50.

19. Gailbert P, Deramond H, Rosat P, et al. Preliminary note on the treatment of vertebral angioma by percutaneous acrylic vertebroplasty. Neurochirurgie. 1987;33:166-8.

20. Eck JC, Nachtigall D, Humphreys SC, et al. Comparison of vertebroplasty and balloon kyphoplasty for treatment of vertebral compression fractures: a meta-analysis of the literature. Spine J. 2008;8:488-97.

21. Bae H, Hatten HP, Linovitz R, et al. A prospective randomized FDA-IDE trial comparing Cortoss to PMMA for vertebroplasty: a comparative effectiveness research study with 24-months follow-up. Spine. 2012;37(7):544-50.

22. Gao M, Lei W, Wu Z, et al. Biomechanical evaluation of fixation strength of conventional and expandable pedicle screw with or without calcium based cement augmentation. Clin Biomech (Bristol, Avon). 2011;26(3):238-44.

23. Hasegawa T, Inufusa A, Imai Y, et al. Hydroxyaptite-coating of pedicle screws improves resistance against pull-out force in the osteoporotic canine lumbar spine model: a pilot study. Spine J. 2005;5(3):239-43.

24. Ponnusamy KE, Iyer S, Gupta G, et al. Instrumentation of the osteoporotic spine: biomechanical and clinical considerations. Spine J. 2011;11(1):54-63.

25. Vishnubhotla S, McGarry WB, Mahar AT, et al. A titanium expandable pedicle screw improves initial pullout strength as compared with standard pedicle screws. Spine J. 2011;11(8):777-81.

17

Spinal Infections

☞ INTRODUCTION

Fortunately, infections of the spine are relatively uncommon, but they are increasing in frequency. This increase in prevalence of spinal infections is likely due to an increase in invasive spinal procedures, increasing age of the population and increased rate of immunocompromised patients. Spinal infections can be difficult to diagnose due to their insidious onset and initial vague symptoms. This often leads to a delay in diagnosis. As a result a high level of suspicion is necessary for prompt diagnosis and initiation of the appropriate treatment.

There are numerous methods to classify spinal infection based on different factors, including pathogen, anatomic location and patient's age. The pathogen-based classification of spinal infections is the most common. Most bacteria cause a pyogenic response that result from either a hematogenous spread or contiguous/direct spread. In contrast, a granulomatous reaction occurs with infections from *Mycobacterium*, fungi, *Brucella* and syphilis. Categorizing spinal infection based on their anatomic location is also common. Infection of the disk space is referred to as discitis, infection of the vertebral body is vertebral osteomyelitis and a combination of both is called spondylodiscitis or vertebral osteodiscitis. An epidural abscess occurs in the epidural space and has the greatest propensity for neurologic symptoms. The final criterion used to classify spinal infection is the patient's age. This method separates infections for children versus adults due to their variation in pathogenesis and treatment.

This chapter reviews the important features of spinal infection including patho-physiology, patient presentation and evaluation, and nonoperative and operative management options. A clear understanding of this information will allow the clinician to recognize and appropriately manage this patient population.

☞ PATHOPHYSIOLOGY

The majority of spinal infections are pyogenic infections that spread to the spine either through a hematogenous or direct route. Hematogenous spread results from bacteremia from a distant and unrelated infection spreading through the bloodstream to the spine.

Table 1: Summary of bacterial pathogens associated with pyogenic spinal infections	
Pathogen	Findings
Staphylococcus aureus	Most common (methicilin resistance becoming more common)
Pseudomonas	More common in intravenous drug users
Escherichia coli	More frequent from genitourinary spread
Klebsiella	More frequent from genitourinary spread
Proteus	More frequent from genitourinary spread
Salmonella	More frequent in patients with sickle cell disease or acute intestinal infection
Bartonella henselae	More frequent in children with cat-scratch disease
Staphylococcus epidermidis	More frequent in cases with instrumentation of/from normal skin flora
Streptococcus	More frequent in cases with instrumentation
Acinetobacter	More frequent in cases with instrumentation

There are numerous distant sources for infection that have been implicated in causing spinal infections, including dental caries, oral surgery, indwelling catheters, spinal injections or discography, urologic procedures, respiratory tract infections, soft tissue infections and intravenous drug use. Despite numerous potential sources of infection, in up to 37% of cases, the underlying source cannot be identified.[1] Numerous bacterial pathogens have been reported in spinal infections as summarized in Table 1.[2,3]

The majority of spinal infections occur in the lumbar spine, followed in frequency by the thoracic spine, and most rare in the cervical spine. Despite occurring less frequently in the cervical and thoracic spine, these patients more often present with neurologic findings due to compression of the spinal cord.

The suspected method by which hematogenous spread of bacteria occurs to the spine is directly related to the complex vascular supply to the spine. In children there is a much more abundant arterial supply to the disk space than in adults. This is thought to allow a more direct access to the disk for hematogenous spread of bacteria in children and explain their increased risk of discitis. In adults the nucleus is relatively avascular and receives its nutrition primarily through diffusion across the endplates.[4] The adult vertebral bodies have a rich vascular anastomosis. Spinal arteries have been shown to enter the spinal canal through the foramen at the level of the disk with branches ascending and descending to the neighboring vertebral bodies.[5] Bacteria can enter the vertebral bodies through the metaphyseal regions by this route and spread to neighboring vertebral bodies around the avascular disk through these anastomoses.

Neurologic symptoms related to spinal infections can occur from direct compression from purulent material or epidural abscess, the formation of granulation tissue, or from compression by bone or disk fragments that can occur from associated pathologic fracture. Ischemic injury to the nerves or spinal cord can also occur with spinal infections.[1]

Postoperative spinal infection can occur from seeding of the surgical site at the time of surgery or through spread of bacteria from remote sites. In cases involving placement of spinal instrumentation the bacteria can form a glycocalyx that allows for adherence to the metal and helps protect it from antibiotic treatment. Different metals have been reported to have increased rates of bacterial adherence. Stainless steel implants have been reported to develop higher rates of infection in animal studies with direct bacterial inoculation as compared to titanium implants.[6]

Epidural abscess refers to a spinal infection that leads to an accumulation of purulent fluid or granulation tissue in the epidural space. This is more common in adults and relatively rare in children. It occurs most commonly in the thoracic spine followed in frequency in the lumbar spine and least commonly in the cervical spine.[7] This is likely due to the large potential epidural space found in the thoracic spine compared to the other regions.

The other main category of spinal infections is granulomatous infections. These organisms include *Mycobacterium*, fungi, *Brucella* and syphilis. The most common granulomatous infection is caused by *Mycobacterium tuberculosis*. Approximately, 10% of patients with tuberculosis (TB) develop infections in the bones or joints, with half of those involving the spine.[8,9] Fortunately, due to improved worldwide public health efforts, the incidence of TB is decreasing. The pathogenesis of these infections is similar to pyogenic infection and can occur through hematogenous or direct spread to the spine. There are three main types of spinal involvement with TB. These include paradiscal, central and anterior. Involvement of the posterior elements is much less common. In patients with paradiscal TB the infection enters the vertebral body at the metaphysis and spreads under the anterior longitudinal ligament (ALL) to the adjacent level, sparing the intervening disk. With central involvement the infection enters the middle of the vertebral body and remains isolated to a single vertebra. With anterior involvement the infection spreads under the ALL but spares the vertebral bodies.

PATIENT PRESENTATION

Due to the often insidious onset and mild initial symptoms, there is frequently a delay in diagnosis of spinal infections. Less than one-third of patients are diagnosed within the first month, and the median time until diagnosis is 1.8 months.[10] The most common presenting complaint for patients with spinal infection is a vague back pain. The back pain is typically constant and achy initially. It is often worse at night, but it can be exacerbated with activity as well. Constitutional symptoms including fevers, chills and weight loss can be present. Severe muscle spasms are commonly found. There is often decreased range of motion of the spine, loss of lumbar lordosis and hamstring tightness. An associated psoas abscess can cause painful flexion and extension of the hip. Torticollis may be present with cervical osteomyelitis.

In more advanced cases, destruction of the disks and vertebral bodies can lead to a progressive kyphotic deformity due to pathologic fracture. Neurologic deficits are reported in 17% of cases.[1] In severe cases, patients may present with paralysis. Risk factors for this include diabetes, rheumatoid arthritis, older age and more cephalad level of involvement.[11]

Children with spinal infections differ in presentation compared to adults. Infants can present with high temperatures and septicemia. Young children often present with irritability and difficulty or refusal to ambulate. Older children have more localized tenderness and spinal rigidity.

Postoperative spinal infection typically presents within 1–2 weeks of surgery with increasing back pain that is not controlled by the patient's previous medication plan.

Table 2: Risk factors for developing a spinal infection
Acquired immunodeficiency syndrome (AIDS)
Alcohol abuse
Cancer
Diabetes
Immunosuppression
Indwelling catheters
Male gender
Malnutrition
Obesity
Renal disease
Rheumatoid arthritis
Smoking
Steroid use
Transplant
Trauma

Initially there may be no constitutional symptoms, and the wound may look benign. With further time, the wound will become erythematous, fluctuant and develop drainage. Delayed presentation of up to years after surgery has been reported, but this is rare.

Patients should undergo a complete medical history and physical examination. Potential risk factors for spinal infection can be identified in the medical history and are summarized in Table 2. Physical examination should evaluate for posture and spinal alignment, the presence of any new or progressive deformity, areas of localized tenderness, spinal and hip range of motion and gait pattern. A neurologic examination should look for any deficits.

If spinal infection is suspected, laboratory studies should be obtained, including white blood cell (WBC) count, erythrocyte sedimentation rate (ESR) and C-reactive protein (CRP) level. The WBC count provides little useful information as it is elevated in only a third of patients with a spinal infection. However, it is more commonly elevated in cases of an epidural abscess.[12] The ESR is much more commonly elevated than the WBC, but it is a nonspecific test for inflammation. It can be elevated in cases of pregnancy, malignancy, connective tissue disorders and remote infections. The ESR can become elevated within several days of the onset of infection and peaks at 7–8 days. The ESR should be used cautiously in the postoperative period as it remains elevated for 4–6 weeks after surgery. As a result it has less benefit in identifying postoperative infections. The CRP is also nonspecific and can be elevated with other conditions similar to the ESR. The CRP typically normalizes within 6–10 days following surgery, so it is often a better measure of postoperative infections than the ESR. Blood cultures should also be obtained with suspected infections as there is a high association between blood culture and vertebral culture results.[13]

Biopsy specimens can be obtained from the disk space or vertebral body under computed tomography (CT) guidance. Antibiotics should be withheld until positive blood or tissue cultures have been obtained to determine the most appropriate treatment except in cases of sepsis.

IMAGING STUDIES

The use of imaging studies for the patient with a suspected spinal infection typically begins with plain radiographs. During the initial period the radiographs may be negative as it can take up to 12 weeks to demonstrate changes in adults. In children, however, radiographic change can occur within several weeks with loss of disk height being present. The earliest signs of infection on plain radiographs of spinal infection include loss of disk height and endplate sclerosis (Fig. 1A). Vertebral body destruction or pathologic fracture and kyphotic deformity are late findings.

Computed tomography scan can provide additional osseous detail and identify earlier changes than traditional plain radiographs (Figs 1B to D). It can also be utilized for surgical planning and for guidance with biopsies.

Magnetic resonance imaging (MRI) provides improved visualization of the soft tissues and neurologic structures. It is very sensitive in detecting spinal infection, which leads to endplate and vertebral edema, loss of disk height, canal compromise and vertebral collapse (Fig. 1E). In more advanced cases, patients may develop pathologic fractures with severe kyphotic deformity and canal compromise (Figs 2A to D). MRI is the study of choice in cases of neurologic findings or suspected epidural abscess to determine the degree of canal compromise and cord compression (Figs 3 and 4). Postoperative wound infections can be evaluated with MRI to reveal the presence of a large posterior fluid collection at the site of the surgery (Fig. 5).

Various nuclear medicine imaging studies including technetium-, gallium- and indium-labeled WBC scans can be performed to evaluate for infection, but they are much less commonly performed than the more traditional studies described above.

NONOPERATIVE TREATMENT

Nonoperative treatment for patients with spinal infection can be effective in many cases. In children, intravenous antibiotic therapy is typically started empirically prior to obtaining culture results. In adults, antibiotic treatment should be delayed until positive blood or biopsy cultures have been obtained to allow for more appropriate treatment. In most cases of adult primary spinal infection intravenous antibiotics are continued for at least 4–6 weeks and in some cases for up to 12 weeks. Consultation with an infectious disease specialist is recommended. Immobilization with a spinal orthosis can be beneficial for both pain relief and to maximize antibiotic effectiveness.

Historically, an epidural abscess was considered a surgical emergency without a role for nonoperative treatment. This trend has changed, and epidural abscesses without progressive neurologic change or spinal deformity can be initially managed with intravenous antibiotics and close neurologic monitoring. Postoperative spinal infections are more commonly treated surgically.

Cases involving TB of spine should involve an infectious disease specialist and typically receive a combination of isoniazid, rifampin, pyrazinamide and streptomycin for 6–12 months.

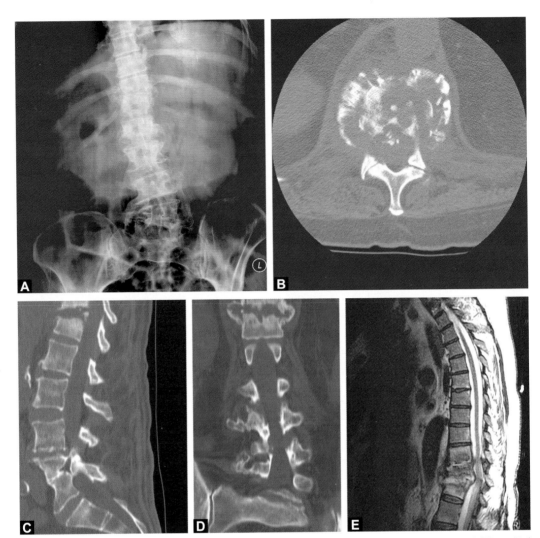

Figs 1A to E: (A) Anteroposterior radiograph; (B) Axial, (C) lateral and (D) coronal CT scan; and (E) sagittal MRI of a patient with thoracic spondylodiscitis revealing loss of disk height and endplate sclerosis at the T11-T12 level

Response to treatment is determined by a decrease in the patient's reports of back pain, improvement of any constitutional signs, and decreasing ESR and CRP levels. Repeated MRI scans are recommended in the setting of new neurologic changes but have limited value in most other cases as there will be chronic changes on these scans despite effective treatment and eradication of the infection.

☞ OPERATIVE TREATMENT

Indications for surgery in the treatment of spinal infection include a progressive neurologic deficit, failure to obtain a closed biopsy specimen, failure of conservative treatment, progressive spinal deformity from pathologic fracture, recurrent infection despite conservative treatment and intractable pain.

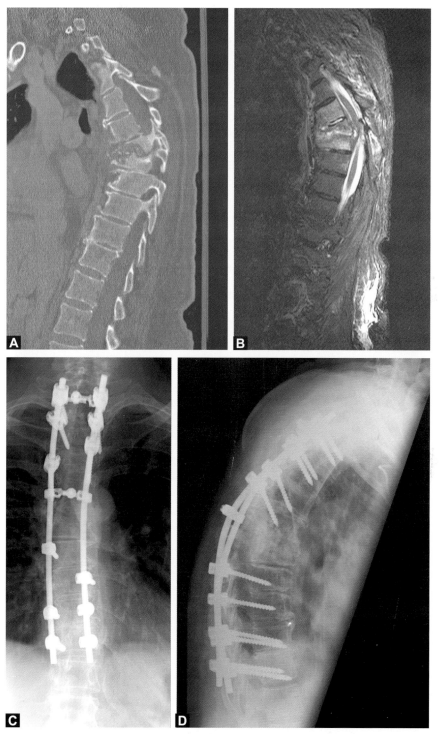

Figs 2A to D: (A) Sagittal CT and (B) MRI scan of a patient with severe spondylodiscitis, pathologic fracture and kyphotic deformity at T5-T8 causing progressive myelopathy; (C) Postoperative anteroposterior (AP) and (D) lateral radiographs showing the partial T6-T7 corpectomy and T2-T11 posterior instrumented fusion

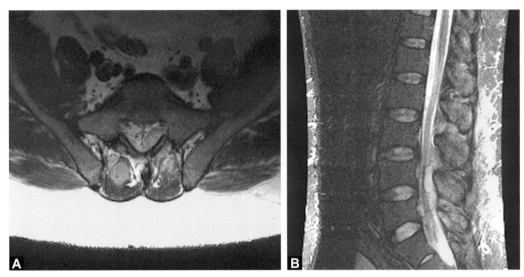

Figs 3A and B: (A) Axial and (B) sagittal MRI scan of a patient with a lumbar epidural abscess showing large fluid collection on to the posterior and left of the dural sac from L3-S1

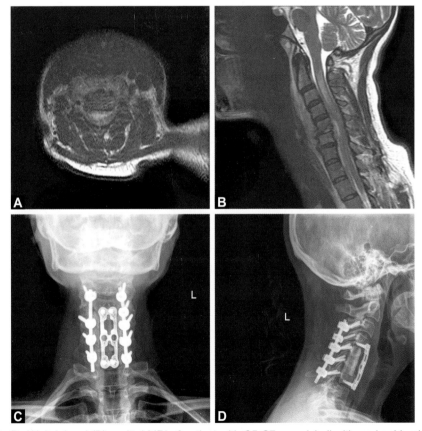

Figs 4A to D: (A) Axial and (B) sagittal MRI of patient with C5-C7 spondylodiscitis and epidural abscess with severe spinal cord compression from intravenous drug use causing progressive paralysis; (C) Postoperative anteroposterior (AP) and (D) lateral radiographs show C5-C6 corpectomy and anterior/posterior C4-C7 instrumented fusion

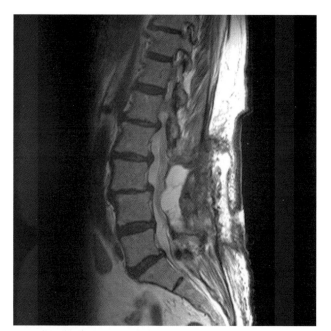

Fig. 5: Sagittal MRI of a patient that developed a wound infection following an L2-L4 decompression for spinal stenosis

The goals of surgical management of spinal infections are to debride infected material, decompress the neurologic structures, stabilize the spine and obtain tissue for culture. Depending on the patient's symptoms and location of the infection there are various surgical options and approaches available.

Lumbar epidural abscesses can often be effectively managed with posterior lumbar laminectomy, and irrigation and debridement of the infected material without the need for fusion as was case for the patient in Figures 3A and B. In more advanced infections with significant bony destruction or pathologic fracture it may be necessary to debride additional vertebral bone through a partial corpectomy and stabilize the spine with an instrumented fusion as in the case shown in Figures 1A to E. This patient had a T11-T12 spondylodiscitis that underwent a posterior extracavitary approach for a T11-T12 partial vertebrectomy and T9-L2 posterior instrumented fusion (Figs 6A and B). An alternative option would have utilized a combined anterior and posterior approach.

A progressive neurologic deficit with deformity from a pathologic fracture as in the patient from Figures 2A to D often requires a wide decompression and stabilization procedure. The patient presented with progressive signs of myelopathy from a T5-T8 spondylodiscitis with kyphotic deformity. The patient underwent a T6-T7 corpectomy and T2-T11 posterior instrumented fusion (Figs 2C and D). In some cases this technique needs to be combined with a pedicle subtraction osteotomy or vertebral column resection for greater sagittal plane correction.

Operative treatment of cervical spine epidural abscesses with neurologic deficits is recommended. The choice of an anterior versus posterior approach is based on the location of the abscess with respect to the spine cord. The patient from Figure 4 presented with an

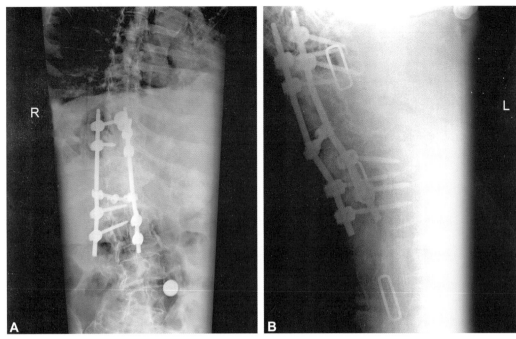

Figs 6A and B: (A) Postoperative anteroposterior (AP) and (B) lateral radiographs of the same patient as in Figure 1 show the partial corpectomy at T11-T12 and posterior instrumented fusion from T9-L2

incomplete paralysis from a ventral epidural abscess at C5-C6. The patient underwent an anterior C5-C6 corpectomy with C4-C7 fusion and delayed posterior C4-C7 instrumented fusion (Figs 4C and D). In cases with a posterior epidural abscess a posterior decompression and instrumented fusion is a good option.

Indications for surgery in the treatment of granulomatous infections are similar as for pyogenic infections. In general, these are more insidious infections and the most common reason for surgery is a progressive neurologic deficit in more advanced cases.

In most cases postoperative wound infections are treated operatively with irrigation and debridement of infected material. Small, superficial wound infections can be managed with antibiotic treatment and are closely monitored.

Postoperative intravenous antibiotics are provided following surgical management of spinal infections. The duration of the antibiotic treatment is based on the severity of the infection, patient risk factors, presence of spinal instrumentation and response to treatment.

👉 REFERENCES

1. Sapico FL, Montgomerie JZ. Pyogenic vertebral osteomyelitis: report of nine cases and review of the literature. Rev Infect Dis. 1979;1:754-76.
2. Carragee EJ. Pyogenic vertebral osteomyelitis. J Bone Joint Surg Am. 1997;79:874-80.
3. Sapico FL, Montgomerie JZ. Vertebral osteomyelitis. Infect Dis Clin North Am. 1990;4:539-50.
4. Brown MD, Tsaltas TT. Studies on the permeability of the intervertebral disc during skeletal maturation. Spine. 1976;1:240-4.

5. Wiley AM, Trueta J. The vascular anatomy of the spine and its relationship to pyogenic vertebral osteomyelitis. J Bone Joint Surg Br. 1959;41:796-809.

6. Arens S, Schlegel U, Printzen G, et al. Influence of materials for fixation implants on local infection. An experimental study of steel versus titanium DCP in rabbits. J Bone Joint Surg Br. 1996;78: 647-51.

7. Danner RL, Hartman BJ. Update on spinal epidural abscess: 35 cases and review of the literature. Rev Infect Dis. 1987;9:265-74.

8. Govender S, Charles RW, Naidoo KS, et al. Results of surgical decompression in chronic tuberculous paraplegia. S Afr Med J. 1988;74:58-9.

9. Tuli SM, Srivastava TP, Varma BP, et al. Tuberculosis of the spine. Acta Orthop Scand. 1967;38: 445-58.

10. McHenry MC, Easley KA, Locker GA. Vertebral osteomyelitis: long-term outcome for 253 patients from 7 Cleveland-area hospitals. Clin Infect Dis. 2002;34:1342-50.

11. Eismont FJ, Bohlman HH, Soni PL, et al. Pyogenic and fungal vertebral osteomyelitis with paralysis. J Bone Joint Surg Am. 1983;65:19-29.

12. Sampath P, Rigamonti D. Spinal epidural abscesses: a review of epidemiology, diagnosis, and treatment. J Spinal Disord. 1999;12:89-93.

13. O'Daly BJ, Morris SF, O'Rourke SK. Long-term functional outcome in pyogenic spinal infection. Spine. 2008;33:E246-53.

CHAPTER

18

Spinal Tumors

☞ INTRODUCTION

Establishing a definitive diagnosis is the most important first step in the management of spinal neoplasms. Spinal neoplasms are categorized into many subtypes. A spine tumor should first be classified as either a primary spinal tumor or secondary metastasis. Metastatic spinal neoplasms comprise the majority of spinal tumors diagnosed each year.[1] Primary spinal tumors are typically then classified as "primary benign neoplasms" or "primary malignant neoplasms". The principles and goals of treatment can be both overlapping and distinct. For metastatic spinal tumors the goals of treatment include preservation or restoration of spinal stability and neurologic function as well as to reduce pain. Most metastatic spinal tumors cannot be fully cured but are typically "managed" to meet these outlined goals. In rare cases, surgical resection of solitary spinal metastases can be curative. This concept is evolving and not widely accepted as standard at this point.[2,3] The treatment of primary spine tumors also shares the aforementioned goals. Benign primary neoplasms may be treated conservatively or operatively depending on the extent of symptoms and invasiveness. Once a lesion becomes aggressive (whether benign or malignant) the goal shifts to complete eradication of the tumor. This is most important when dealing with tumors that have potential to recur or metastasize.

☞ GENERAL PRINCIPLES OF EVALUATION, CLASSIFICATION AND STAGING FOR ALL SPINAL NEOPLASMS

There are four key principles that form the foundation of initial assessment of spinal metastases:

1. Maintain a high index of suspicion: For example, when a patient with a known primary cancer presents with back pain or radicular findings, the clinician is obligated to consider metastasis until proven otherwise.

2. Establish a diagnosis and perform proper staging: Once a spinal metastasis has been identified, (for instance, in the thoracic spine) the surgeon should obtain magnetic resonance imaging (MRI) (preferred) or computed tomography (CT) myelogram imaging of the entire spine. This constitutes "local staging" of the spinal metastatic disease. Systemic

staging of spinal metastases should be performed in conjunction with the medical oncology team and is dependent on the primary tumor origin. Typically CT of the chest, abdomen and pelvis is the first choice among other laboratory tests such as complete blood cell count, erythrocyte sedimentation rate, C-reactive protein, lactate dehydrogenase and alkaline phosphatase. Various tumor markers may also be helpful in assessing disease burden. Technetium bone scan or skeletal survey may be of benefit in identifying distant skeletal metastases. Hematologic and urinary studies such as serum or urine protein electrophoresis may also be helpful in identifying protein chains that are characteristic of hematologic malignancies such as myeloma. Bone marrow biopsy can also help identify the nature and extent of hematologic malignancies.

3. Use of consistent terminology: Use of consistent terminology can take many forms. For physical examination, it is important to adhere to consistent grading standards to assess neurologic function. This is perhaps the most important common language that surgeons and other clinicians need to develop because the timing of surgery can be influenced heavily by the time course of neurologic deterioration. The authors prefer the use of the American Spinal Injury Association standard neurologic examination classification.[4,5] It is also important to adhere to a common language of staging tumors as well as surgical resection techniques. Multiple scoring systems have been developed to assess tumor location and respectability, patient prognosis and spinal stability.[4,6-8]

4. Lastly a multidisciplinary approach should be maintained: The treatment of patients with metastatic (or primary) neoplastic disease requires a cohesive approach by medical oncologists and radiation oncologists to maintain a multidisciplinary approach.

The improvement in technology and medications to treat tumors has lead to longer life expectancy and has contributed to a broader utilization of surgical treatment of spinal neoplasms.

The history and physical examination are the key components of the spine surgeon's initial assessment that should establish a suspicion for metastatic spinal disease. Other symptoms such as unexplained weight loss, constitutional symptoms, radiculopathy and myelopathy are important features to identify.

☛ PATHOPHYSIOLOGY

The pathophysiology of every type of spine tumor is beyond the scope of this chapter. However, there are key points that all surgeons should understand regarding the pathophysiology of spinal tumors. Spinal tumors arise as uncontrolled cellular proliferation of either primary spinal/paraspinal tissue or from tissue that has seeded (metastasized) to the spine from a distant site. Primary spinal tumors may be benign or malignant, and their treatments depend on the histologic behavior of those tissues as well as how they are affecting surrounding structures such as bone or neural elements. Metastatic tumors can arise from almost any type of tissue in the body. Treatment choice is very dependent on histologic behavior of the tumor as this has a direct bearing on patient prognosis. Tokuhashi et al. have developed a scoring system to help predict prognosis of patients with spinal tumors. One of the main factors in the scoring system is the primary site of cancer. Tumors that derive from thyroid, kidney, uterus, breast and prostate tend to have a favorable prognosis whereas lung, osteosarcoma, stomach, pancreas and bladder tend to have much poorer prognosis due to the more aggressive nature of these tumors.[8]

The basis for obtaining any spine tumor diagnosis is by direct tissue biopsy. If it is safe and feasible, most spine tumors should be biopsied in the least invasive way possible. This will help guide treatment. Decisions on how to perform biopsy are made on a case by case basis and should respect tissue planes that may be contaminated by biopsy tracts if clean margin surgery is potentially necessary. Some patients present with progressive paralysis and instability, and thus delaying surgical treatment is not always possible to accommodate percutaneous biopsy. There are a multitude of histologic subtypes of spinal tumors. They often present more commonly in specific age ranges and gender and may or may not be related to specific genetic conditions or anomalies. This chapter will address a spectrum of primary and secondary (metastatic) spinal tumors. However, it is beyond the scope of this chapter to give a complete comprehensive review of all pertinent points concerning all known spine tumor subtypes.

☞ PATIENT PRESENTATION

There are common symptoms and presentations for the majority of tumors that affect the spine. Common symptoms include biologic (or "tumor related") pain, mechanical pain, radicular pain, motor or sensory dysfunction or generalized weight loss and constitutional symptoms.[1] Biological/tumor pain tends to occur at night and early in the morning and is related to tumor induced inflammatory mediators. It is often an early sign of metastatic disease or pain confined to the bone.[1] Mechanical pain is related to movement and worsens when the patient goes from recumbent to upright position.[1,6] Mechanical pain is broadly defined as pain with movement or pain with spinal loading. Symptoms of radiculopathy often develop as tumors invade the epidural space. Nerve root and spinal cord compression can lead to motor and sensory dysfunction. Symptoms of myelopathy, such as gait disturbance and proprioceptive disruption can also occur.[1] These signs are important indicators to the clinician to perform three-dimensional axial imaging of the spine. Specific tumor subtypes may present more commonly to certain patient populations and in more specific fashions.

Metastatic Spinal Disease

The spine is the most common site for bone metastasis.[3] Up to 40% of cancer patients develop spinal metastases and upwards of 10–20% of these develop spinal cord compression.[2,3] The most common sources for metastatic spinal disease include prostate, renal, lung, thyroid, prostate, colorectal, melanoma and lymphoma.[8,9] Approximately 50% spinal metastases originate from the prostate, lung or breast.[2,3] Most patients with spinal metastases present with back or neck pain as a symptomatic complaint.[1,10] Advances in imaging technology have made it increasingly common to detect asymptomatic spinal metastases in routine screening examinations (typically when known primary tumors exist).

Primary Spine Tumors

The Leeds Bone Tumor Registry was reviewed and a total of 2,750 cases of bone tumors and tumor-like cases were analyzed. Primary bone tumors of the osseous spine constituted only 126 of the 2,750 cases (4.6%). Chordoma was the most frequent tumor in the cervical and sacral regions, while the most common diagnosis overall was multiple myeloma and plasmacytoma. Osteosarcoma ranked third. The mean age of presentation was 42 years, and pain was the most common presenting symptom, occurring in 95% of malignant and 76% of benign tumors. Neurological involvement occurred in 52% of malignant tumors and usually meant a poor prognosis.[11]

Benign Primary Spinal Neoplasms

Spinal hemangioma is typically asymptomatic. Hemangiomas are vascular intraosseous lesions. They are incredibly common and often identified incidentally on radiographic imaging. They may occur in up to 10% of individuals.[12] Aggressive hemangiomas can be painful and may lead to neurologic symptoms such as radiculopathy or neurogenic claudication. These aggressive lesions can cause pathologic fracture.

Osteoid osteomas are bone forming tumors that range from 15 mm to 20 mm in size. They have limited growth potential. They typically cause pain and account for approximately 10% of primary bone tumors. Approximately 10% of osteoid osteomas occur in the vertebrae, primarily in the posterior elements.[12] Patients with osteoid osteoma commonly present with back pain that is worse at night. The majority of patients present with osteoid osteoma in their late teens, and males are more commonly affected than females. Osteoid osteoma is the most common reason for painful scoliosis in adolescents.[12] Osteoblastoma is a benign bone forming neoplasm similar to osteoid osteoma, but it is larger and clinically more aggressive. Spinal osteoblastomas typically arise in the posterior elements, although extension into the vertebral body is common in larger tumors. They occur most often in the lumbar spine.[12] They presents with dull back pain or with symptoms of neurologic compression. Symptoms typically are not different at night and respond poorly to nonsteroidal anti-inflammatory drugs. The average age at presentation is 20–24 years. Males are twice as commonly affected as females. Scoliosis is also known to occur in spinal osteoblastoma, but less frequently than with osteoid osteoma.

Aneurysmal bone cyst (ABC) makes up about 15% of all primary spine tumors.[12] They occur most commonly in the second decade of life and present with gradual onset of pain over several months. The patient may have a palpable mass, and they may notice it change in size with recumbence. Laboratories are typically not elevated.

Osteochondroma primarily occurs in the posterior elements with almost 50% of these lesions occurring at C2 because of an osteocartilaginous proliferation at a growth plate.[12] Patients tend to present with pain and/or swelling in region of the lesion. Average age of onset is in the early 30s.[12]

Giant cell tumors (GCTs) are rare. They account for approximately 2–4% of spine tumors.[12] They tend to present between 20 years and 50 years of age. They affect all regions of the spine equally and tend to favor the vertebral body. They typically present with back pain, and about half may have neurologic compromise.[13]

Eosinophilic granuloma (EG) typically occurs in children less than 10 years old, more commonly in boys.[12,14] They often affect vertebral bodies in the thoracic spine. Multilevel spinal involvement occurs in more than one-third of cases.[12,14] Patients with EG present with persistent back pain and restricted range of motion. Deformity such as kyphosis, scoliosis, and/or torticollis may also occur.

Malignant Primary Spinal Neoplasms

Malignant primary spinal neoplasms can present in a similar fashion to many of the above described tumors. Back pain, especially at night or at rest is typical. Other red flags, including night sweats, fever and chills may masquerade as infection but may be signs of Ewing's sarcoma or lymphoma.[15] Due to the predilection for malignant primary spine tumors to affect children, there may be challenges in assessing the neurologic examination. Babies and toddlers are often unable to articulate the particular problem, so neurologic deficit is often ascertained by observation of asymmetry in activity of limb use or failure of the patient to achieve developmental milestones. Neurologic deficit occurs in over 50% of patients with malignant primary spine tumors.[15]

Chordoma deserves special mention among primary malignant tumors of the spine. Chordomas are the most common primary malignant tumor of the mobile spine and of the sacrum. They are most common in older men.[16] Although considered not to possess significant metastatic potential, such lesions are locally aggressive, leading to neurologic compromise and lytic destruction of bone.[16] Because of the neoplasm's origin in the embryonic notochord, most chordomas occur in the midline of the body, involving the clivus (50%), the sacrum (35%) and the remainder of the spine (15%). Though chordoma is a relatively slow-growing tumor, it is associated with a high incidence of local recurrence and with a poor long-term prognosis. Sacral chordoma is a rare, low to intermediate-grade tumor that is often diagnosed late because of the insidious onset of symptoms and a location deep within the pelvic cavity. For these reasons, many sacral tumors are quite large at the time of diagnosis and may involve adjacent neurovascular structures and vital organs. In general, chordoma has been considered primarily a local disease, although the authors of previously published reports have noted that the incidence of metastasis has ranged from 5% to 40%.[16-18]

☞ IMAGING

Magnetic resonance imaging is the gold standard for evaluation of epidural neoplastic disease, but in patients who are unable to undergo MRI, CT myelogram should be considered. Assessment of rectal and urinary sphincter function is important as well.

Hemangioma

Aggressive hemangiomas may sometimes cause pathologic fracture or even spontaneous epidural bleeding.[12] Diagnosis can be made with plain radiographs or CT and usually yields a "jailbar" type pattern. MRI is hyperintense on both T1- and T2-weighted sequences.

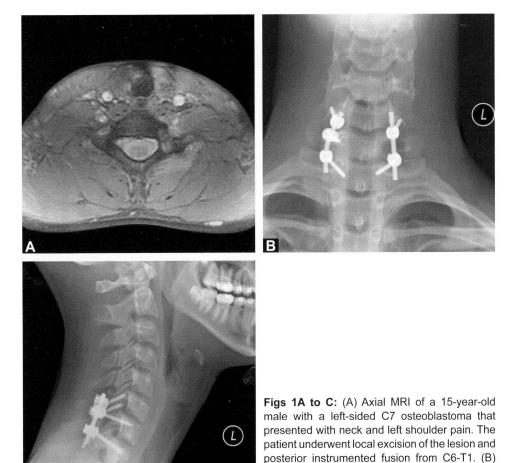

Figs 1A to C: (A) Axial MRI of a 15-year-old male with a left-sided C7 osteoblastoma that presented with neck and left shoulder pain. The patient underwent local excision of the lesion and posterior instrumented fusion from C6-T1. (B) Postoperative anteroposterior (AP) and (C) lateral radiographs are shown

Osteoid Osteoma

Plain X-ray may be negative because the lesion is typically in the posterior elements and less than 20 mm. On CT scan it is typified by sclerosis surrounding a radiolucent nidus.[19] MRI is typically used to aid in preoperative planning to determine proximity to neurologic structures.[19]

Osteoblastoma

Radiographic evaluation is similar to that of osteoid osteomas. The exception is that the nidus is more than 20 mm in diameter. Osteoblastoma lesions commonly have multiple calcifications, aggressive bony destruction, and infiltration into surrounding tissues. Preoperative CT is useful for precisely defining the location of the tumor and extent of osseous involvement. The appearance on MRI is generally nonspecific and may overestimate the size of the lesion due to local inflammation and edema; however, MRI helps determine the effect of the tumor on neural elements as well as soft-tissue changes (Figs 1A to C).

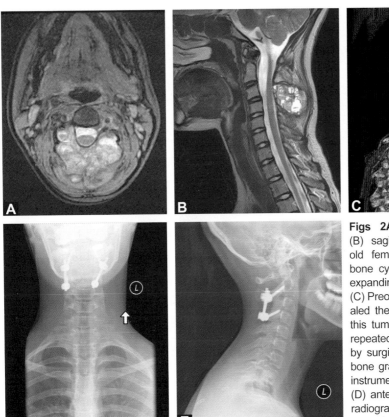

Figs 2A to E: (A) Axial and (B) sagittal MRI of an 11-year-old female with C2 aneurysmal bone cyst that presented with an expanding posterior neck mass; (C) Preoperative angiography revealed the highly vascular nature of this tumor. The patient underwent repeated embolization followed by surgical excision of the lesion, bone grafting and C2-C4 posterior instrumented fusion. Follow-up (D) anteroposterior and (E) lateral radiographs reveal solid fusion with no evidence of recurrence

Aneurysmal Bone Cyst

Imaging such as plain radiographs, CT typically show a lytic expansile lesion with erosion and expansion of the cortex. There are usually fluid-fluid levels on MRI that are demarcated by intralesional separations (Figs 2A to E). The differential diagnosis of ABC includes malignant fibrous histiocytoma, GCT, and EG and telangiectatic osteosarcoma (Fig. 3).[12] When an ABC is suspected it is critical to make the differentiation between primary ABC and another tumor with secondary changes that mimic it. Management and surveillance of the other lesions can differ substantially. Though rare, a telangiectatic osteosarcoma may appear identical to a common spinal ABC. The prognosis for the former is much worse and has a high potential for local recurrence, metastasis and early death. Its treatment requires neoadjuvant chemotherapy and where feasible, en bloc resection.

Osteochondroma

The hallmark of an osteochondroma is the cartilage cap at the end of a stalk, which is attached to the parent bone without underlying cortex.[12] This can be visualized on CT and MRI.

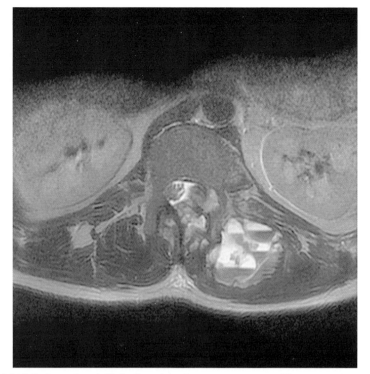

Fig. 3: Axial MRI of a patient initially thought to have an aneurysmal bone cyst that was proven by biopsy to be a telangiectatic osteosarcoma

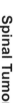

Giant Cell Tumor

Plain radiographs reveal an expansile, lytic lesion without a sclerotic rim.[12-14] Associated compression fractures may occur as a result of bone destruction. CT and MRI aid in defining bone, marrow, and soft-tissue involvement. Chest CT can aid in diagnosing pulmonary metastases. The radiographic differential diagnosis is brown tumor of hyperparathyroidism, metastases, hematologic malignancies, ABC, giant cell reparative granuloma, malignant fibrous histiocytoma and chordoma. Work up should involve open biopsy to differentiate between the above possibilities.

Eosinophilic Granuloma

On radiographic evaluation, EG typically appears as lytic lesion in the vertebral body or rarely, on the posterior elements. Approximately 40% of cases present as vertebra plana. Technetium Tc-99m bone scan is recommended to identify other affected areas because of the high frequency of multiple skeletal lesions. Differential diagnosis includes leukemia, lymphoma, infection, Ewing sarcoma, osteosarcoma, and ABC.[12-14] If radiographic and MRI findings are classically those for EG (i.e. vertebral collapse, disk space maintained, no extraspinal spread or soft-tissue mass), then close follow-up is recommended, and unnecessary biopsy can be avoided. If atypical features are present (i.e. soft-tissue mass, disk involvement, neurologic symptoms), then biopsy is indicated.[12-14]

Metastatic Spinal Disease

Metastatic disease of the spine remains a common problem, and its incidence is increasing as detection methods improve. Treatments for primary cancers allows patients with active disease to have a longer life expectancy.[3] It has been well demonstrated that patients with metastatic epidural cord compression who undergo surgical decompression and reconstruction followed by radiation have superior outcomes.[20] Ambulatory function and pain relief are superior.[20] It has also been shown that timing of surgery in relation to radiation treatment is critical in limiting wound complications.[21] It important to develop treatment plans for patients with spinal metastases via a multidisciplinary approach between medical oncologists, radiation oncologists and spine surgeons. Surgical treatment decisions for spinal metastases are broadly based on a series of factors including neurology, spinal stability and patient-specific factors that include patient health, prognosis and tumor histology.[1,6,8] The concept of spinal instability, however, remains critical in the surgical decision-making process.[6] The Spine Oncology Study Group (SOSG) defines spine instability as loss of spinal integrity as a result of a neoplastic process that is associated with movement-related pain, symptomatic or progressive deformity, and/or neural compromise under physiologic loads.[6] The Spine Instability Neoplastic Score (SINS) was developed and validated to assess spinal instability in metastatic spinal lesions.[6] SINS is a comprehensive classification system based on patient symptoms and radiographic criteria of the spine. The classification system includes global spinal location of the tumor, type and presence of pain, bone lesion quality, spinal alignment, extent of vertebral body collapse, and posterolateral spinal element involvement. By analyzing the six criteria, the clinician can assign a score and have a relative determination of spinal stability. The scoring system is outlined in Table 1.

The SINS is generated by tallying each score from the six individual components. The minimum score is 0, and maximum is 18. Scores of 0–6 denote "stability", scores of 7–12 denote "indeterminate (possibly impending) instability", and scores of 13–18 denote "instability". Patients with SINS scores of 7–18 warrant surgical consultation.

Tokuhashi et al. have devised a staging system to handle prognostic concerns.[8] Since the decision to operate on patients with metastatic disease is so closely tied to patient prognosis, this system deserves consideration in the evaluation of patients with metastatic spinal disease. Metastatic spinal disease is considered a systemic disease, and the main purposes of treatments are pain relief and the improvement of neurology as well as activities of daily living.[8] The value of surgery may be lost if complications develop during or after surgery. Therefore, utilization of a treatment strategy, based on life expectancy and pretreatment prognosis evaluation, is critically important in determining treatment methods including surgical procedures.[8]

The Tokuhashi score utilizes information that is readily available to the clinician including primary tumor histology, general patient condition, neurologic status, number of skeletal and visceral metastases and number of vertebral metastases. By calculating a

Element of Spine Instability Neoplastic Score (SINS)	Score
Table 1: Scoring system for determining spinal stability in cases of metastatic spinal disease	
Location	
Junctional (occiput-C2, C7-T2, T11-L1, L5-S1)	3
Mobile spine (C3-C6), L2-L4)	2
Semi-rigid (T3-T10)	1
Rigid (S2-S5)	0
Pain relief with recumbency and/or pain with movement/loading of the spine	
Yes	3
No (occasional pain but not mechanical)	1
Pain-free lesion	0
Bone lesion	
Lytic	2
Mixed (lytic/blastic)	1
Blastic	0
Radiographic spinal alignment	
Subluxation/translation present	4
De novo deformity (kyphosis/scoliosis)	2
Normal alignment	0
Vertebral body collapse	
> 50% collapse	3
< 50% collapse	2
No collapse with > 50% body involved	1
None of the above	0
Posterolateral involvement of the spinal elements [(facet, pedicle or costovertebral (CV) joint fracture or replacement with tumor)]	
Bilateral	3
Unilateral	1
None of the above	0

score utilizing information from Table 2, a reasonable idea of patient prognosis can be determined.[8] Tokuhashi et al. use the score to help assign a treatment protocol which is outlined in Figure 4.[8]

Benign Primary Spinal Neoplasms

Benign neoplasms can be classified according to the Enneking classification which helps the clinician judge tumor behavior and guide treatment (Table 3). The Enneking classification system can help guide the surgeon to determine the extent o surgical resection necessary so as to offer the best chance possible at preventing local recurrence.

Malignant Primary Spinal Neoplasms

The most widely accepted staging system for malignant primary spinal neoplasms is the Weinstein-Biagini-Boriani (WBB) classification.[7] It accomplishes two goals. The first

Table 2: Tokuhashi scoring system to determine patient prognosis	
Characteristic	*Score*
General condition (performance status)	
Poor (PS 10–40%)	0
Moderate (PS 50–70%)	1
Good (PS 80–100%)	2
No. of extraspinal bone metastases foci	
≥ 3	0
1–2	1
0	2
Metastases to the major internal organs	
Unremovable	0
Removable	1
No metastases	2
Primary site of the cancer	
Lung, osteosarcoma, stomach, bladder, esophagus, pancreas	0
Lever, gallbladder, unidentified	1
Others	2
Kidney, uterus	3
Rectum	4
Thyroid, breast, prostate, carcinoid tumor	5
Palsy	
Complete (Frankel A, B)	0
Incomplete (Frankel C, D)	1
None (Frankel E)	2

Criteria of predicted prognosis: Total score (TS) 0–8 = > 6 mo; TS 9–11 = ≤ 6 mo; TS 12–15 = ≤ 1 year.

Table 3: Enneking classification for benign primary spinal neoplasms	
Stage	*Description*
1	Latent: Usually asymptomatic
2	Active: Locally symptomatic
3	Aggressive: Symptomatic with local invasion and/or destruction of tissues with potential for metastasis

is a reproducible characterization of the lesion in terms of its extent. In the axial plane, the tumor extent is defined by 12 equal radiating zones centered about the spinal canal and numbered from 1 to 12 in a clockwise fashion, with 12 o'clock located at the spinous process (Fig. 5).[7,22] The tumor is further classified into one or more of five concentric layers that are centered about the dural sac and that range from the location of the tumor in the paravertebral extraosseous soft tissue (A) to tumor involvement of the dura (E). Finally, the longitudinal extent of the tumor is recorded according to the vertebral levels involved. The second goal of the classification is to guide the surgical resection which entails a combined

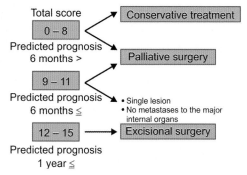

Fig. 4: Diagram of the use of the Tokuhashi score to help guide surgical treatment protocols for patients with metastatic spine disease

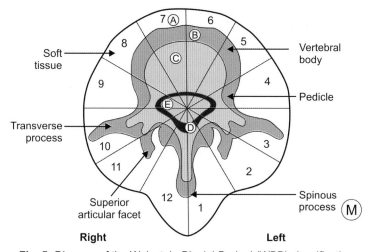

Fig. 5: Diagram of the Weinstein-Biagini-Boriani (WBB) classification

approach vertebrectomy for tumors spanning zones 4–8 or 5–9, a combined approach sagittal resection for tumors in zones 2–5 or 7–11, and posterior arch resection for tumors limited to the posterior arch (zones 10–3).[7,22]

☞ NONOPERATIVE TREATMENT

Spinal Metastases

Nonoperative treatment plays an important role in the management of spinal metastases. It is beyond the scope of this chapter to provide a fully detailed outline of all nonoperative treatment modalities for spinal metastases. But basic principles should be understood. Radiation therapy plays a significant role in the treatment of the majority of metastatic spinal tumors.[3] It is especially effective in "radiation sensitive" histologic subtypes and is utilized as a first-line treatment when no neurologic deficit or spinal instability exists. Intensity modulated radiation therapy (IMRT) and stereotactic radiotherapy utilize sophisticated computer-guided image planning available to deliver higher doses of radiation to the target. This appears to be a safer way to deliver treatment around sensitive neural structures.[3,10]

The rationale and role for corticosteroid treatment should also be understood by the spine surgeon. There is strong evidence to support the use of steroids in patients with spinal metastatic disease causing spinal cord compression. Dexamethasone is the most widely used agent with a loading dose of 10–100 mg and four times per day dosing regimen of 4–24 mg per dose with a taper over a few weeks. Higher doses are associated with more complications, and it appears that a 10 mg loading dose with routine dosing of 4–8 mg per dose is reasonable.[3,10]

Bisphosphonates also play a role in preventing bone resorption from metastatic disease. This can help prevent fracture and decrease pain from metastatic skeletal disease.[3]

Benign Primary Spinal Neoplasms

Benign tumors in the spine include osteoid osteoma, osteoblastoma, ABC, osteochondroma, neurofibroma, GCT of bone, eosinophilic granuloma and hemangioma. Although some are incidental findings, some cause local pain, radicular symptoms, neurologic compromise, spinal instability and deformity. Appropriate treatment may be observational (e.g. eosinophilic granuloma) or ablative (e.g. osteoid osteoma, neurofibroma, hemangioma), but generally is surgical, depending on the level of pain, instability, neurologic compromise and natural history of the lesion.

Management of vertebral osteoid osteoma lesions without associated spinal deformity or neurologic compression is typically conservative.[12] Anti-inflammatory medications are the first-line defense. If this does not work, then the lesions are usually effectively treated with percutaneous radiofrequency thermal ablation (RFA) or laser photocoagulation.[12] The mainstay for management of ABCs used to be surgical resection either en bloc or marginal for a complete resection.[12] However, it has been shown that serial embolizations of spinal ABCs offers the safest and probably the most consistent results for cure and complete healing of lesions.[23] The use of serial embolization has been shown to allow most patients to heal without surgery and with minimal complications.[23] For those that fail, surgery is recommended. Osteochondromas that are causing neurologic deficit should be completely surgically resected. This is typically curative. The use of instrumentation and spinal reconstruction should be tailored to the instability that may be generated. Malignant degeneration is rare and may occur in about 2.5% of cases.[12]

Eosinophilic granuloma of the spine often improves spontaneously, achieving variable degrees of vertebral body height reconstitution. As a result, surgery is rarely required. Management is usually symptomatic, with rest and analgesics/anti-inflammatory drugs. Orthoses are useful for pain and may help prevent kyphosis. Intralesional CT-guided steroid injection may be helpful for symptomatic solitary EGs of the spine. Low-dose radiation therapy has been used for cases with neurologic compromise. Rarely, surgical curettage with stabilization may be needed if neurologic defects or spinal instability is observed.

Malignant Primary Spinal Neoplasms

The role for nonoperative care in patients with malignant primary spine tumors is based on tumor histology, staging and prognosis. Typically, hematologically-derived cancers such as lymphoma can be treated with chemotherapy and/or radiation. Surgery is typically reserved

Table 4: Enneking classification of resection	
Intralesional	Margins are entirely within the tumor (i.e., incisional biopsy)
Marginal	Margins are situated at the immediate extent of the tumor only (i.e., excisional biopsy)
Wide	Margins include the tumor and a cuff of normal tissue
Radical	Margins include the tumor and the entire compartment in which the tumor is contained

for patients with spinal instability and/or neurologic compromise. Patients with Ewing's sarcoma typically benefit from radiation and chemotherapy as well, while those with osteosarcoma require neoadjuvant chemotherapy without radiation.[15] Surgical treatment for Ewing's sarcoma and osteosarcoma is meant to increase patient survival and to provide palliative relief of pain. If a patient has extensive disease burden (extensive metastasis), is not physiologically fit enough and/or has a poor (typically less than 3–6-month prognosis) then surgical treatment is not considered. Corticosteroids can be utilized to help manage tumor pain and occasionally can diminish the neurologic effects of tumor edema.

OPERATIVE TREATMENT

Some general considerations about terminology should be identified. In the literature there is often inconsistency in terms used to describe the surgical management of tumors. Terms like "en bloc", "gross total resection", and "radical resection" are sometimes used indiscriminately, not representing the actual procedure performed.[22] Similarly, histologic margins and surgical margins are interchanged. It is essential for the oncologic spine surgeon to completely assimilate the original definitions of the terms as described by Enneking.[4,22] Using the surgical principles dictated by the Enneking classification is possible as it pertains to intralesional, marginal, and wide resection of spine tumors. However, the complete adaptation of the classification to spine surgery is limited. This is attributed to the fact that radical resection of tumors in the spine is never feasible because of the fact that the epidural space is one continuous compartment extending from occiput to sacrum, and its excision to perform true radical resections as described by Enneking is simply not possible in the spine. It is important, therefore, to differentiate between surgical margins in the spine that can be intralesional (leaving tumor behind), marginal (leaving the reactive zone of the tumor behind), or wide (removing the tumor with a cuff of healthy tissue), as well as to distinguish between the different surgical techniques used to achieve these margins. The latter can be either piecemeal (curettage being a prominent example) or en bloc in which the tumor is removed in one piece regardless of the surgical margins. Finally, the accurate analysis of the histologic margins serves as the final verdict for the surgeon regarding his or her success at achieving the planned surgical margins (intralesional, marginal or wide).[4,22] Table 4 lists the definitions that apply to the Enneking classification for surgical resection of skeletal neoplasia.

Spinal Metastases

The goals of surgical treatment for spinal metastases need to be understood and clearly communicated to patients and other health care providers. They include maintaining or restoring spinal stability, and preserving and/or recovering neurologic function. In some cases, operative treatment for spinal metastasis may prolong survival, but this has not been fully proven and is an area of active research. The prognosis of a patient with metastatic disease is primarily governed by the histology and staging of the tumor.[1,10] The assessment of life expectancy is a critical component of decision making for surgery.[2,8,24] Complication rates can be 20–32%.[21,25-27]

Surgical techniques can vary widely. It is the authors' preference to utilize a single stage all posterior approach when performing spinal decompression and reconstruction for the majority of thoracic and lumbar metastatic cases. Because most metastatic disease involves the vertebral bodies and pedicles, most of the patients require augmentation of both anterior and posterior spinal columns. Frequently, epidural compression of the spinal cord is circumferential. Anterior approaches generally require an access surgeon for exposure, and although they have the advantages of good visualization and the potential for excellent ventral decompression, the neural elements to be decompressed, however, are usually visualized late in the decompression process.[28] Posterior instrumentation is almost always required and thus requires a second, separate procedure. Thus the patient is exposed to all of the risks inherent in a thoracic or thoracoabdominal approach in addition to the further risks of a posterior procedure. Posterolateral approaches allow excellent decompression with early visualization of the tumor and neural structures. With bilateral costotransversectomies, it is possible to perform a nearly complete spondylectomy if needed, but this is rarely necessary to achieve the goals of surgery. Because the chest and abdominal cavities are not opened, the risk of damage to the contents of these cavities is also minimized, as is the risk of pulmonary dysfunction.[28]

Benign Primary Spinal Neoplasms

If a hemangioma is symptomatic (aggressive) and causes neurologic compromise or instability, it may warrant surgical treatment that addresses these concerns. For lesions simply causing pain, less invasive treatments may include sequential arterial embolization, radiation or vertebroplasty.[12] Most osteoid osteomas are treated nonsurgically. However, en bloc excision is recommended in patients with osteoid osteoma with associated fixed spinal deformity, with neurologic compression, or if RFA is deemed unsafe due to the anatomic location or has been previously unsuccessful.[12] With complete surgical excision, a cure is expected. Associated spinal deformity can resolve if the lesion is resected within 15 months of onset of deformity.[12,29] Osteoblastomas are managed surgically because of both pain and the increasing size that can cause bony destruction, neurologic compression, spinal deformity or destabilization.[12] Treatment consists of resection and fusion when instability is present. En bloc resection is preferred but if complete resection is not possible due to neurologic safety concerns, then intralesional curettage and cementation or bone grafting may be performed.[12] Prognosis is based on completeness of the resection, with a reported recurrence rate of 10–24%. Larger lesions and those locally more aggressive tend to have higher rates of recurrence. Surgery is no longer seen as a first-line treatment and is reserved for cased of spinal instability and neurologic deterioration.[23] In these cases, angiography should be used to embolize lesions preoperatively and reduce intraoperative blood loss. GCTs are often locally aggressive, and surgery is required for Enneking stage II and III lesions. En bloc resection should be considered for Enneking stage III GCTs of the mobile spine. The choice of en bloc resection must be balanced with the inherent risks of the procedure. Intralesional resection of Enneking stage II tumors provides adequate local control. Use of adjuvant treatments intraoperatively may include polymethylmethacrylate (PMMA), phenol and cryotherapy. Systemic corticosteroid and newer antibody treatments are also being used as supplemental treatments.[12-14] Patients should be followed for at least 5 years because local relapse can occur late.[13]

Malignant Primary Spinal Neoplasms

The principles of Enneking should be employed when undertaking surgical resection of malignant primary spinal tumors. Proper staging using the WBB system can aid in surgical planning. Where technically and safely feasible and when medically appropriate according to patient prognosis and health considerations, primary malignant spine tumors should

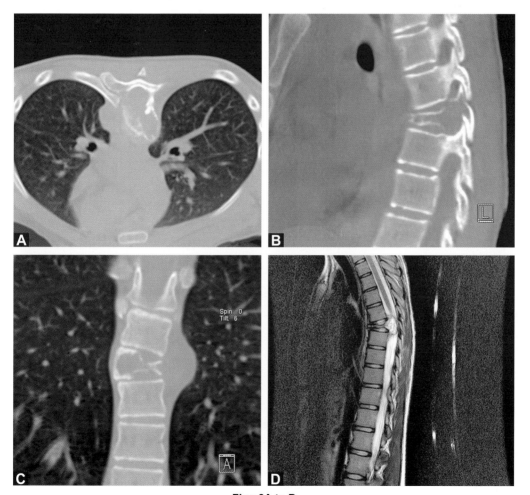

Figs 6A to D

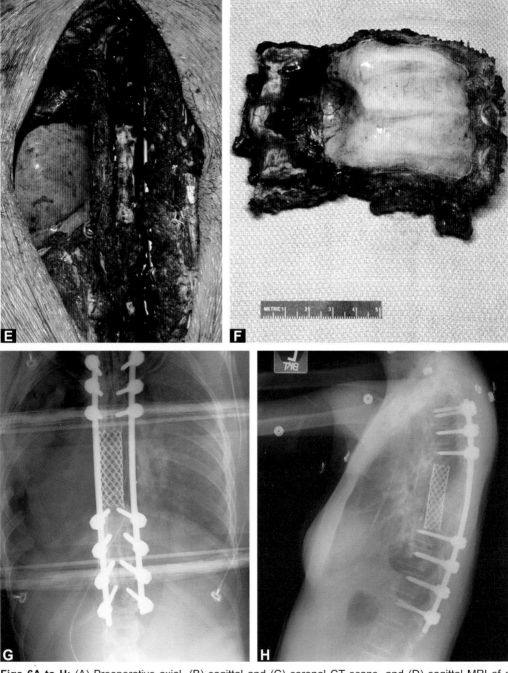

Figs 6A to H: (A) Preoperative axial, (B) sagittal and (C) coronal CT scans, and (D) sagittal MRI of a 15-year-old female with an osteosarcoma at T7. The patient underwent an en bloc excision of T6-T8 with posterior instrumented fusion T2-T12, vascularized rib graft, and T5-T9 anterior cage reconstruction through a posterior approach; (E and F) Intraoperative figures are shown as well as (G) postoperative anteroposterior and (H) lateral radiographs be resected with the goal of complete eradication. En bloc wide or marginal resections are usually the treatment of choice for tumors such as chordoma, osteosarcoma and Ewings sarcoma. Unfortunately, the treatment of malignant primary spinal neoplasms, especially ones such as chordoma may be an arduous clinical undertaking (Figs 6A to H). They require a multidisciplinary approach and attention to detail from the outset. Despite aggressive well-planned surgical management and adherence to strict surveillance protocols, recurrence and the late onset of metastatic disease are to be expected in a substantial proportion of patients. Adequate surgical treatment may result in substantial functional preservation; however, numerous complications can be expected.[15,16,18]

REFERENCES

1. Bilsky M, Smith M. Surgical approach to epidural spinal cord compression. Hematol Oncol Clin North Am. 2006;20:1307-17.
2. Bilsky MH, Laufer I, Burch S. Shifting paradigms in the treatment of metastatic spine disease. Spine (Phila Pa 1976). 2009;34:S101-7.
3. Klimo P Jr, Kestle JR, Schmidt MH. Clinical trials and evidence-based medicine for metastatic spine disease. Neurosurg Clin N Am. 2004;15:549-64.
4. Enneking WF. A system of staging musculoskeletal neoplasms. Clin Orthop Relat Res. 1986:9-24.
5. Maynard FM Jr, Bracken MB, Creasey G, et al. International Standards for Neurological and Functional Classification of Spinal Cord Injury. American Spinal Injury Association. Spinal Cord. 1997;35:266-74.
6. Fisher CG, DiPaola CP, Ryken TC, et al. A novel classification system for spinal instability in neoplastic disease: an evidence-based approach and expert consensus from the Spine Oncology Study Group. Spine (Phila Pa 1976). 2010;35:E1221-9.
7. Chan P, Boriani S, Fourney DR, et al. An assessment of the reliability of the Enneking and Weinstein-Boriani-Biagini classifications for staging of primary spinal tumors by the Spine Oncology Study Group. Spine (Phila Pa 1976). 2009;34:384-91.
8. Tokuhashi Y, Matsuzaki H, Oda H, et al. A revised scoring system for preoperative evaluation of metastatic spine tumor prognosis. Spine. 2005;30:2186-91.
9. Tomita K, Kawahara N, Kobayashi T, et al. Surgical strategy for spinal metastases. Spine. 2001;26:298-306.
10. Bilsky MH, Boakye M, Collignon F, et al. Operative management of metastatic and malignant primary subaxial cervical tumors. J Neurosurg Spine. 2005;2:256-64.
11. Kelley SP, Ashford RU, Rao AS, et al. Primary bone tumours of the spine: a 42-year survey from the Leeds Regional Bone Tumour Registry. Eur Spine J. 2007;16:405-9.
12. Thakur NA, Daniels AH, Schiller J, et al. Benign tumors of the spine. J Am Acad Orthop Surg. 2012;20:715-24.
13. Boriani S, Bandiera S, Casadei R, et al. Giant cell tumor of the mobile spine: a review of 49 cases. Spine (Phila Pa 1976). 2012;37:E37-45.
14. Harrop JS, Schmidt MH, Boriani S, et al. Aggressive "benign" primary spine neoplasms: osteoblastoma, aneurysmal bone cyst, and giant cell tumor. Spine (Phila Pa 1976). 2009;34: S39-47.
15. Kim HJ, McLawhorn AS, Goldstein MJ, et al. Malignant osseous tumors of the pediatric spine. J Am Acad Orthop Surg. 2012;20:646-56.
16. Sciubba DM, Chi JH, Rhines LD, et al. Chordoma of the spinal column. Neurosurg Clin N Am. 2008;19:5-15.

17. Boriani S, Chevalley F, Weinstein JN, et al. Chordoma of the spine above the sacrum. Treatment and outcome in 21 cases. Spine (Phila Pa 1976). 1996;21:1569-77.

18. Hulen CA, Temple HT, Fox WP, et al. Oncologic and functional outcome following sacrectomy for sacral chordoma. J Bone Joint Surg Am. 2006;88:1532-9.

19. Hosalkar HS, Garg S, Moroz L, et al. The diagnostic accuracy of MRI versus CT imaging for osteoid osteoma in children. Clin Orthop Relat Res. 2005:171-7.

20. Patchell RA, Tibbs PA, Regine WF, et al. Direct decompressive surgical resection in the treatment of spinal cord compression caused by metastatic cancer: a randomised trial. Lancet. 2005;366: 643-8.

21. Ghogawala Z, Mansfield FL, Borges LF. Spinal radiation before surgical decompression adversely affects outcomes of surgery for symptomatic metastatic spinal cord compression. Spine. 2001;26:818-24.

22. Fisher CG, Saravanja DD, Dvorak MF, et al. Surgical management of primary bone tumors of the spine: validation of an approach to enhance cure and reduce local recurrence. Spine (Phila Pa 1976). 2011;36:830-6.

23. Amendola L, Simonetti L, Simoes CE, et al. Aneurysmal bone cyst of the mobile spine: the therapeutic role of embolization. Eur Spine J. 2012 ;21(10):2003-10.

24. Bilsky MH, Shannon FJ, Sheppard S, et al. Diagnosis and management of a metastatic tumor in the atlantoaxial spine. Spine. 2002;27:1062-9.

25. Street JT, Lenehan BJ, DiPaola CP, et al. Morbidity and mortality of major adult spinal surgery. A prospective cohort analysis of 942 consecutive patients. Spine J. 2012;12:22-34.

26. Sundaresan N, Sachdev VP, Holland JF, et al. Surgical treatment of spinal cord compression from epidural metastasis. J Clin Oncol. 1995;13:2330-5.

27. Tzortzidis F, Elahi F, Wright D, et al. Patient outcome at long-term follow-up after aggressive microsurgical resection of cranial base chordomas. Neurosurgery. 2006;59:230-7.

28. Street J, Fisher C, Sparkes J, et al. Single-stage posterolateral vertebrectomy for the management of metastatic disease of the thoracic and lumbar spine: a prospective study of an evolving surgical technique. J Spinal Disord Tech. 2007;20:509-20.

29. Pettine KA, Klassen RA. Osteoid-osteoma and osteoblastoma of the spine. J Bone Joint Surg Am. 1986;68:354-61.

CHAPTER

19

Bone Grafting

Bone graft substitutes are frequently utilized in spine surgery. The reasons are varied, but ultimately they are used to achieve fusion (eliminate motion across spinal motion levels) and to reconstruct defects left from bone or disk removal. Spinal reconstruction is often required to stabilize the spine from the effects of trauma, tumors, infection, deformity and neurologic decompression.

It is important to first review how bone healing occurs. As an example, the posterior intertransverse region is a difficult area in which to achieve fusion. The bone healing process has been well documented in animal models. It occurs in three distinct and overlapping phases: (1) inflammatory, (2) reparative and (3) remodeling. In the case of the posterior intertransverse model of healing (Fig. 1), there are two defined zones: (1) the outer and (2) central zone.[1,2] The outer zones heal first in a "bone to bone" intramembranous fashion. Intramembranous ossification is bone formation produced by the direct differentiation of mesenchymal cells into osteoblasts. Mesenchymal cells group together and are typically recruited from the surrounding muscle tissue, bone and bone marrow. Osteogenic cells deposit bone matrix and secrete osteoid which leads to the formation of trabeculae. These fuse and form woven bone. There is no cartilage intermediate. The central zone of an intertransverse fusion heals through endochondral ossification (Fig. 1). This means that there is a cartilaginous intermediary that first forms and is then replaced by bone. This type of bone formation lags intramembranous bone formation by 3–4 weeks.

From a molecular standpoint there are distinct processes occurring in the different phases of bone healing. In the inflammatory phase (generally week 1–3), collagen I and II, osteopontin, osteonectin, bone morphogenetic proteins (BMP) 4 and 6 and alkaline phosphatase are elevated. BMP-2 peaks around week 3 as well.[2] In the reparative phase (generally weeks 4–5), the central zone of healing is active and BMP-2, 4 and 6 are elevated, and osteonectin and osteocalcin peak. In the remodeling phase (weeks 6–10), most gene upregulation and protein signaling molecules return to baseline except BMP-6.[2]

The anterior spine presents a different biomechanical environment to the posterior intertransverse region. Structural interbody or vertebral body replacement grafts are typically chosen. These grafts are placed and are meant to heal under compressive loads. This is typically a favorable environment for bone healing.

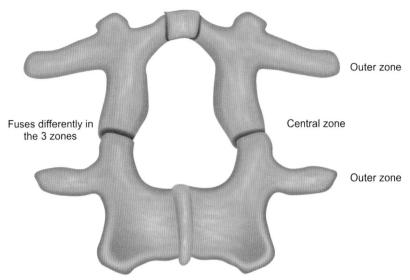

Fig. 1: Diagram of the areas of fusion achieved during a posterior inter-transverse process fusion

The gold standard for bone grafting in spine surgery is autograft. It has become the standard to which all other graft substitutes are compared. Autograft used in spinal fusion can be divided into two main categories:

1. Bone harvested from an extraspinal site, e.g. iliac crest bone graft (ICBG).
2. Salvaged bone removed during spinal decompression, osteotomy or vertebrectomy (typically referred to as local bone graft).

The advantage of local bone graft over ICBG is that it does not require a separate harvest; therefore, it requires less surgical time and avoids complications associated with bone graft harvest.[3] Complications associated with ICBG harvest include persistent pain, surgical site infection, wound dehiscence and neuroma. Several studies on fusion rates using local bone have reported rates comparable to those achieved with ICBG, especially for single-level fusions.[3-5] Local bone graft often cannot provide the volume needed for larger thoracolumbar surgeries, and it is often combined with synthetic products or "bone extenders or allograft".[3] In patients who have undergone a prior laminectomy or in-revision surgeries, quantities of local bone graft may be in limited quantity. At this point, harvest of iliac crest or use of bone graft extenders or expanders may be sought.

The iliac crest is typically the best "reservoir" upon which to draw for autologous donated bone when local bone is not adequate in volume. It offers a large surface area and volume of cortical and cancellous bone. The bone may be harvested in structural form to a limited degree without destabilizing the pelvis. The iliac crest can be harvested for spine patients concomitantly while undergoing an anterior, lateral or posterior approach. All approaches can yield structural, cancellous and corticocancellous graft. Special anatomic considerations should be considered for each approach. For a patient in the supine position, undergoing anterior iliac crest bone harvest, the lateral femoral cutaneous nerve is the most common

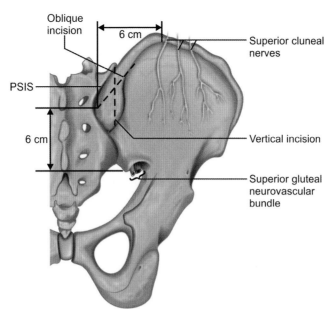

Fig. 2: Diagram of the nerve potentially at risk of injury during harvest of iliac crest bone graft

structure that generates potential adverse outcomes. It typically crosses the ilium beneath the anterior superior iliac spine (ASIS), but variations may occur up to 2.5 cm lateral and posterior to it. Therefore, it is recommended that anterior iliac crest harvest start at least 3 cm posterolateral to the ASIS.[6] Posterior harvest should avoid the cluneal nerves which run over the ilium approximately 6 cm from the posterior superior iliac spine (PSIS). The superior gluteal artery and nerve may also be injured if harvest extends toward the greater sciatic notch (Fig. 2).[6]

Harvested bone contains osteoblasts, bony matrix, and factors such as BMPs and transforming growth factor (TGF)-β. However, because TGF-β is found in relatively small quantities, autograft implanted within soft tissue will not generate new bone unlike recombinant human bone morphogenetic protein (rhBMP), leading some to question the long-standing belief that autograft should be considered osteoinductive.[3] However, one can debate the merits of this test alone. Autograft cells possess the ability to act in an autocrine and paracrine fashion to upregulate and downregulate signaling cascades for the purposes of bone formation as needed in the physiologic scenario. Other benefits of autograft include lack of disease transmission potential, tissue compatibility and no added cost.

The use of autograft has been shown to achieve high rates of fusion, and these rates vary based on the location, surgical technique, the use of instrumentation, volume of graft used, preparation of fusion bed, and the method used to assess whether bony fusion has been achieved.[3] In a retrospective comparative study of 76 patients treated with instrumented posterolateral fusion, Sengupta et al. reported overall fusion rates of 75% (27 of 36 patients) with ICBG and 65% (26 of 40 patients) with local bone graft.[5] However, when only multilevel fusions were included in the analysis, fusion rates for ICBG and local bone were only 66% and 20% respectively.[5]

Despite decreased rates of fusion, no significant difference in overall clinical outcome was noted between the two groups. ICBG can be harvested anteriorly or posteriorly, depending on the procedure. Harvest typically requires a separate incision; however, bone graft can be harvested through the same incision made for the approach to the spine, particularly in patients undergoing posterior lumbar procedures. Pain is the most common reported complication for patients who have undergone ICBG, but hematomas, paresthesias and wound complications can occur as well. Studies have been done in which patients were interviewed about donor site pain. It has been generally reported that chronic pain at the donor site occurs in about 25% of those patients.[3] However, patients who had unsatisfactory relief of back pain following fusion tend to have significantly higher donor site pain than did those with satisfactory pain relief; this may indicate a psychological component to donor site pain.[3] Other, more recent studies question whether iliac crest donor site pain may be overestimated.[7] Delawi et al. studied trauma patients that had fusion and ICBG. They found that in patients with a fusion of high levels (above L3), the donor site pain was significantly lower compared with patients with fusion of low levels (below L2). They concluded that patients probably cannot differentiate between donor site pain and residual low back pain. The reported incidence of pain related to posterior ICBG harvesting may therefore be overestimated. A subgroup analysis of the Spine Patient Outcomes Research Trial (SPORT) investigated the clinical outcomes of patients after the use of ICBG for degenerative spondylolisthesis of the lumbar spine. The outcome scores associated with the use of posterior ICBG for lumbar spinal fusion were not significantly lower than those after fusion without iliac crest autograft.[8] Conversely, iliac crest bone grafting was not associated with an increase in the complication rates or rates of reoperation. On the basis of these results, the authors recommend that surgeons choose to use ICBG on a case-by-case basis for lumbar spinal fusion.[8]

The grafting material provided by autologous bone has been described as having three properties that promote proper bone healing and fusion. Autograft bone is osteoconductive, osteoinductive and osteogenic. If bone graft is osteogenic that means it provides viable cells that promote bone healing. These cells can be either precursor cells that eventually mature and give rise to bone forming cells or differentiated cells. Osteoinductivity means that a bone graft has the ability to stimulate surrounding mesenchymal stem cells to induce cartilage and bone formation. This occurs through molecular signaling pathways. Osteoinductive substances can act either in an endocrine or paracrine fashion to recruit or differentiate cells to the fusion site to aid in fusion.

Through this process, a true osteoinductive agent can stimulate bone production anywhere in the body.[3] Osteoconductivity is a property by which the bone graft provides a mechanical support or "microscaffold" to allow attachment for cells, growth factors and mineralization to occur. It also promotes vascular ingrowth to support bone nutrition. This property allows the bone to form in a manner that is referred to as "creeping substitution". The main properties attributable to ICBG are sought after in bone graft substitutes. Most substitutes possess at least one or two of the three essential properties to promote bone healing. As bone graft substitutes are discussed, the attributes and extent of these properties will be illustrated for each class.

The supply of autologous bone, whether it is from the patient's pelvis or other sources like the fibula, is not unlimited. Also, its harvest is not without morbidity. The goal in utilizing "bone graft substitutes" and "bone graft extenders" is to replace or enhance autograft for spinal reconstruction and fusion. There are a multitude of fusion material options that are commercially available to add to or replace ICBG for spinal fusion. They all possess at least one of the three main components of bone healing promotion (osteoconduction, osteoinduction and osteogenesis).

☛ ALLOGRAFT

Allograft bone is frequently used as a bone graft extender in posterior spinal fusion surgery. It can come in fresh, fresh-frozen or freeze-dried forms, and is typically utilized as corticocancellous or cancellous morsels. Allograft is also prepared and utilized as structural grafting material, typically for anterior spinal arthrodesis. In these applications, it may be used alone. Allograft is osteoconductive and can be partly osteoinductive depending on the preparation. Freeze-dried allograft does not retain any cells or active proteins, but fresh-frozen allograft may have varying amounts of biologic activity from cellular and protein components. There is good evidence to suggest that allograft bone can have strong osteoinductive properties, but there may be significant donor variability.[9] It has also been shown that fresh-frozen allograft bone typically retains cells that are viable even after processing.[10] This suggests that these grafts may offer some osteogenic potential as well.

Allograft bone is highly available compared to autograft. It does, however, rely on harvest from allogeneic donors. A large commercial industry exists to procure and process these tissues. Unfortunately, despite rigorous industry regulation and meticulous processing protocols, the potential for disease transmission from these tissues still exists. In a retrospective review of US Food and Drug Administration data regarding recalled allograft tissue, Mroz et al. reported that 59,476 musculoskeletal allograft tissue specimens were recalled from 1994 to 2007. Improper donor evaluation, contamination, and recipient infections were the primary reasons for the recall. Despite these concerns, there have been no reports of bacterial disease transmission in spine surgery using allograft bone, and only one case of viral transmission to a spine patient (HIV transmission to a spine patient in 1988).[3,11]

Allograft bone is readily available and avoids the complications associated with harvest of autograft bone; however, concerns exist regarding the efficacy of allograft usage alone for fusion in the lumbar spine.[3] However, Gibson et al. reported similar clinical results in 69 patients who received either fresh-frozen allograft or ICBG during instrumented posterolateral lumbar fusion.[12] They utilized a plain radiographic measure of fusion and admittedly noted that clinical outcomes do not necessarily correlate with fusion.[12] They also noted that donor site morbidity of ICBG could be avoided with allograft. Their choice of graft was fresh-frozen allograft.

Structural allograft has been heavily studied in the anterior cervical spine. Without plating, allograft has been shown to be effective but slightly inferior to autograft, especially so, with multiple level cases.[13] However, in a comparison of allograft versus autograft [even in multilevel anterior cervical discectomy and fusion (ACDF)] with instrumentation, there have been reported fusion rates of 94.3% and 100% for allograft and autograft respectively.[14] It appears that fibula allograft may be the allograft of choice for ACDF due to the structural properties. Though it is slightly less osteoconductive than iliac crest allograft, due to its high cortical bone content, it has a lower resorption and failure rate.[13] There is mixed data to support smoking as a driver for nonunion with allograft. Some reports appear to confirm the higher nonunion potential while others refute this.[13] Overall, allograft long bone cross sections appear to have excellent utility in anterior spinal arthrodesis surgery. Fibula is well suited for cervical and femur for lumbar fusions, because of the biomechanical and osteoconductive/osteoinductive properties that they provide.

☞ DEMINERALIZED BONE MATRIX

Demineralized bone matrix (DBM) is derived from human allograft tissue. It is an osteoinductive agent. It is a potent stimulator of differentiation of osteoprogenitor cells into the bone-forming cells, osteoblasts.[15] The active element of DBM that confers its osteoinductive property is a group of low-molecular-weight glycoproteins adherent to its organic phase of which the BMPs are the most potent. Buried within the mineralized matrix of cortical bone, these osteoinductive proteins are exposed by decalcification process. DBM is primarily composed of collagen (93%), which contributes as an osteoconductive surface. Roughly 5% of DBM is comprised of soluble osteoinductive proteins such as BMPs, with residual mineralized matrix accounting for the additional 2%.[15] It is a family of commercially available products with varying degrees of osteoconductive as well as osteoinductive properties based on the composition of carriers and additives.[3] Because DBM is derived from human tissue, its disease transmission rates are similar to those of allograft bone. However, because of the proprietary nature of the demineralization process, the actual techniques used are not published, and these processes are not regulated. Therefore, significant variation in the actual concentrations of BMPs exists when comparing preparations to each other and even within various lots of the same preparation.[3] Animal studies support the ability of DBM preparations to serve as fusion adjuncts.

The efficacy of a DBM as a bone-graft substitute or extender is influenced by many factors, including the sterilization process, carrier, the quantity of BMP in the sample, and the osteoconductivity of the demineralized bone matrix-carrier complex, which affects migration of osteoprogenitor cells to the fusion site. This has been reflected in animal studies that have shown significant variability among DBM products.[15]

The most significant drawback to DBM may be the difference between and within products. In a rat model, Bae et al. observed significant lot-to-lot variability of a single DBM product with regard to BMP concentrations and in vivo fusion rates.[16] It has also been shown that the variability of BMP concentrations among different lots of the same DBM formulation, or intra-product variability, was higher than the inter-product variability or concentrations among different DBM formulations. Furthermore, donor variability in terms of age, sex and lifestyle habits determine the type of bone available for the preparation of DBM.[17]

Several animal and human studies suggest that DBM can successfully act as a bone graft extender or enhancer in spinal fusion surgery. However, very few prospective controlled trials exist on this topic. To date, the highest level of evidence studies have been performed using DBM in posterolateral lumbar fusion, and suggest that DBM can be used successfully as a graft extender. DBM has been successfully combined with iliac crest autograft, local bone autograft and bone marrow to facilitate fusion.[15] A number of studies have evaluated the use of DBM used in conjunction with various interbody devices typically made of polyetheretherketone (PEEK) used in anterior cervical fusions. Fusion rates from 88.9% to 97% have been achieved when cages were packed with DBM in anterior cervical discectomy and fusion.[15] Studies have also focused on the effectiveness of DBM in lumbar intertransverse fusion in humans. Most have shown favorable results when DBM has been used as a "graft extender". Cammisa et al. demonstrated that DBM can be used in a 2:1 ratio with ICBG in posterolateral lumbar fusion.[18] Fusion rates were strictly classified and demonstrated approximately 55% rate in both ICBG and DBM, and ICBG only groups.[18] Kang et al. had more favorable results in a randomized prospective trial that compared ICBG to DBM and local bone.[19] Fusion rates were comparable and over 85% in both groups. Use of ICBG caused greater blood loss and operative time.[19] The conclusion for DBM is that it appears to function as a bone graft extender with either ICBG or local bone. It has also been used a supplement to cancellous allograft bone in long fusions for spinal deformity and has demonstrated success in cohort trials.[15]

☞ BONE MORPHOGENETIC PROTEIN

The bone morphogenetic proteins play a role in the differentiation, proliferation, growth inhibition, and arrest of a wide variety of cells, with various actions dependent on the cellular microenvironment and interactions with other regulatory factors.[3] A review of the molecular signaling and molecular biology of the BMP family is beyond the scope of this chapter. The basic science is quite complex, and new signaling pathways continue to be discovered. By the time, this chapter is published, some of today's information about the BMP signaling cascades is likely to seem out of date. But a brief summary can be outlined as follows. BMPs bind to and act via serine-threonine kinase receptors found on the surface of target cells and then via the SMAD and Ras/Raf protein families. Cells affected by BMPs often express large numbers of BMP receptors of various types (up to 2,500 per cell); variability within these receptors, as well as heteromeric complex formation of these receptors, allows BMPs to induce numerous response cascades.[3] BMP-2 and BMP-7 have been widely studied in animals and in vitro. They have been shown to induce ectopic bone formation in rats as well as enhance spinal arthrodesis in rabbit models.[1-3]

Bone morphogenetic proteins have been approved for usage in humans in two forms: (1) rhBMP-2 (InFUSE, Medtronic Sofamor Danek) and (2) BMP-7 (osteogenic protein-1, Stryker). The US Food and Drug Administration approved the use of rhBMP-2 in spine surgery as a medical device used in conjunction with the LT-Cage tapered fusion device (Medtronic Sofamor Danek) for anterior lumbar interbody fusions of L4-S1.[3] BMP-7 was approved via a humanitarian device exemption for use in revision posterolateral lumbar spinal fusion, in "compromised hosts", or in those in whom bone graft harvest is not feasible or is not expected to promote fusion (e.g. patients with osteoporosis or diabetes and those who smoke).[3]

There are a multitude of studies utilizing BMP-2 for spinal fusion in physician directed (off-label) capacities, for a variety of types of operations including ACDF, transforaminal lumbar interbody fusion, and posterolateral cervical, thoracic and lumbosacral fusion.[3,20-28] These studies typically overwhelmingly support the use of BMP-2 for its ability to generate fusion, even in challenging environments. Results tend to be as good as or better than ICBG, and adverse events reporting were often quite low and appeared inconsequential.[3,20-28] It is important to bear in mind that the majority of these studies were industry funded. It should also be reiterated that BMP-2 was approved as a "device" and not as a drug. The dosing of BMP-2 on the collagen sponges appears to have been worked out for anterior lumbar fusion, but there is still much to learn. It is really not yet well understood what the minimum doses should be to generate fusion and minimize side-effects in off-label usage. This is a subject of considerable current interest.

The subject of dosing BMP-2 has come to the forefront most likely because a series of independent reviews have recently been completed on complications associated with BMP-2.[29] Over the last few years, significant attention has been placed upon the adverse events related to the usage of BMP-2 in spinal fusion. While demonstrating significant potential to generate bony union, the use of BMP-2 has been associated with a long list of complications that are likely (though not yet well determined to be) dose dependent. Complications include seroma formation, neuritis, increased pain and swelling, osteolysis, retrograde ejaculation, ectopic bone formation and life-threatening airway complications.[27,29-35] The authors feel strongly that the use of BMP-2 in the anterior cervical spine generates risk that is likely not worth the potential benefit that BMP-2 provides. The US Food and Drug Administration has made strong warnings against usage in the anterior cervical spine due to the high rate of swelling complications that have had life-threatening consequences.[3,35] Other reports have suggested that BMP-2 has tumorigenic capabilities and have warned against its usage in patients with known malignancy. Compared with rhBMP-2, rhBMP-7 (osteogenic protein-1) has been far less heavily studied. Its clinical application and market share appear to be less widespread relatively speaking. In a prospective, randomized, controlled, multicenter pilot study, 36 patients with lumbar spondylolisthesis underwent lumbar laminectomy and noninstrumented fusion with either rhBMP-7 or iliac crest autograft. Osteogenic protein-1 (OP-1) putty was demonstrated to be statistically equivalent to autograft with respect to the primary end point of modified overall success. The use of OP-1 putty when compared to autograft was associated with statistically lower intraoperative blood loss and shorter operative times.[36] OP-1 putty was determined to be a safe and effective alternative to autograft in the setting of uninstrumented posterolateral spinal arthrodesis.[36,37] In a 4-year follow-up the ICBG and OP-1 groups appeared to maintain equivalence in clinical and radiographic outcomes.[36] The fusion rates for BMP-7 have been less than stellar in well-designed studies. Though clinical results appear equivalent to ICBG, fusion rates have been reported as low as 63% (lower than the control ICBG group).[38] BMP-7 has also been studied in the anterior cervical spine, and though it had similar fusion rates to the control cage group, there was significantly more anterior cervical swelling.[39] There is a paucity of literature to support the use of BMP-7/OP-1 in spinal fusion surgery. One might postulate that there is a selection or publication bias in the literature to publish more frequently when results are favorable toward a particular treatment and avoid publishing when results are not.

Usage of biologics such as BMP-2 and -7 has exploded in frequency over the last decade. With advances in science, comes responsibility to evaluate the best science available to make informed shared decisions with and for our patients. These biologics demonstrate promise in medication of the bone healing cascade and may even tip the odds in our favor. But with all potential favorable results, comes the potential for adverse consequences. As this chapter is being written, further studies are taking place to help refine the indications, patient factors and dosing that are most appropriate for each challenging scenario in which these drugs may be called upon.

☛ SYNTHETIC BONE GRAFTS

Ceramics are a class of bone graft substitutes that have been engineered to mimic the mineral phase of bone. They have been designed to maximize bone ingrowth. They offer osteoconductive properties. They are readily available in large quantities, are inexpensive to manufacture, and carry no risk of disease transmission. Many different preparations are available. The resorption rate of these ceramics is important to consider. Calcium sulfate is absorbed within weeks of implantation, and tricalcium phosphate (TCP) is absorbed over several months, whereas hydroxyapatite (HA) is absorbed over the course of years.[15] TCP and HA are most widely used due to their resorption times.

Clinical studies in humans have shown near equivalence when comparing ICBG and TCP and local bone for single level lumbar posterior fusions.[15,40] TCP and coralline HA have been shown to generate fusion at high rates in posterior lumbar operations for degenerative conditions when used alone.[23] Silicated calcium phosphates and HA preparations have been shown in retrospective case series to act as bone graft substitutes in fusion cases of three or fewer levels.[41,42] Overall the quality of studies are lacking to support the use of ceramics as complete bone graft substitutes, especially in demanding surgeries such as long fusions for spinal deformity. A systematic review on the subject has been performed, and the authors made these statements, "Osteoconductive bone graft extenders, combined with local spine autograft and/or bone marrow aspirate have comparable fusion rates, similar functional outcomes, lower complication rates, and a lower risk of donor site pain than ICBG. Caution should be taken in interpreting these findings, given the low quality of the studies and the heterogeneity in the results. Randomized controlled studies using blinded assessments are required to help elucidate more conclusive evidence".[43]

☛ OSTEOPROMOTIVE AGENTS

Grabowski et al. used the term "osteopromotive agents" to identify products that assist in de novo bone formation despite these agents not distinctly being classified as osteogenic, osteoinductive or osteoconductive.[3] Platelet gels fall into this category. These contain platelets and growth factors and are generated intraoperatively by drawing a patient's own blood and then processing it to extract the buffy coat from the platelet-poor plasma. It is combined with thrombin and calcium chloride to produce the gel.[3] Though animal studies have shown some promise, human application of this technique has resulted in high nonunion rates.[44,45] Not all studies have shown increased nonunion rates, but there is certainly not statistical evidence to support platelet gel use as an adjunct to bone grafting in spinal fusion.[3]

REFERENCES

1. Boden SD. Biology of lumbar spine fusion and use of bone graft substitutes: present, future, and next generation. Tissue Eng. 2000;6:383-99.
2. Boden SD. Overview of the biology of lumbar spine fusion and principles for selecting a bone graft substitute. Spine (Phila Pa 1976). 2002;27:S26-31.
3. Grabowski G, Cornett CA. Bone graft and bone graft substitutes in spine surgery: current concepts and controversies. J Am Acad Orthop Surg. 2013;21:51-60.
4. Rihn JA, Kirkpatrick K, Albert TJ. Graft options in posterolateral and posterior interbody lumbar fusion. Spine (Phila Pa 1976). 2010;35:1629-39.
5. Sengupta DK, Truumees E, Patel CK, et al. Outcome of local bone versus autogenous iliac crest bone graft in the instrumented posterolateral fusion of the lumbar spine. Spine (Phila Pa 1976). 2006;31:985-91.
6. Ebraheim NA, Elgafy H, Xu R. Bone-graft harvesting from iliac and fibular donor sites: techniques and complications. J Am Acad Orthop Surg. 2001;9:210-8.
7. Delawi D, Dhert WJ, Castelein RM, et al. The incidence of donor site pain after bone graft harvesting from the posterior iliac crest may be overestimated: a study on spine fracture patients. Spine (Phila Pa 1976). 2007;32:1865-8.
8. Radcliff K, Hwang R, Hilibrand A, et al. The effect of iliac crest autograft on the outcome of fusion in the setting of degenerative spondylolisthesis: a subgroup analysis of the Spine Patient Outcomes Research Trial (SPORT). J Bone Joint Surg Am. 2012;94:1685-92.
9. Bormann N, Pruss A, Schmidmaier G, et al. In vitro testing of the osteoinductive potential of different bony allograft preparations. Arch Orthop Trauma Surg. 2010;130:143-9.
10. Simpson D, Kakarala G, Hampson K, et al. Viable cells survive in fresh frozen human bone allografts. Acta Orthop. 2007;78:26-30.
11. Mroz TE, Joyce MJ, Steinmetz MP, et al. Musculoskeletal allograft risks and recalls in the United States. J Am Acad Orthop Surg. 2008;16:559-65.
12. Gibson S, McLeod I, Wardlaw D, et al. Allograft versus autograft in instrumented posterolateral lumbar spinal fusion: a randomized control trial. Spine (Phila Pa 1976). 2002;27:1599-603.
13. Chau AM, Mobbs RJ. Bone graft substitutes in anterior cervical discectomy and fusion. Eur Spine J. 2009;18:449-64.
14. Samartzis D, Shen FH, Matthews DK, et al. Comparison of allograft to autograft in multilevel anterior cervical discectomy and fusion with rigid plate fixation. Spine J. 2003;3:451-9.
15. Aghdasi B, Montgomery SR, Daubs MD, et al. A review of demineralized bone matrices for spinal fusion: The evidence for efficacy. Surgeon. 2013;11:39-48.
16. Bae HW, Zhao L, Kanim LE, et al. Intervariability and intravariability of bone morphogenetic proteins in commercially available demineralized bone matrix products. Spine (Phila Pa 1976). 2006;31:1299-306.
17. Bae H, Zhao L, Zhu D, et al. Variability across ten production lots of a single demineralized bone matrix product. J Bone Joint Surg Am. 2010;92:427-35.

18. Cammisa FP Jr, Lowery G, Garfin SR, et al. Two-year fusion rate equivalency between Grafton DBM gel and autograft in posterolateral spine fusion: a prospective controlled trial employing a side-by-side comparison in the same patient. Spine (Phila Pa 1976). 2004;29:660-6.

19. Kang J, An H, Hilibrand A, et al. Grafton and local bone have comparable outcomes to iliac crest bone in instrumented single-level lumbar fusions. Spine (Phila Pa 1976). 2012;37:1083-91.

20. Carreon LY, Glassman SD, Djurasovic M, et al. RhBMP-2 versus iliac crest bone graft for lumbar spine fusion in patients over 60 years of age: a cost-utility study. Spine (Phila Pa 1976). 2009;34:238-43.

21. Dimar JR 2nd, Glassman SD, Burkus JK, et al. Two-year fusion and clinical outcomes in 224 patients treated with a single-level instrumented posterolateral fusion with iliac crest bone graft. Spine J. 2009;9:880-5.

22. Even J, Eskander M, Kang J. Bone morphogenetic protein in spine surgery: current and future uses. J Am Acad Orthop Surg. 2012;20:547-52.

23. Glassman SD, Carreon L, Djurasovic M, et al. Posterolateral lumbar spine fusion with INFUSE bone graft. Spine J. 2007;7:44-9.

24. Glassman SD, Carreon LY, Campbell MJ, et al. The perioperative cost of Infuse bone graft in posterolateral lumbar spine fusion. Spine J. 2008;8:443-8.

25. Glassman SD, Carreon LY, Djurasovic M, et al. RhBMP-2 versus iliac crest bone graft for lumbar spine fusion: a randomized, controlled trial in patients over sixty years of age. Spine (Phila Pa 1976). 2008;33:2843-9.

26. Lee KB, Taghavi CE, Hsu MS, et al. The efficacy of rhBMP-2 versus autograft for posterolateral lumbar spine fusion in elderly patients. Eur Spine J. 2010;19:924-30.

27. Ong KL, Villarraga ML, Lau E, et al. Off-label use of bone morphogenetic proteins in the United States using administrative data. Spine (Phila Pa 1976). 2010;35:1794-800.

28. Thawani JP, Wang AC, Than KD, et al. Bone morphogenetic proteins and cancer: review of the literature. Neurosurgery. 2010;66:233-46.

29. Carragee EJ, Hurwitz EL, Weiner BK. A critical review of recombinant human bone morphogenetic protein-2 trials in spinal surgery: emerging safety concerns and lessons learned. Spine J. 2011;11:471-91.

30. Anderson CL, Whitaker MC. Heterotopic ossification associated with recombinant human bone morphogenetic protein-2 (infuse) in posterolateral lumbar spine fusion: a case report. Spine (Phila Pa 1976). 2012;37:E502-6.

31. Choudhry OJ, Christiano LD, Singh R, et al. Bone morphogenetic protein-induced inflammatory cyst formation after lumbar fusion causing nerve root compression. J Neurosurg Spine. 2012;16:296-301.

32. Crawford CH 3rd, Carreon LY, McGinnis MD, et al. Perioperative complications of recombinant human bone morphogenetic protein-2 on an absorbable collagen sponge versus iliac crest bone graft for posterior cervical arthrodesis. Spine (Phila Pa 1976). 2009;34:1390-4.

33. Glassman SD, Howard J, Dimar J, et al. Complications with recombinant human bone morphogenic protein-2 in posterolateral spine fusion: a consecutive series of 1037 cases. Spine (Phila Pa 1976). 2011;36:1849-54.

34. Lindley EM, McBeth ZL, Henry SE, et al. Retrograde ejaculation after anterior lumbar spine surgery. Spine (Phila Pa 1976). 2012;37:1785-9.

35. Perri B, Cooper M, Lauryssen C, et al. Adverse swelling associated with use of rh-BMP-2 in anterior cervical discectomy and fusion: a case study. Spine J. 2007;7:235-9.

36. Vaccaro AR, Lawrence JP, Patel T, et al. The safety and efficacy of OP-1 (rhBMP-7) as a replacement for iliac crest autograft in posterolateral lumbar arthrodesis: a long-term (>4 years) pivotal study. Spine (Phila Pa 1976). 2008;33:2850-62.

37. Vaccaro AR, Patel T, Fischgrund J, et al. A pilot study evaluating the safety and efficacy of OP-1 Putty (rhBMP-7) as a replacement for iliac crest autograft in posterolateral lumbar arthrodesis for degenerative spondylolisthesis. Spine (Phila Pa 1976). 2004;29:1885-92.

38. Delawi D, Dhert WJ, Rillardon L, et al. A prospective, randomized, controlled, multicenter study of osteogenic protein-1 in instrumented posterolateral fusions: report on safety and feasibility. Spine (Phila Pa 1976). 2010;35:1185-91.

39. Leach J, Bittar RG. BMP-7 (OP-1) safety in anterior cervical fusion surgery. J Clin Neurosci. 2009;16:1417-20.

40. Dai LY, Jiang LS. Single-level instrumented posterolateral fusion of lumbar spine with beta-tricalcium phosphate versus autograft: a prospective, randomized study with 3-year follow-up. Spine (Phila Pa 1976). 2008;33:1299-304.

41. Jenis LG, Banco RJ. Efficacy of silicate-substituted calcium phosphate ceramic in posterolateral instrumented lumbar fusion. Spine (Phila Pa 1976). 2010;35:E1058-63.

42. Nagineni VV, James AR, Alimi M, et al. Silicate-substituted calcium phosphate ceramic bone graft replacement for spinal fusion procedures. Spine (Phila Pa 1976). 2012;37:E1264-72.

43. Alsaleh KA, Tougas CA, Roffey DM, et al. Osteoconductive bone graft extenders in posterolateral thoracolumbar spinal fusion: a systematic review. Spine (Phila Pa 1976). 2012;37:E993-1000.

44. Castro FP Jr. Role of activated growth factors in lumbar spinal fusions. J Spinal Disord Tech. 2004;17:380-4.

45. Tsai CH, Hsu HC, Chen YJ, et al. Using the growth factors-enriched platelet glue in spinal fusion and its efficiency. J Spinal Disord Tech. 2009;22:246-50.

Index

Page numbers followed by *f* refer to figure and *t* refer to table